Eminently practical and useful, this belongs on the desks of campus-based a and drug counselors, college administ developmental psychologists, and resea.c.. ers in the fields of substance abuse and adolescent psychology/psychiatry. Graduate students will find it a uniquely informative supplemental text for courses on substance use and addictions.

Helene Raskin White, PhD, is Professor II of Sociology, with joint appointments in the Center of Alcohol Studies and the Department of Sociology, and Deputy Director of the Center for Behavioral Health Services and Criminal Justice Research at Rutgers, The State University of New Jersey. Her research focuses on the etiology, development, consequences, and comorbidity of substance use and other problem behaviors (e.g., violence, crime, and mental health problems) over the life course. She also develops, implements, and evaluates brief substance use interventions for college students.

David L. Rabiner, PhD, is Associate Director of the Center for Child and Family Policy and Director of Undergraduate Studies in the Department of Psychology and Neuroscience at Duke University. His recent work focuses on interventions to improve academic performance in children with attention difficulties and a variety of other issues related to attention-deficit/hyperactivity disorder (ADHD), including the nonmedical use of ADHD medications by college students.

COLLEGE DRINKING AND DRUG USE

Duke Series in Child Development and Public Policy

Kenneth A. Dodge and Martha Putallaz, *Editors*

Aggression, Antisocial Behavior, and Violence among Girls:
A Developmental Perspective
Martha Putallaz and Karen L. Bierman, Editors

Enhancing Early Attachments: Theory, Research, Intervention, and Policy
Lisa J. Berlin, Yair Ziv, Lisa Amaya-Jackson, and Mark T. Greenberg, Editors

African American Family Life: Ecological and Cultural Diversity
Vonnie C. McLoyd, Nancy E. Hill, and Kenneth A. Dodge, Editors

Deviant Peer Influences in Programs for Youth: Problems and Solutions
Kenneth A. Dodge, Thomas J. Dishion, and Jennifer E. Lansford, Editors

Immigrant Families in Contemporary Society
Jennifer E. Lansford, Kirby Deater-Deckard, and Marc H. Bornstein, Editors

Understanding Peer Influence in Children and Adolescents
Mitchell J. Prinstein and Kenneth A. Dodge, Editors

Preventing Child Maltreatment: Community Approaches
Kenneth A. Dodge and Doriane Lambelet Coleman, Editors

Depression in Adolescent Girls: Science and Prevention
Timothy J. Strauman, Philip R. Costanzo, and Judy Garber, Editors

Gene–Environment Interactions in Developmental Psychopathology
Kenneth A. Dodge and Michael Rutter, Editors

College Drinking and Drug Use
Helene Raskin White and David L. Rabiner, Editors

College Drinking and Drug Use

Edited by
HELENE RASKIN WHITE
DAVID L. RABINER

THE GUILFORD PRESS
NEW YORK   LONDON

© 2012 The Guilford Press
A Division of Guilford Publications, Inc.
72 Spring Street, New York, NY 10012
www.guilford.com

Printed in the United States of America

This book is printed on acid-free paper.

Last digit is print number: 9 8 7 6 5 4 3 2 1

Library of Congress Cataloging-in-Publication Data

College drinking and drug use / edited by Helene Raskin White, David L. Rabiner.
    p. cm. — (Duke series in child development and public policy)
  Includes bibliographical references and index.
  ISBN 978-1-60623-995-7 (hardback : acid-free paper)
  1. College students—Substance use—United States.   2. College students—
Alcohol use—United States.   3. Substance abuse—United States—Prevention.
4. Alcoholism—United States—Prevention.   I. White, Helene Raskin, 1949–
I. Rabiner, David L.
  HV4999.Y68C65 2012
  362.2′91208420973—dc23
                                                              2011040019

In memory of G. Alan Marlatt

for his numerous achievements in the
alcohol and drug field and his groundbreaking
contributions to reducing the harm
associated with college student heavy drinking

He was an inspiration to all who knew him or his
work, and a great friend, collaborator, and mentor.
His kindness, generosity, and loyalty to the people
around him have set the standard that so many of us
try to model in our work with colleagues and students.

Alan was a true visionary
and he will be greatly missed.

About the Editors

Helene Raskin White, PhD, is Professor II of Sociology, with joint appointments in the Center of Alcohol Studies and the Department of Sociology, and Deputy Director of the Center for Behavioral Health Services and Criminal Justice Research at Rutgers, The State University of New Jersey. Her research focuses on the etiology, development, consequences, and comorbidity of substance use and other problem behaviors (e.g., violence, crime, and mental health problems) over the life course. She also develops, implements, and evaluates brief substance use interventions for college students.

David L. Rabiner, PhD, is Associate Director of the Center for Child and Family Policy and Director of Undergraduate Studies in the Department of Psychology and Neuroscience at Duke University. His recent work focuses on interventions to improve academic performance in children with attention difficulties and a variety of other issues related to attention-deficit/hyperactivity disorder (ADHD), including the nonmedical use of ADHD medications by college students.

Contributors

Shannon K. Bailie, MSW, Health and Wellness, Division of Student Life, University of Washington, Seattle, Washington

Marsha E. Bates, PhD, Center of Alcohol Studies, Rutgers, The State University of New Jersey, Piscataway, New Jersey

Carol J. Boyd, PhD, Substance Abuse Research Center and Institute for Research on Women and Gender, University of Michigan, Ann Arbor, Michigan

Jennifer F. Buckman, PhD, Center of Alcohol Studies, Rutgers, The State University of New Jersey, Piscataway, New Jersey

Philip J. Cook, PhD, Sanford School of Public Policy, Duke University, Durham, North Carolina

James A. Cranford, PhD, Substance Abuse Research Center and Addiction Research Center, University of Michigan, Ann Arbor, Michigan

Jessica M. Cronce, PhD, Department of Psychiatry and Behavioral Sciences, University of Washington, Seattle, Washington

James C. Fell, MS, Pacific Institute for Research and Evaluation, Calverton, Maryland

Kim Fromme, PhD, Department of Psychology, University of Texas at Austin, Austin, Texas

Maeve E. Gearing, BA, Sanford School of Public Policy, Duke University, Durham, North Carolina

Mark S. Goldman, PhD, Department of Psychology and Alcohol and Substance Use Research Institute, University of South Florida, Tampa, Florida

Jason R. Kilmer, PhD, Center for the Study of Health and Risk Behaviors, Department of Psychiatry and Behavioral Sciences, and Health and Wellness, Division of Student Life, University of Washington, Seattle, Washington

Lisa Laitman, MSEd, LCADC, Rutgers Health Services, Rutgers, The State University of New Jersey, New Brunswick, New Jersey

Mary E. Larimer, PhD, Department of Psychiatry and Behavioral Sciences and Addictive Behaviors Research Center, University of Washington, Seattle, Washington

Christine M. Lee, PhD, Department of Psychiatry and Behavioral Sciences, University of Washington, Seattle, Washington

Krista M. Lisdahl, PhD, Department of Psychology, University of Cincinnati, Cincinnati, Ohio

Matthew P. Martens, PhD, Department of Educational, School, and Counseling Psychology, University of Missouri, Columbia, Missouri

Sean Esteban McCabe, PhD, Substance Abuse Research Center and Institute for Research on Women and Gender, University of Michigan, Ann Arbor, Michigan

Megan E. Patrick, PhD, Institute for Social Research, University of Michigan, Ann Arbor, Michigan

Patrick D. Quinn, BA, Department of Psychology, University of Texas at Austin, Austin, Texas

David L. Rabiner, PhD, Center for Child and Family Policy and Department of Psychology and Neuroscience, Duke University, Durham, North Carolina

Richard R. Reich, PhD, College of Arts and Sciences, University of South Florida, Sarasota–Manatee, Florida

Robert F. Saltz, PhD, Prevention Research Center, Berkeley, California

John E. Schulenberg, PhD, Survey Research Center, Institute for Social Research, University of Michigan, Ann Arbor, Michigan

Kenneth J. Sher, PhD, Department of Psychological Sciences, University of Missouri, Columbia, Missouri

Lea P. Stewart, PhD, Livingston College and Department of Communication, Rutgers, The State University of New Jersey, New Brunswick, New Jersey

Susan Tapert, PhD, VA San Diego Healthcare System and Department of Psychiatry, University of California, San Diego, La Jolla, California

Christian J. Teter, PharmD, Substance Abuse Research Center, University of Michigan, Ann Arbor, Michigan, and College of Pharmacy, University of New England, Portland, Maine

Alvaro Vergés, MA, Department of Psychological Sciences, University of Missouri, Columbia, Missouri

Denise D. Walker, PhD, School of Social Work, University of Washington, Seattle, Washington

Scott T. Walters, PhD, School of Public Health, University of North Texas, Fort Worth, Texas

Helene Raskin White, PhD, Center of Alcohol Studies and Department of Sociology, Rutgers, The State University of New Jersey, Piscataway, New Jersey

Series Editors' Note

Virtually every college in the United States now offers an orientation to incoming students about the dangers of binge drinking. Although it is not clear that this orientation is effective, college leaders know that they must try to address the problem. Colleges are searching for solutions. They have been extraordinarily diverse in their responses, ranging from hard-and-fast public sanctions to privately wishing that the problem would simply go away. Colleges have likewise been diverse in their success, although the relation between response and success is not obvious.

Part of the challenge is that since the early 1980s, when states were enticed by the federal government to enact laws making alcohol consumption illegal for anyone under the age of 21, college leaders have not been publicly able to tolerate drinking in moderation, and they cannot implement experiences in the learning of "drinking in moderation." In 2006, Congress passed the Sober Truth on Preventing (STOP) Underage Drinking Act, which further solidified a zero-tolerance approach to the problem. Adolescents are not allowed to drink, but when they turn 21 they are suddenly given full license to consume alcohol without any preparation. Not surprisingly, many 21-year-olds fail miserably. Also not surprisingly, many college students under age 21 drink to excess.

Some college presidents have called for open discussion and innovative solutions, even to the point of wondering whether laws should be amended to allow for on-campus drinking. To other college leaders, the very suggestion of allowing drinking on campus is sacrilegious and tantamount to opening the flood gates.

The goal of this volume is to bring developmental and prevention science to bear on this unsolved problem. The volume had its origins in discussions with officials at the National Institute on Drug Abuse. It developed further during discussions with Duke University President Richard Brodhead, who understood both the magnitude of the national problem and the challenge in solving it. In May 2010, we held the conference "College Student Drinking and Drug Use: Multiple Perspectives on a Complex Problem" at the Center for Child and Family Policy at Duke University, during which 200 scholars, college administrators, and practitioners assembled for 2 days to examine what is known about the development and ecology of college drinking and other substance use problems, and ways to intervene. This volume compiles the research of speakers at that conference.

This volume brings to a close the Duke Series in Child Development and Public Policy. The series has brought the highest-quality research in the vibrant field of child development to bear on important problems in clinical practice and public policy facing children and families. Each volume in the series has grown out of a national conference held at Duke's Center for Child and Family Policy. Participants across conferences have included nationally renowned scholars from multiple disciplines, officials in public service who are charged with improving the lives of families and children, and students who are learning how to integrate scholarship with service. We are grateful to those who have attended. Reflecting the goal of intersecting basic behavioral science with public policy, the series itself has been a partnership between Duke's Center for Child and Family Policy and the Department of Psychology and Neuroscience, with Series Editors Kenneth A. Dodge and Martha Putallaz, respectively, anchoring these two groups. Each volume in the series also follows the model of an editorial partnership between a scholar at Duke and a leading scholar at another university. This volume's editors, Duke's David L. Rabiner, a clinical psychologist, and Rutgers University's Helene Raskin White, a sociologist, are leading scholars of college substance abuse. We are grateful for their leadership of the conference and volume. They have assembled a fascinating, engaging, and rigorous analysis of the problem that offers innovative solutions, policies, and programs.

KENNETH A. DODGE, PhD
MARTHA PUTALLAZ, PhD

Acknowledgments

We would like to thank all of the authors for their contributions to the success of the 2010 conference at Duke University and for their excellent chapters that make up this book. Generous support for the conference was provided by the Center for Child and Family Policy, under the directorship of Kenneth A. Dodge, and by the Office of the Provost, under the leadership of Provost Peter Lang and Vice Provost Susan Roth. This support enabled us to bring together researchers, practitioners, and college administrators to discuss the important issue of college drinking and drug use and to open the event to a diverse audience interested in learning about the latest developments in the field.

We appreciate the support of Duke University President Richard Brodhead, who has been a vocal advocate of public debate about the problem of college-age drinking and a staunch supporter of the importance of scientific research as a guide to policy.

Special thanks go to Center for Child and Family Policy Associate Director Barbara Pollock and her administrative staff for their help in making the conference run smoothly. In particular, we would like to recognize the invaluable contributions of Erika Layko at the Center for overseeing all organizational details and Suzanne Valdivia for her editorial assistance in completing the manuscript. Finally, we would like to thank those who attended the conference and whose insightful questions and comments contributed greatly to what both presenters and attendees were able to learn from the event.

Contents

College Drinking and Drug Use

Introductory Comments

Helene Raskin White *and* David L. Rabiner

A substantial number of youth experience significant increases in their substance use as they transition from high school to college (Bachman, Wadsworth, O'Malley, Johnston, & Schulenberg, 1997). Many leave their homes, parents, and old friends and these changes lead to new freedoms, including more free time, and reductions of informal social controls. The freedoms associated with this transitional period can contribute to an increase in alcohol and drug use (Arnett, 2005; Maggs, 1997; White & Jackson, 2004/2005). Youth also face more challenges as they enter college, such as paying for college, balancing academic demands and social pressures, taking on new roles, and developing new friendships. Each of these challenges may be stressful, and some students turn to alcohol and drugs to cope with this stress and associate with other students who also use substances to cope, thereby reinforcing such behavior (Paschall & Flewelling, 2002). In addition, many students enter college with perceptions that heavy drinking and drug use are normative behaviors among college students, that substance use has a facilitative effect on making new friends, and that substance use is a symbol of maturity (Maggs, 1997; Paschall & Flewelling, 2002; Schulenberg & Maggs, 2002; White & Jackson, 2004/2005). Therefore, there may be both positive (e.g., to be social) and negative (e.g., to cope with the stresses and challenges or to conform to misperceived norms) reasons associated with increases in substance use during the transition to college.

Despite some potentially positive benefits of drinking for college students (e.g., socializing), excessive drinking and drug use among college students are associated with negative consequences that can have long-term ramifications (White & Jackson, 2004/2005). In 2005, 1,825 U.S. college student deaths and 599,000 injuries among college students were directly or indirectly alcohol related (Hingson, Zha, & Weitzman, 2009). Excessive drinking and drug use by college students is associated with increased risks of injury, academic failure, unsafe sexual behavior, and violence perpetration and victimization (Goldman, 2002; Presley, Meilman, & Cashin, 1996; Wechsler, Lee, Kuo, & Lee, 2000; Wechsler, Lee, Nelson, & Lee, 2001). In addition, other students and residents of local neighborhoods are often affected (e.g., by vandalism, insults, and sleep disturbances; Wechsler et al., 2001).

Approximately 31% of U.S. college students report symptoms of alcohol abuse and 6% report symptoms of dependence (Knight et al., 2002). Most of these students, however, will outgrow problematic drinking and drug use without treatment (Marlatt et al., 1998; Schulenberg, O'Malley, Bachman, Wadsworth, & Johnston, 1996; Weingardt et al., 1998). Nevertheless, they are still in danger of negative consequences during their college years when their substance use peaks. Therefore, there is a need for effective prevention and intervention programs to help students make it safely through this risky period (Dimeff, Baer, Kivlahan, & Marlatt, 1999). Furthermore, for a subset of youth, problem use is quite stable from the early to late 20s and can develop into more serious problems following college (O'Neill, Parra, & Sher, 2001). Therefore, heavy drinking and drug use among college students represents an important concern for campus policymakers and practitioners.

This concern led to the organization of a national meeting held at Duke University on May 18 and 19, 2010, to discuss the issues surrounding college student drinking and drug use. This 1½-day meeting brought together researchers, clinicians, and college administrators interested in addressing this problem. The presentations at the conference provided multiple perspectives on this complex problem and form the basis for the chapters in this book. Our hope is that you will find that these chapters not only represent comprehensive reviews of the most up-to-date scientific information on college student alcohol and drug use, but that they also include a number of useful suggestions for how this information can be applied today to address this issue on college campuses. By integrating the latest scientific information with suggestions for how this information can be applied, our goal is to provide a volume that has utility for the diverse range of audiences that were represented at the conference.

The first section of the book presents information on the nature and extent of substance use on college campuses. First, Schulenberg and Patrick summarize national trends in 30-day drinking, binge drinking, marijuana use, and other illicit drug use using multiple waves of data from the Monitoring the Future Study. They argue that patterns of substance use vary over time due to both historical and developmental shifts in use. Whereas rates of 30-day alcohol use among college students have shown only modest linear declines from the 1970s to today, and rates of binge drinking have been amazingly constant over time, rates of marijuana and other illicit drug use have shown wide cyclical trends. In general, college students binge-drink more often than their non-college peers but are less likely to use hard drugs. Both groups, however, have experienced the same historical changes in use patterns. Schulenberg and Patrick also show how developmental trajectories of substance use differ between college students and their non-college peers, and between those who graduate from college and those who drop out. Finally, they demonstrate that even within a college sample, there is wide variation in patterns of binge drinking over time. Predicting in advance which youth will follow which trajectory—something that would have important prevention implications—is quite difficult.

Next, McCabe and colleagues focus on prescription medication use. After marijuana use, nonmedical use of prescription drugs is the most prevalent form of illicit drug use among college students. And, in contrast to longitudinal trends in the rates of illicit drug use among college students, which have shown substantial declines, the rate of nonmedical use of prescription drugs has been increasing. McCabe and colleagues discuss the prevalence of prescription medication diversion and nonmedical misuse of prescription medications (including scheduled opioid, stimulant, sedative/anxiolytic, and sleeping medications). They also cover other critical issues related to nonmedical misuse of prescription medications, such as routes of administration, co-ingestion with other drugs, motivations for using, and the negative consequences of use. Their chapter closes with a number of thoughtful suggestions for college/university administrators and heath professionals who wish to address this issue on their campus.

The second section of the book explores biological and neuropsychological effects of, and contributions to, substance use. Lisdahl and Tapert report findings from their research that show how heavy drinking and marijuana use among adolescents and college students impair brain structure and functioning. Specifically, certain parts of the brain are still maturing during the college years and use of alcohol and drugs can interfere with this maturation. They argue that the effects of alcohol and drugs on the developing brain may partially account for the lower academic achievement of heavy drinkers and drug users compared to their nonusing peers. This information may be quite useful for clinicians working with college populations. Bates and Buckman discuss emotional dysregulation and how it affects drinking behavior. They suggest that some students may use alcohol and drugs to regulate their emotions, and that such use may be biologically determined. In other words, students who have greater difficulty regulating their emotional arousal may be at heightened risk for persistent substance use. Bates and Buckman summarize results from their own research demonstrating heterogeneity in students' physiological modulation of emotional arousal and suggest that interventions designed to help students regulate their emotional arousal may be beneficial for reducing hazardous drinking and drug use, particularly among the subset of students who are prone to become dysregulated.

Psychological and social aspects of substance use are explored in the third section of the book. First, Reich and Goldman discuss how expectancies surrounding alcohol affect student behavior. They argue that young people expect social and sexual benefits from drinking and that these expectations may consciously and unconsciously influence their decision to drink. Reich and Goldman present data from their laboratory showing that similar expectancies are held by both college students and their non-college peers. Their research suggests that there are developmental processes that are common to all young people during this life period, regardless of college attendance. Reich and Goldman focus their chapter on two of these developmental characteristics, which are strongly related to drinking: risk taking and elevated social motivation. Expectancies regarding the effects of alcohol on these processes are significantly related to drinking behavior. Their research demonstrates the importance of both explicit (conscious) and implicit (unconscious) alcohol expectancies for predicting drinking behavior.

Next, also focusing in part on alcohol expectancies, Fromme and Quinn discuss the associations between heavy drinking and other problematic behaviors including aggression, risky sexual behaviors, sexual assault, and illicit drug use. They highlight several theoretical models that can account for these associations and then present results from their own laboratory and survey research. Their research clearly demonstrates that heavy drinking increases the risk for engagement in many types of high-risk behaviors. Overall, their studies support an expectancy-mediated pharmacological model in which alcohol intoxication contributes to behavioral risk taking by reducing negative outcome expectancies. Their laboratory and daily diary studies suggest that risk taking may not only be a function of how much alcohol a student consumes but also his or her actual and subjective response to that alcohol. Their findings have particularly interesting implications for "light" drinkers who exceed their typical level of intoxication, a group that may not be served well by current universal prevention programs.

Fromme and Quinn's discussion of underlying traits ties directly to Vergés and Sher's chapter, which examines how personality and environmental influences affect drinking behavior. These authors summarize data from national studies, as well as data from their own longitudinal research on college students. Several environmental factors strongly influence drinking among college students, including the characteristics of the campus and student population (e.g., size, racial/ethnic makeup), class schedules, where students live, and fraternity and sorority membership. Nevertheless, there are also individual factors that predict heavy drinking, such as personality traits and motives/expectancies. Vergés and Sher's research highlights the importance of paying greater attention to the interaction of individual and environmental factors in efforts to address college student drinking and drug use.

The fourth section of the book focuses on preventive strategies. First, Cronce and Larimer discuss brief interventions to reduce heavy drinking. Previously, Larimer and Cronce (2002, 2007) reviewed outcomes of randomized controlled trials of individually focused preventive interventions published between 1984 and early 2007 and showed that there is a significant body of research supporting the efficacy of brief motivational interventions and personal feedback interventions. In their chapter, they update those earlier reviews by including studies published from 2007 to 2010. This latter body of research adds more support for these types of individualized approaches as well as some support for cognitive-behavioral skills-based approaches. The limitations of these approaches are also noted.

Marijuana is used by more than half of all college students (Johnston, O'Malley, Bachman, & Schulenberg, 2010) and can have negative effects on learning (Medina et al., 2007). Therefore, specific interventions are needed to address college student marijuana use, although few have been implemented and even fewer have been evaluated. Walters, Lee, and Walker argue that despite the documented negative consequences associated with marijuana use, most students perceive that marijuana use is not very harmful. They also discuss the individual and environmental predictors of marijuana use among college students, which are quite similar to those highlighted by Vergés and Sher for heavy drinking. Finally, they summarize the interventions that exist for marijuana use. Because of the scarcity of college-based programs that address marijuana use, they describe interventions for adults in general. They conclude their chapter by discussing issues surrounding implementation of interventions for marijuana use on college campuses; highlighting two promising approaches: personal feedback interventions and motivational enhancement interventions. Interestingly, according to Cronce and Larimer, these two types of interventions are also the most promising for reducing heavy drinking.

Martens then discusses the unique issues facing college student-athletes who generally report higher levels of binge drinking than other students. He first summarizes studies that have compared alcohol use among college athletes to their non-athlete peers. Next, he highlights risk factors that might account for the high rates of binge drinking among college students, including personality traits, stress, competition, and social opportunities. He then discusses the various interventions available for athletes, such as skills building interventions, social marketing interventions, and personalized feedback interventions. Because of the lack of rigorous research on this population, Martens is hesitant to make a definitive statement about which interventions are most effective. Nevertheless, he and his colleagues have recently completed an interesting study with college athletes that demonstrates promising results for personal feedback interventions.

Whereas the three preceding chapters focused primarily on individual-level interventions, Saltz focuses on community and environmental interventions. He argues that reducing college student drinking should be framed within a public health perspective, and that individually oriented preventive interventions should be part of a more comprehensive program aimed at reducing drinking at the broader community level. Saltz notes that there are many more light and moderate drinkers than heavy drinkers, and that the former two groups are responsible for the majority of alcohol-related problems. Thus, one needs universal, population-level interventions to reduce drinking and related problems, rather than focusing efforts exclusively on heavy drinkers. He provides examples of three successful community interventions that could be adopted for college campuses and then summarizes recent multicomponent, comprehensive prevention interventions that he and his colleagues designed, implemented, and evaluated. As you will see, evaluations of these programs clearly demonstrate that community-level environmental interventions can reduce college student drinking and related problems.

In agreement with Saltz, Kilmer and Bailie argue that more comprehensive programs are needed. They claim that college student substance use is frequently embedded in a host of other mental health problems, such as depression and stress, and that all these problems need to be addressed concurrently. Kilmer and Bailie note that more than half of the students who need help for mental health and substance use problems are not receiving help. Therefore, more screening and outreach is needed to identify students with mental health problems. The authors end their chapter by describing the comprehensive Health and Wellness program being run at the University of Washington campus that represents an innovative method for addressing this pressing need.

Most college student problem drinking and drug use is time limited, and the main purpose of the preventive interventions described above is to help students reduce their substance use and the risks associated with it during their peak using years. Nonetheless, a growing proportion of college students have substance use disorders, which require more intensive interventions. Furthermore, there is a group of students who are in recovery from substance use disorders when they first enter college, and another group who end up in recovery at some point during their college careers. Laitman and Stewart discuss the special challenges these students face on college campuses, given the extent of alcohol and drug use in the immediate environment. They also highlight the need to offer recovery support programs for these students. Laitman and Stewart describe the elements necessary to develop and maintain recovery support programs on college campuses (strikingly few such programs exist today) and summarize results from evaluations of such programs. They end their chapter by describing the existing program at Rutgers University, which was the first college campus in the United States to provide recovery housing for students.

The fifth and final section of the book focuses on policy changes to address college student drinking. Specifically, Cook and Gearing present an argument for lowering the current minimum legal drinking age (MLDA) from 21 to 18. First, they argue that the current MLDA is an infringement on liberty. Second, it interferes with a broader, potentially more effective approach to reducing alcohol abuse. Third, it interferes with experimentation with potentially effective alternative prevention and policy approaches, especially on college campuses. Cook and Gearing concede that lowering the MLDA could lead to more traffic fatalities and alcohol-related deaths and accidents among 18- to 20-year-olds, and to increased drinking by this age group and possibly younger adolescents. Nevertheless, they argue that the benefits, especially greater liberty for young adults and an understanding that college drinking is embedded in the broader problem of adult drinking, outweigh the potential costs. Furthermore, if drinking among college students were legal, then lawmakers and college administrators would have the opportunity to adopt innovative regulations and policies and to study how they work. Cook and Gearing also argue that making it illegal for 18- to 20-year-olds to drink pushes drinking "underground" and limits monitoring of drinking behavior.

In response, Saltz and Fell argue that lowering the drinking age would not only increase traffic fatalities but would also increase drinking at earlier ages. That is, if the drinking age were lowered to 18, youth would start drinking at younger ages because it would be much easier for younger students to obtain alcohol from their 18-year-old peers still in high school. Saltz and Fell present evidence showing that the age 21 MLDA law significantly reduced traffic accidents and fatalities for drivers under age 21, as well as reduced homicides, suicides, and unintentional injuries by 18- to 20-year-olds. They also argue that in other countries with lower drinking ages than the United States, youth suffer from alcohol-related problems as great as or greater than those in the United States.

We present both sides of the MLDA argument in an effort to provide an objective account of this ongoing and important debate. It is hoped that these two chapters and the other chapters in this book will provide information that will promote continued dialogue about college student drinking and drug use, and contribute to the search for more cost-effective methods for dealing with the problems associated with this issue. As Berg (2010) suggests, real progress toward reducing substance use problems on college campuses will not occur without institutionwide support for prevention, and input and support from key stakeholders across campuses. At present, she argues, prevention of alcohol use problems is not an institutional priority on many campuses due to a lack of leadership from senior administrators, lack of consistent funding for such efforts, and the absence of institutionwide accountability for performance on student health and wellness. Berg suggests that an effective way to make alcohol prevention a priority for a university is to highlight the connections between high-risk drinking and "mission-critical" priorities including enrollment and retention, academic excellence, student engagement, revenue generation, cost reduction, and protecting the value of the brand. Further, she estimates that alcohol use costs the average university more than $500,000 a year in terms of attrition, counseling, adjudication, nonbillable property damage, and public safety. Making the financial and retention issues related to student substance use more visible to campus leaders may be a good strategy for increasing universitywide commitment to alcohol and drug prevention. It will take a concerted effort to reduce the problems associated with college student drinking and drug use. This book highlights some of the approaches that can be used to move us in that direction.

REFERENCES

Arnett, J. J. (2005). The developmental context of substance use in emerging adulthood. *Journal of Drug Issues, 35,* 235–254.

Bachman, J. G., Wadsworth, K. N., O'Malley, P. M., Johnston, L. D., & Schulenberg, J. (1997). *Smoking, drinking and drug use in young adulthood: The impacts of new freedoms and new responsibilities.* Mahway, NJ: Erlbaum.

Berg, C. (2010, May). *Institutionalizing alcohol prevention: Broadening alcohol prevention beyond student affairs.* Paper presented at the Duke University conference College Student Drinking and Drug Use: Multiple Perspectives on a Complex Problem, Durham, NC.

Dimeff, L. A., Baer, J. S., Kivlahan, D. R., & Marlatt, G. A. (1999). *Brief Alcohol Screening and Intervention for College Students (BASICS): A harm reduction approach.* New York: Guilford Press.

Goldman, M. S. (2002). Introduction. *Journal of Studies on Alcohol* (Suppl. 14), 5.

Hingson, R. W., Zha, W., & Weitzman, E. R. (2009). Magnitude of and trends in alcohol-related mortality and morbidity among U.S. college students ages 18–24, 1998–2005. *Journal of Studies on Alcohol and Drugs, 16,* 12–20.

Johnston, L. D., O'Malley, P. M., Bachman, J. G., & Schulenberg, J. E. (2010). *Monitoring the Future national survey results on drug use, 1975–2009: Vol. II. College students and adults ages 19–50* (NIH Publication No. 10-7585). Bethesda, MD: National Institute on Drug Abuse.

Knight, J., Wechsler, H., Kuo, M., Seibring, M., Weitzman, E., & Schuckit, M. (2002). Alcohol abuse and dependence among U.S. college students. *Journal of Studies on Alcohol, 63,* 263–270.

Larimer, M. E., & Cronce, J. M. (2002). Identification, prevention and treatment: A review of individual-focused strategies to reduce problematic alcohol consumption by college students. *Journal of Studies on Alcohol, 14,* 148–163.

Larimer, M. E., & Cronce, J. M. (2007). Identification, prevention, and treatment revisited: Individual-focused college drinking prevention strategies 1999–2006. *Addictive Behaviors, 32,* 2439–2468.

Maggs, J. L. (1997). Alcohol use and binge drinking as goal-directed action during the transition to postsecondary education. In J. Schulenberg, J. L. Maggs, & K. Horrelmann (Eds.), *Health risks and developmental transitions during adolescence* (pp. 345–371). New York: Cambridge University Press.

Marlatt, G. A., Baer, J. S., Kivlahan, D. R., Dimeff, L. A., Larimer, M. E., Quigley, L. A., et al. (1998). Screening and brief intervention for high-risk college student drinkers: Results from a 2–year follow-up assessment. *Journal of Consulting and Clinical Psychology, 66,* 604–615.

Medina, K. L., Hanson, K., Schweinsburg, A. D., Cohen-Zion, M., Nagel, B. J., & Tapert, S. F. (2007). Neuropsychological functioning in adolescent marijuana users: Subtle deficits detectable after 30 days of abstinence. *Journal of the International Neuropsychological Society, 13*(5), 807–820.

O'Neill, S., Parra, G., & Sher, K. J. (2001). Clinical relevance of heavy drinking during the college years: Cross-sectional and prospective perspectives. *Psychology of Addictive Behaviors, 15,* 350–359.

Paschall, M., & Flewelling, R. L. (2002). Postsecondary education and heavy drinking by young adults: The moderating effect of race. *Journal of Studies on Alcohol, 63,* 447–455.

Presley, C. A., Meilman, P. W., & Cashin, J. R. (1996). *Alcohol and drugs on American campuses: Use, consequences, and perceptions of the campus environment: Vol. 4. 1992–1994.* Carbondale, IL: CORE Institute, Southern Illinois University.

Schulenburg, J. E., & Maggs, J. L. (2002). A developmental perspective on alcohol use and heavy drinking during adolescence and the transition to young adulthood. *Journal of Studies on Alcohol* (Suppl. No. 14), 54–70.

Schulenberg, J., O'Malley, P. M., Bachman, J. G., Wadsworth, K. M., & Johnston, L. D. (1996). Getting drunk and growing up: Trajectories of frequent binge drinking in the transition to young adulthood. *Journal of Studies on Alcohol, 57,* 289–304.

Wechsler, H., Lee, J. E., Kuo, M., & Lee, H. (2000). College binge drinking in the 1990s: A continuing problem: Results of the Harvard School of Public Health 1999 College Alcohol Study. *Journal of American College Health, 48,* 199–210.

Wechsler, H., Lee, J. E., Nelson, T. F., & Lee, H. (2001). Drinking levels, alcohol problems, and secondhand effects in substance-free college residences: Results of a national study. *Journal of Studies on Alcohol, 62,* 23–31.

Weingardt, K. R., Baer, J. S., Kivlahan, D. R., Roberts, L. J., Miller, E. T., & Marlatt, G.A. (1998). Episodic heavy drinking among college students: Methodological issues and longitudinal perspectives. *Psychology of Addictive Behaviors, 12,* 155–167.

White, H. R., & Jackson, K. M. (2004/2005). Social and psychological influences on emerging adult drinking behavior. *Alcohol Health and Research, 28,* 182–190.

PART I

THE SCOPE
OF THE PROBLEM

Historical and Developmental Patterns of Alcohol and Drug Use among College Students

Framing the Problem

John E. Schulenberg *and* Megan E. Patrick

How do we best frame the problem of college student alcohol and drug use? Is it a problem that has been getting worse or better in recent years? Have the historical changes been specific to college students or more generally true of all in the 18- to 22-year-old age group? Indeed, is it more productive to view age 18–22 substance use as a college-specific issue or more of a time-of-life issue? What are the developmental trajectories of alcohol and drug use across the college years? How do these trajectories vary for those who drop out of, or never enroll in, college? And do the trajectories matter in terms of psychosocial adjustment? In this chapter, we consider these "big picture" questions, providing empirical evidence based on national multicohort panel data from the Monitoring the Future (MTF) study (Johnston, O'Malley, Bachman, & Schulenberg, 2010) to frame college student substance use both historically and developmentally.

We begin by providing an overview of historical variations, considering trends in several indices of substance use across three decades (1980–2009) as a function of college student status among national samples of young people 1 to 4 years post-high school. Then, after considering the developmental context that surrounds college transitions, we examine developmental trends in the two most common substances of abuse—alcohol and marijuana—from the senior year of high school through age 25 as a function of college status and of dropping out of college. Next, we examine different developmental trajectories of frequent heavy drinking (i.e., binge drinking), with particular attention given to college students who were not binge drinkers in high school. In the final section, we discuss theoretical and practical implications.

HISTORICAL TRENDS IN COLLEGE STUDENT AND NON-COLLEGE PEER SUBSTANCE USE, 1980–2009

One truism regarding the epidemiology of substance use is that indices are best thought of as moving targets across historical time. Rarely does a substance use index stay steady across multiple years (Johnston et al., 2010), making it important to know the years of assessment to place substance use within the broader historical context. In describing historical trends, we can conceptualize three types (Schulenberg, Bachman, Johnston, & O'Malley, 1995): (1) cyclical change, represented as a wave-like function (e.g., shifts between political conservatism and liberalism); (2) unidirectional change, represented as a linear function (e.g., the place of computers in our lives); and (3) no change, represented as a constant function (e.g., the desire of parents to give their children a better life). Of course, given sufficient time, it is possible that unidirectional and no-change trends are eventually realized as cyclical change.

Reasons for historical variation in substance use are multiple and complex, relating to drug supply and demand, which are cast in broader cultural, political, and societal trends. Much of what we have seen in substance use over the past half century has been cyclical trends (Johnston et al., 2010). To help explain such cyclical trends, one important consideration is what Johnston (1991) terms "generational forgetting," whereby the dangers of a given drug take center stage for many years, resulting in a decline in use of the drug, followed by a reduction in preventive attention paid to the drug, resulting in a subsequent increase in use. In regard to linear historical trends in drug use, mechanisms pertain to the slow but constant amassing of evidence indicating the dangers (or lack of dangers). The rarity of constant historical trends suggests countervailing forces that oppose the mechanisms of historical change. One leading edge of historical trends in substance use relates to attitudes about the dangers of the given drug, which have shown remarkable prognostic power regarding use of the given drug (e.g., Johnston et al., 2010).

Any consideration of historical variation must contend with possible age-related, cohort (i.e., history-graded), and period (i.e., secular trend) effects. Because we hold age constant (ages 19–22) in this section, we do not attend to age-related changes, and we cannot disentangle cohort and period effects. The historical trends we show could be due to lasting individual differences dependent on one's birth cohort, or to more generalized social-cultural effects experienced by all regardless of cohort. Because our emphasis is descriptive, we do not delve into determining cohort versus period effects (for more on such distinctions, see Johnston et al., 2010).

Monitoring the Future (MTF) Study Data

Data for this chapter come from the MTF study, an ongoing study of adolescents and adults (Johnston et al., 2010). MTF was initiated in 1975 with the primary purpose of understanding the epidemiology and etiology of substance use among American youth. Two design components of the larger project are important for results shown in this chapter: (1) nationally representative samples of high school seniors are surveyed each year; and (2) a subset of individuals is randomly selected for biennial follow-up into adulthood. We briefly summarize MTF design and procedures (for more details, see Bachman, Wadsworth, O'Malley, Johnston, & Schulenberg, 1997; Johnston et al., 2010; Schulenberg, Wadsworth, O'Malley, Bachman, & Johnston, 1996; Schulenberg et al., 2005).

Each year, approximately 17,000 high school seniors in approximately 135 public and private high schools representative of the 48 coterminous states participate in the MTF survey. Self-administered questionnaires are given each spring during school hours. Beginning with the class of 1976, approximately 2,400 respondents have been randomly selected for biennial follow-up from each cohort through mail surveys. One random half of each cohort is surveyed 1 year after high school (modal age 19) and the other random half is surveyed 2 years after high school (modal age 20); each half is followed biennially thereafter. The sample retention rates between wave 1 (age 18) and waves 3 (ages 21–22) and 4 (ages 23–24) (age coverage of primary interest in this chapter) have been between 60% and 70% (which is quite favorable given that MTF is a low-cost national survey study, rather than a more in-depth smaller-scale interview study, which typically gets better retention rates). Previous MTF attrition analyses have shown that, compared with those lost to follow-up, those retained are more likely to be female and white, to have higher parent education levels and GPAs, and to have lower levels of senior-year truancy and substance use (Schulenberg et al., 1996, 2005).

Our emphasis in this section is on the historical variation across three decades (1980–2009) in prevalence rates for four substance use indices as a function of college student status, defined as being enrolled full-time in March of the given year in a 2- or 4-year college at wave 2 (modal ages 19–20) or wave 3 (modal ages 21–22). Thus, the college student group includes those ages 19–22 enrolled full-time; the non-college comparison group includes those ages 19–22 engaged in other pursuits. Between 1980 and 2009, sample sizes per year ranged from 1,000 to 1,500 for college students and 800 to 1,300 for non-college peers. Substance use prevalence rates were based on two indices of occasions of alcohol use (past 30-day use, past 2-week binge drinking) and two indices of occasions of illicit drug use (12-month marijuana use, 12-month illicit drug use other than marijuana) (see Johnston et al., 2010, for details about these measures).

Historical Trends in Alcohol Use

As shown in Figure 1.1a, 30-day alcohol use has shown mostly linear decline across the past three decades, with most change occurring from the early 1980s to the mid-1990s. As is clear, rates have been consistently higher by about 5 percentage points for college students than for non-college youth. For college students, rates went from 81% in 1980 to 64% in 2009; for non-college youth, rates went from 76% in 1980 to 58% in 2009. In general, 30-day alcohol use has been more frequent among young men than young women, but in recent years, rates have not always differed by gender (see Johnston et al., 2010).

A similar historical trend is revealed for binge drinking, as shown in

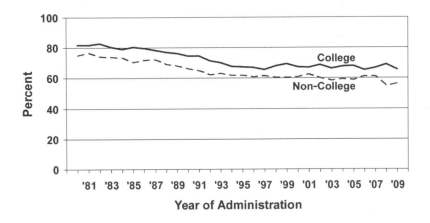

FIGURE 1.1a. Historical trends in 30-day prevalence of alcohol use: College students versus non-college youth (ages 19–22).

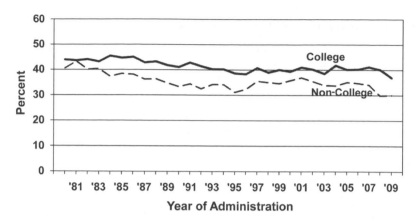

FIGURE 1.1b. Historical trends in 2-week prevalence of binge drinking: College students versus non-college youth (ages 19–22).

Figure 1.1b. Rates have dropped for both college and non-college youth with most of the decline occurring from the early 1980s to the mid-1990s. Rates have been consistently higher for college students than non-college youth by an average of 5 to 6 percentage points. The decline has not been large, however, especially for college students: their rates went from 42% in 1980 to 37% in 2009; for non-college youth, rates went from 40% in 1980 to 30% in 2009. Indeed, despite the slight decline in binge drinking for college students, the rate has been 40% plus/minus 2 percentage points for the past three decades. Gender differences have been consistent, with rates being 15 to 20 percentage points higher for young men than for young women. (This difference would be smaller if we defined binge drinking as four-plus drinks for women [Wechsler, Dowdall, Davenport, & Rimm, 1995]).

Thus, it is clear that alcohol use has been consistently higher for college students than for non-college youth over the past three decades. This pattern is due to numerous causes, including the fact that full-time college enrollment typically involves living away from parents and with like-minded peers (Bachman et al., 1997), as well as being immersed in a culture of excessive drinking, which is common at many colleges (Schulenberg & Maggs, 2002). The modest historical decline in alcohol use is consistent with the general population decline in alcohol use, making this more of a secular trend than a cohort effect (Johnston et al., 2010). It is noteworthy that binge drinking among college students has changed little across the past three decades, hovering around 40%.

Historical Trends in Illicit Drug Use

In contrast to the largely linear and modest declines in alcohol use, the historical change in 12-month marijuana use has been cyclical and extensive as shown in Figure 1.1c. In addition, rates have not differed consistently between college students and non-college youth. For both groups, rates dropped linearly and rapidly (by about 50%) from the early 1980s through the early 1990s, increased modestly until the late 1990s–early 2000s, and decreased inconsistently since then. Between 1980 and 2009, rates of 12-month marijuana use declined from 51% to 33% for college students, and from 49% to 34% for non-college youth. As for gender differences, prevalence rates of 12-month marijuana use have consistently been higher for men than for women, with the difference being 3 to 8 percentage points (Johnston et al., 2010).

Historical trends in use of illicit drugs other than marijuana (OTM) are shown in Figure 1.1d. The cyclical trends are consistent with those found for marijuana use, but OTM rates have been consistently lower by 3 to 5 percentage points for college students than for non-college youth. For both groups, OTM rates dropped by about 60% between the early 1980s and early 1990s, then increased inconsistently into the mid-2000s, and have declined inconsistently since then. Between 1980 and 2009 there was an overall decline from 32% to 17% for college students, and from 36% to 21% for non-college youth. Young men have shown consistently higher rates of OTM use than young women (3 to 8 percentage point differences).

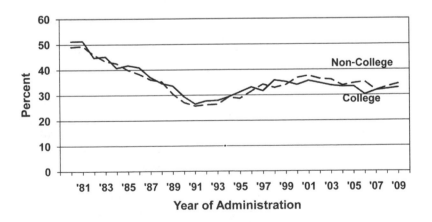

FIGURE 1.1c. Historical trends in annual prevalence of marijuana use: College students versus non-college youth (ages 19–22).

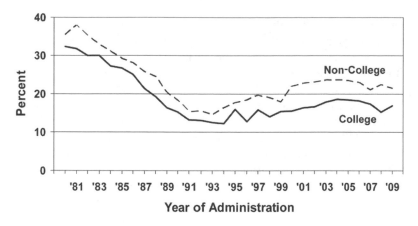

FIGURE 1.1d. Historical trends in annual prevalence of use of any illicit drug other than marijuana: College students versus non-college youth (ages 19–22).

Thus, for illicit drug use, historical trends have shown uneven cyclical trends. The cycles of decline and increase are consistent with Johnston's (1991) notion of generational forgetting discussed earlier. The fact that annual prevalence of marijuana use has been similar for college students and non-college youth suggests that such use is more of an age-of-life matter rather than a college status one. However, as we see below, when considering developmental trends, 30-day marijuana use is more common among those not in college. The annual prevalence of OTM illicit drugs has been consistently higher for non-college youth. Annual marijuana use can be viewed as not particularly deviant or unconventional, but the same is not true for OTM illicit drugs (or for frequent marijuana use), suggesting that, on average, those who attend college are less deviant than non-college youth. Importantly, differences between college students and non-college youth have not changed in any systematic fashion over the past three decades.

COLLEGE AND DEVELOPMENTAL TRENDS IN SUBSTANCE USE

The pursuit of postsecondary education can be a transformative experience. College attendance, particularly if full-time and residential, propels young people into new and unique social contexts variously focused on academic and social activities (Carter, Brandon, & Goldman, 2010; Patrick, Schulenberg, Maggs, & Maslowsky, in press; Schulenberg &

Maggs, 2002). Although more self-direction is required than in high school, college prolongs the availability of innumerable institutional supportive structures for students. These same structures, however, are generally unavailable to those not enrolled. Students are surrounded with age-mates, motivated by cultural beliefs extolling the college years as a time of exploration and experimentation, and buffered by environments relatively tolerant to youthful infractions (Maggs, 1997; Schulenberg & Maggs, 2002). Given these conditions, it is perhaps unsurprising that college students show increased rates of heavy drinking (Johnston et al., 2010). As the college experience ends, and young people make transitions into full-time work and typically more serious romantic relationships, substance use tends to subside (e.g., Bachman et al., 1997; Leonard & Homish, 2005; Staff et al., 2010; White, Labouvie, & Papadaratsakis, 2005), though clearly not for all.

Changes in substance use typically co-vary with changes in the individual and surrounding contexts, making it important to view age-related changes in substance use vis-à-vis other developmental changes. Developmental transitions include major transformations in individuals, in their contexts, and in the relations between individuals and their contexts across the life course (Schulenberg & Maggs, 2002). They often are viewed globally as the connections between major life periods (e.g., transition to adolescence, transition to adulthood), and include a series of specific changes that are internally based (e.g., biological, cognitive) and externally based (e.g., starting college, getting married) (Rutter, 1996). The period between the end of high school and the beginning of full adulthood constitutes the most potentially dynamic decade in the life span in terms of internally based and especially socially based transitions (Arnett, 2000; Patrick et al., 2010; Schulenberg & Maggs, 2002; Shanahan, 2000).

Issues of continuity and discontinuity are central to understanding the power of major developmental transitions. Transitions can contribute to discontinuity in ongoing trajectories of substance use in several ways, such as by overwhelming coping capacities, by changing the person–context match, or by increasing vulnerability to chance events (Schulenberg & Maggs, 2002). By providing "shocks to the system," transitions serve as proximal effects that can counteract developmentally distal (e.g., childhood) effects. The result of such shocks can range from turning points to developmental disturbances (Schulenberg & Zarrett, 2006). Turning points are represented by long-term changes in the course of ongoing trajectories (Rutter, 1996). For example, the transition into marriage relates to declines in substance use, even among those who were heavily involved in alcohol and other drug use (Bachman et al., 1997; Bartholow, Sher, & Krull, 2003).

Developmental disturbances, in contrast, are momentary perturbations followed by resumption of the prior ongoing trajectory (Schulenberg & Zarrett, 2006). In such cases, transitions may simply result in some normative short-term deviance—such as excessive drinking—that is neither predictable in advance nor predictive of future functioning. Of course, despite major life transitions, important contexts sometimes change little. In particular, if one does not leave the parental home after high school and thus maintains similar relationships (good or bad) with family members and peers, then the person–context match (or mismatch) may be maintained across the transition, contributing to some continuity in substance use trajectories (Bachman et al., 1997; Staff et al., 2010; White, Fleming, Kim, Catalano, & McMorris, 2008).

An important non-normative transition embedded within the college experience is dropping out or leaving without a degree. In the United States, one out of every four college freshmen fails to return for a second year, and only 56% of students seeking a bachelor's degree are successful in doing so within 6 years (National Center for Education Statistics, 2010). The association between substance use and dropping out of college is not a clear or consistent one. Although there is some evidence that binge drinking is positively associated with dropping out of college (Jennison, 2004; Perkins, 2002), the evidence about causal connections is mixed (Williams, Powell, & Wechsler, 2002). We suspect that part of the complexity here is that binge drinking can reflect peer bonding and engagement in the college experience, if not the academic part of the experience (Maggs, 1997).

Questions and Data

We examine developmental trends in binge drinking and 30-day marijuana use as a function of college student status and gender. Alcohol and marijuana use are the most common psychoactive substances, and binge drinking during a 2-week period and marijuana use during a 30-day period reflect relatively serious involvement compared to more experimental use. We also show how dropping out relates to substance use trajectories.

We draw from the MTF national panel data described earlier, following young people from senior year in high school (age 18) to age 25 (senior-year cohorts 1976–2000). We limit analyses to the half sample that was surveyed a year after high school (modal age 19), then biennially at modal ages 21, 23, and 25. This allows us to examine the freshman year transition and to consider dropouts between the first and third years of college. College students here are defined as being enrolled full-time in a 4-year college at wave 2 (modal age 19; weighted $N \approx 6,000$ college students, $N \approx 8,000$ non-college youth). College dropouts were enrolled full-time in a 4-year college at wave 2 and then not enrolled full-time in a 4-year college at any of the subsequent waves ($N \approx 600$); college stay-ins were enrolled full-time in a 4-year college at waves 2 and 3 ($N \approx 4,400$); we excluded other small subgroups such as stop-outs.

To test the parameters of the trajectories, we use piece-wise latent growth modeling to represent the five waves of observed data as three latent variables: an intercept (age 18 level), slope 1 (describing the direction and rate of change across ages 18 to 21), and slope 2 (direction and rate of change across ages 21 to 25). This allows us to divide the overall age 19–25 trajectories into two meaningful slopes, with the break (age 21) co-occurring with the typical peak in binge drinking (Patrick & Schulenberg, 2011). We use multigroup modeling to determine whether subgroup differences in intercepts and slopes are significant. We illustrate findings in terms of observed means to describe the average trajectories and note subgroup differences.

Developmental Trajectories by College Student Status and Gender

As shown in Figure 1.2a, when in the senior year of high school, those who are college bound have lower levels of binge drinking than those

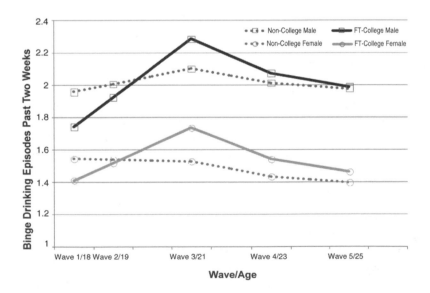

FIGURE 1.2a. Developmental trends in binge drinking: Full-time college students versus non-college youth by gender.

who are not college bound (for males and females, the intercept is significantly lower for youth who will attend college). Then, college students
quickly escalate to surpass non-college youth in rates of binge drinking
by age 21 (slope 1 is increasing and is significantly greater for college students). From ages 21 to 25, college students decrease their binge drinking
at a faster rate than do non-college youth (slope 2 is decreasing and is
significantly greater for college students). By age 25, there is no significant difference in level of binge drinking as a function of previous college
status. Thus, the pattern of steep escalation and decline from senior year
in high school through the mid-20s is far more distinctive of full-time college students (consistent with White et al., 2005), providing support for
characterizing the college experience, for many, as immersion in a culture
of heavy drinking (Schulenberg & Maggs, 2002). These developmental
trends and group differences have not varied historically.

This distinctive escalation–decline pattern for college students is
also evident for 30-day marijuana use, as illustrated in Figure 1.2b. At
senior year of high school (age 18), college-bound students have significantly lower levels of marijuana use than those not college bound. Then,
between ages 18 and 21, marijuana use increases for college students and
declines for non-college youth (slope 1 is significant for all groups, positive for college students and negative for non-college youth). Marijuana

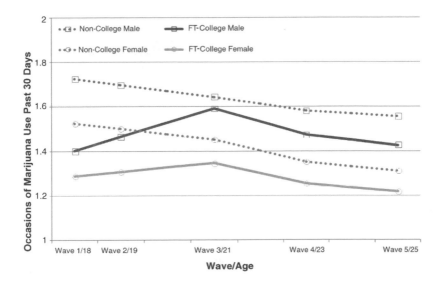

FIGURE 1.2b. Developmental trends in 30-day marijuana use: Full-time college
students versus non-college youth by gender.

use peaks at age 21 for college students and at age 18 for non-college youth. Between ages 21 and 25, marijuana use declines for all groups (slope 2 is significant and negative for all groups); for males, the rate of decline is faster for college than non-college (slope 2 is significantly greater for college males); for females, the rate of decline is similar for college and non-college. Thus, as is true for binge drinking, the trajectory of 30-day marijuana use for college students is characterized as quick escalation out of high school, a peak at age 21, and then a decline to age 25. However, at all ages, marijuana use is higher for non-college youth. These differences and developmental trends have not varied historically.

Developmental Trajectories by College Dropout Status and Gender

We next turn to considering how dropping out of college relates to substance use trajectories. As shown in Figure 1.2c, as seniors in high school, those who eventually drop out have higher rates of binge drinking (significant only for males). Those who dropped out of college (between ages 19 and 21) had significantly *slower* rates of increase than did those who stayed in college during this period; this was true for males and females. That is, *a more rapid increase in binge drinking across the first few years of college was related to staying in, not dropping out of, college*, suggest-

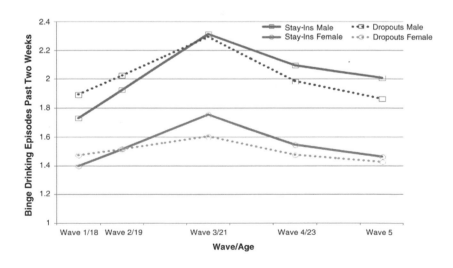

FIGURE 1.2c. Developmental trends in binge drinking: Full-time college student stay-ins versus dropouts by gender.

ing the possible prosocial and peer bonding correlates of binge drinking in college (Maggs, 1997). At age 21, when dropping out had already occurred, stay-in and dropout males had the same level of binge drinking; and then between ages 21 and 25, the level of binge drinking for dropouts declined significantly faster than that for stay-ins. In contrast, for females, stay-ins had a significantly higher level of binge drinking at age 21 and a significantly faster decline between ages 21 and 25 than dropouts. Thus, dropping out of college related to subsequently lower binge drinking, sooner for females and later for males. These differences and developmental trends have not varied historically.

The story is somewhat similar for marijuana use. As shown in Figure 1.2d, those who eventually dropped out of college had higher rates of 30-day marijuana use at age 18. In fact, across the entire age period from 18 to 25, college dropouts had significantly higher rates of marijuana use than stay-ins. For males, dropouts had a significantly slower rate of increase between ages 18 and 21 and a significantly faster rate of decrease between ages 21 and 25 compared to stay-ins. For females, however, there were no differences in the slopes. Thus, only for males' marijuana use do we see the characteristic pattern found for binge drinking: higher intercept, slower positive slope 1, and steeper negative slope 2 for college dropouts compared to stay-ins. These differences and developmental trends have not varied historically.

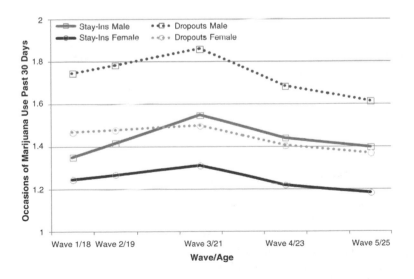

FIGURE 1.2d. Developmental trends in 30-day marijuana use: Full-time college student stay-ins versus dropout by gender.

COLLEGE AND DIFFERENT DEVELOPMENTAL
TRAJECTORIES OF BINGE DRINKING

Building on the findings above, an important question is the extent to which the normative trajectories apply to all. More generally, the question pertains to the heterogeneity of individual trajectories of binge drinking embedded within the total sample. Over the past two decades, developmental science and the study of addictions have recognized the advantages of examining both total sample and individual-level longitudinal trajectories (e.g., Jackson, Sher, & Schulenberg, 2008; Schulenberg & Maggs, 2002; Zucker, 2006).

Questions and Data

In this section, we deconstruct the total sample binge-drinking trajectory described in the previous section, identifying the different embedded developmental trajectory groups. We consider how prevalence of the different binge-drinking trajectory groups varies by college status and college characteristics. We give special attention to college students who were not binge drinkers in high school to see how their trajectories unfold across the college years, attending to psychosocial predictors, correlates, and adulthood outcomes.

MTF national panel data, described extensively above, are used. For the most part, we include four waves of panel data, following young people from senior year of high school through age 24. This time, we use both random halves of each cohort that are followed up (one half starting at age 19 and the other half at age 20, and both followed up biennially thereafter) and combine the two halves such that wave 2 covers modal ages 19–20, wave 3 covers modal ages 21–22, and wave 4 covers modal ages 23–24. We include 23 senior-year cohorts 1976–1998, with weighted $N \approx 20{,}000$. For the long-term follow-up analyses we include panel data up through modal ages 29–30 (cohorts 1976–1995; $N \approx 16{,}000$).

Binge Drinking Trajectory Groups

We have been working with binge drinking (and marijuana use) trajectories for many years, first constructing them with cluster analysis and conceptual groupings followed by growth mixture modeling (e.g., Schulenberg & Maggs, 2002; Schulenberg et al., 1996, 2005). We have consistently found six distinct binge-drinking trajectory groups, as illustrated in Figure 1.3. Clearly, hidden within the total sample trajectory are several distinct longitudinal patterns. The Chronic group, representing 6% of the population (11% of men, 2% of women), had consistently high levels

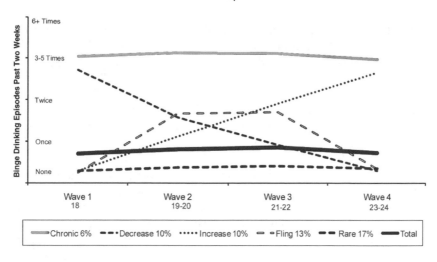

FIGURE 1.3. Developmental trajectories of binge drinking: Mean scores by trajectory group. Adapted from Schulenberg and Maggs (2002). Copyright 2002 by Alcohol Research Documentation, Inc., Rutgers Center of Alcohol Studies, Piscataway, NJ, 08854. Adapted by permission.

of binge drinking between ages 18 and 24, averaging 3–5 binge-drinking episodes per 2-week period. The Decreased group (10% of the population; 11% men, 9% women), had a high level of binge drinking at age 18 (almost as high as the Chronic group), and then dropped consistently across the years to be at a very low level by ages 23–24. Three trajectory groups—Increased, Fling, and Rare—had the same initial level of binge drinking, an average of 0.25 episodes per 2-week period. The Increased group (10% of the population; 14% men, 7% women) showed steadily increasing binge drinking over time, escalating almost to the Chronic group level by ages 23–24. The Fling group (13% of the population; 13% men, 13% women) showed a rapid escalation, rising to an average of over 1.5 episodes of binge drinking per 2-week period at ages 19–20 and 21–22, and then rapidly declining to an average of 0.3 episodes per 2-week period by ages 23–24. The Rare group (17% of the population; 16% men, 18% women) showed consistently low levels of binge drinking across the four waves, averaging 0.3 episodes per 2-week period. The "never" group is not illustrated in Figure 1.3. (It would be a flat line along the *x* axis.) This group represents 38% of the population (26% men, 46% women). Finally, 6% of the population (8% men, 5% women) did not fit into any of the groups.

The number and shape of trajectory groups did not vary by college student status, but prevalence rates of some of the groups did. Significant differences were found for the Decreased group (7% vs. 12% for college and non-college youth, respectively), the Increased group (12% vs. 9%, respectively), and the Fling group (16% vs. 10%, respectively). Thus, college students are more likely to be "late starters," with the Fling group being especially emblematic of college students. Within the college group, there are important differences according to sociodemographics and college experiences. In particular, considering age 19–20 living arrangements (home with parents, in fraternities/sororities, elsewhere), the Chronic, Increased, and Fling groups are most prevalent among fraternity/sorority students and least prevalent among those living with parents; the Never group is most prevalent among students living with parents and least prevalent among fraternity/sorority students. White students have lower rates of the Rare and Never trajectories, and higher rates of the other groups. There were no differences by historical cohort or size of university. Finally, those who eventually dropped out of college had higher rates in the Chronic and Decreased groups, and no differences in the other groups.

College Student Increased versus Fling versus Rare Groups: Predictors and Correlates

The Increased, Fling, and Rare groups offer a natural experiment of sorts because of their initial identical low binge-drinking levels, allowing for the examination of characteristics and experiences that relate to subsequent divergence in trajectories. We consider three questions: (1) can the three groups be distinguished in advance according to age 18 demographic and psychosocial characteristics?; (2) at age 19–20, are there psychosocial differences among the three groups corresponding to the clear binge-drinking differences?; and (3) looking into the future at age 30, are there psychosocial differences among the three trajectory groups?

Numerous predictors and correlates were included in these analyses (for details on the various measures see Bachman et al., 1997; Jackson et al., 2008; McCabe et al., 2005; Schulenberg et al., 1996, 2005; Staff et al., 2010). We used logistic regression analyses to distinguish among the groups based on age 18 predictors, and we used analyses of variance (ANOVAs) to compare the three groups at ages 19–20 and 30.

In predicting trajectory group membership with age 18 measures, it was found that men, whites, those youth who scored higher on drinking to get drunk and evenings out with friends, and those lower on conventionality were more likely to be in the Increased group than in the Rare group; whites and those youth who were higher on evenings out with friends were more likely to be in the Fling group than in the Rare group;

and women were more likely to be in the Fling group than in the Rare group. Especially for the latter two comparisons, these are very short lists of significant predictors, thus highlighting the difficulty in prospectively predicting the divergences, and suggesting that the divergences have more to do with transitional experiences (and perhaps earlier and additional measures).

At ages 19–20 (wave 2), when differences in binge drinking are evident between the groups, there is an abundance of psychosocial differences as well. The Increased and Fling groups, compared to the Rare group, were higher on sensation seeking, risky driving, marijuana and other substance use, drinking to get drunk, evenings out with friends, and fraternity/sorority involvement; they were lower on social conservatism. In addition, the Increased group only (compared to Rare group) was higher on delinquency, social intolerance, proportion of friends who got drunk, and dating; they scored lower on religious importance. These numerous differences between the Increased/Fling groups and the Rare group emerged with the transition to college. Finally, the Increased group, compared to the Fling group, was higher on delinquency and marijuana use and lower on religious importance, suggesting some foreshadowing related to deviance and conventionality of the future divergence in binge drinking in these two groups.

Finally, in terms of psychosocial differences among the three groups at age 30, we found almost no differences in the long list of constructs between the Fling and Rare groups, with the only difference being that the Fling group was significantly higher on self-rated competence as a spouse and parent. Thus, despite their clear differences in binge drinking and psychosocial constructs during college, these two groups were indistinguishable by age 30. Comparing these two groups to the Increased group at age 30 yielded numerous differences: the Increased group was higher on binge drinking, substance use, sensation seeking, risky driving, drinking to get drunk, social intolerance, evenings out with friends, and proportion of friends who got drunk; they were less likely to be married and scored lower on religiosity. The Increased group looked, in relative terms, like they did at age 20. Thus, there appear to be few long-term consequences for the Fling group, yet clear consequences for the Increased group. That these two groups were not especially distinguishable at ages 18 and 19–20 suggests that the emerging and lasting differences had more to do with transitional than preexisting differences.

In relating these findings to what we discussed earlier about discontinuities in substance use, the Increased group reflects a turning point: they experienced a clear and lasting change in course that was difficult to predict in advance (compared to the Rare and Fling groups); that is, they appeared fine at age 18, then increased their binge drinking and related problem behaviors through college, and ended up worse off at age 30. In contrast, the Fling group reflects a developmental disturbance: they experienced a time-limited deviance that was difficult to predict in advance (compared to the Rare and Increased groups) and did not result in future negative consequences (compared to the Rare group). But it would be a mistake to view the Fling group as a salutary trajectory. Although it was time-limited, college students in this group were heavily involved in alcohol use and related deviant activities that could cause themselves and others harm (see Hingson, Heeren, Winter, & Weschler, 2005; Perkins, 2002). Furthermore, recent preliminary evidence suggests male college students in the Fling group were at elevated risk for an alcohol use disorder at age 35 (compared to the Rare group). Finally, because we could not easily distinguish Fling from Increased drinkers at ages 18–20, there is no guarantee that an escalating trajectory of binge drinking is reversible rather than potentially problematic for poorer adult outcomes.

SUMMARY AND IMPLICATIONS

As we have shown, college student substance use is best viewed as a moving target that changes both historically and developmentally. The swings in substance use can be dramatic—for example, prevalence rates of 12-month marijuana use for college students went from 53% in 1981 to 27% in 1991 (a 49% drop in 10 years); developmentally, binge drinking for college males climbs from an average of 0.75 episodes to 1.3 episodes per 2-week period between ages 18 and 21 (a 73% increase in 3 years). Thus, the appropriate frame for the problem of college student substance use includes the historical and developmental context.

Historical Trends

The Monitoring the Future project has monitored historical trends in substance use for over a third of a century, providing the foundation for understanding causes of changes in substance use, and ultimately for reducing substance use (Johnston et al., 2010). For college students across the past three decades, rates of 30-day alcohol use have shown modest linear declines, and rates of illicit drug use (12-month marijuana and other illicit drug use) have shown wide cyclical trends with an overall decline. College student substance use today is not as prevalent as it has been in the past. Compared to historic highs in the last three decades, current rates of monthly alcohol use and annual marijuana and other illicit drug use are all lower. Nonetheless, there is clear room for improvement, and consistent with Johnston, O'Malley, and Bachman's (1995) notion of generational forgetting, easing up on prevention efforts when rates are relatively low can result in subsequent increases.

Constant historical trends are unusual for substance use. Thus, the fact that binge drinking among college students has been nearly constant over the past three decades (hovering around 40%), when all other substances for all other subgroups have varied widely, suggests that powerful countervailing forces keep it locked in place. It would be a mistake to see college binge drinking as an intractable problem, but we must view it as a problem that is multiply determined. That this rate has dropped in the past two years (to 37% in 2009) allows for some optimism. Over the past three decades, compared to non-college youth, college students have been consistently higher in alcohol use (30-day and binge drinking), not consistently different in 12-month marijuana use, and consistently lower in 12-month use of other illicit drugs. The differences between college and non-college youth have generally been consistent (i.e., despite level differences, shapes of the historical trends have been consistent), suggesting that the historical variation is due to forces pertaining to all youth ages 19–22 rather than just to college youth.

Developmental Trends

We show that attending a 4-year college full-time, compared to nonattendance, is related to lower levels of binge drinking and 30-day marijuana use in high school, faster rates of increase in both substances across ages 18 to 21, and then faster rates of decline across ages 21 to 25 such that by age 25, there is little difference in rates for the two groups. Those who eventually drop out of college have higher rates of binge drinking and 30-day marijuana use in high school, suggesting some selection effects; but their rates of increase between ages 18 and 21 (by the time they have dropped out) are actually *slower* than the rates of increase for those who stay in college (except for marijuana use for women), suggesting little relation between escalating substance use during the first few years of college and dropping out.

As we show, embedded within the total sample normative trajectory of binge drinking are several distinct trajectory groups including the Chronic, Decreased, Increased, Fling, Rare, and Never groups. The first two groups (12% of college population) represent the heavy drinkers that colleges "inherit," and the third and fourth groups (38%) represent those who become heavy drinkers with the transition to college. It is instructive to compare the Increased, Fling, and Rare groups, given their common low level of drinking in the senior year of high school. In general, distinguishing the three based on senior-year psychosocial risk factors proved unsuccessful. But at ages 19–20, when most were first- and second-year students, and when their binge drinking started to diverge, the Increased and Fling groups were found to be quite different from the Rare group on many of the same psychosocial risk factors. Then, at age 30, the Fling and Rare groups were found to be nearly indistinguishable, and both were found to be quite distinct from the Increased group, who were slower in taking on adult responsibilities. The Fling group, which represents a prototypical college student trajectory, can be viewed as the result of a developmental disturbance, a time-limited period of deviance that is neither predictable in advance nor predictive of future difficulties. The Increased group can be viewed as having experienced a negative turning point, a clear and long-term change in course that was not predictable in advance. Using this framework to view college student substance use is instructive, but the trajectory groups should be viewed as fluid and not preordained. Although it is tempting to be unconcerned about the Fling group, it is important to note that they are not easily distinguishable in advance from the Increased group who continue to experience problems in adulthood, underscoring the perils of venturing down the path of escalating substance use during the college years.

Prevention and Policy Implications

Several implications follow from the perspective and findings offered in this chapter. First, the transition to college, like other major life transitions, represents a window of opportunity for intervening. Much is already in flux, so the purpose becomes to change something that is already changing, to redirect wayward trajectories. Second, to the extent that difficulties with the transition to college contribute to difficulties with substance use, easing the transition can yield reduced substance abuse (Schulenberg & Maggs, 2002). Third, recognizing that distinct trajectories are embedded within the normative trajectories of binge drinking and marijuana use is important when trying to reduce rates of use (e.g., working to turn Increased trajectories to Fling trajectories). Fourth, common risk factors may be less powerful in college than they are at other ages or in other contexts. The transition to college may be accompanied by substance use that seems to "come out of nowhere" in that those who develop difficulties (e.g., Increased and Fling groups) did not have the well-known risk factors in high school, thus making advanced identification more difficult.

Finally, it must be recognized that important developmental tasks can sometimes be accomplished through substance use (Schulenberg & Maggs, 2002). Indeed, adolescents and young adults typically report that a primary reason for drinking and using illicit drugs is to have a good time with their friends (Patrick & Schulenberg, 2011). According to Chassin, Pitts, and DeLucia (1999), risk taking and even deviance can serve "constructive" as well as "destructive" functions in health and development. As Maggs (1997) demonstrates, alcohol use during the transition to college may help to achieve valued social goals, such as making new friends, although at the same time it may threaten safety and short- and long-term health and well-being. In addition, as we show, staying in college, rather than dropping out, is associated with a more rapid increase in binge drinking, suggesting that such drinking reflects college engagement. Thus, substance use may sometimes reflect success in, or help accomplish, various social and identity tasks; finding alternatives that are equally effective in accomplishing such tasks is an important goal for substance use prevention efforts with college students.

ACKNOWLEDGMENTS

Work on this chapter was funded in part by support from the National Institute on Drug Abuse (Grant No. R01 DA 01411). The content here is solely the responsibility of the authors and does not necessarily represent the official views of the sponsors. We thank Deborah Kloska, Patti Meyer, Adam Burke, and Patricia Berglund for assistance with analyses and figures.

REFERENCES

Arnett, J. J. (2000). Emerging adulthood: A theory of development from the late teens through the twenties. *American Psychologist, 55,* 469–480.

Bachman, J. G., Wadsworth, K. N., O'Malley, P. M., Johnston, L. D., & Schulenberg, J. E. (1997). *Smoking, drinking, and drug use in young adulthood: The impact of new freedoms and new responsibilities.* Mahwah, NJ: Erlbaum.

Bartholow, B. D., Sher, K. J., & Krull, J. L. (2003). Changes in heavy drinking over the third decade of life as a function of collegiate fraternity and sorority involvement: A prospective, multilevel analysis. *Health Psychology, 22,* 616–626.

Carter, A. C., Brandon, K. O., & Goldman, M. S. (2010). The college and noncollege experience: A review of the factors that influence drinking behavior in young adulthood. *Journal of Studies on Alcohol and Drugs, 71,* 742–750.

Chassin, L., Pitts, S. C., & DeLucia, C. (1999). The relation of adolescent substance use to young adult autonomy, positive activity involvement, and perceived competence. *Development and Psychopathology, 11,* 915–932.

Hingson, R., Heeren, T., Winter, M., & Wechsler, H. (2005). Magnitude of alcohol-related mortality and morbidity among U. S. college students ages 18–24: Changes from 1998 to 2001. *Annual Review of Public Health, 26,* 259–279.

Jackson, K. M., Sher, K. J., & Schulenberg, J. E. (2008). Conjoint developmental trajectories of young adult substance use. *Alcoholism: Clinical and Experimental Research, 32,* 1–15.

Jennison, K. M. (2004). The short-term effects and unintended long-term consequences of binge drinking in college: A 10-year follow-up study. *American Journal of Drug and Alcohol Abuse, 30,* 659–684.

Johnston, L. D. (1991). Toward a theory of drug epidemics. In R. L. Donohew, H. Sypher, & W. Bukoski (Eds.), *Persuasive communication and drug abuse prevention* (pp. 93–132). Hillsdale, NJ: Erlbaum.

Johnston, L. D., O'Malley, P. M., & Bachman, J. G. (1995). *National survey results on drug use from the Monitoring the Future Study, 1975–1994: Vol. 1. Secondary school students* (NIH Publication No. 95-4026). Rockville, MD: National Institute on Drug Abuse.

Johnston, L. D., O'Malley, P. M., Bachman, J. G., & Schulenberg, J. E. (2010). *Monitoring the Future national survey results on drug use, 1975–2009: Vol. I. Secondary school students* (NIH Publication No. 10-7584). Bethesda, MD: National Institute on Drug Abuse.

Leonard, K. E., & Homish, G. G. (2005). Changes in marijuana use over the transition into marriage. *Journal of Drug Issues, 45,* 409–429.

Maggs, J. L. (1997). Alcohol use and binge drinking as goal-directed action during the transition to post-secondary education. In J. Schulenberg, J. L. Maggs, & K. Hurrelmann (Eds.), *Health risks and developmental transitions during adolescence* (pp. 345–371). New York: Cambridge University Press.

McCabe, S. E., Schulenberg, J. E., Johnston, L. D., O'Malley, P. M., Bachman, J. G., & Kloska, D. D. (2005). Selection and socialization effects of fraternities and sororities on U. S. college student substance use: A multi-cohort national longitudinal study. *Addiction, 100,* 512–524.

National Center for Education Statistics. (2010). *IPEDS graduation rate survey.* Washington, DC: U.S. Department of Education.

Patrick, M. E., & Schulenberg, J. E. (2011). How trajectories of reasons for alcohol use relate to trajectories of binge drinking: National panel data spanning late adolescence to early adulthood. *Developmental Psychology, 47*(2), 311–317.

Patrick, M. E., Schulenberg, J. E., Maggs, J. L., & Maslowsky, J. (in press). Substance use and peers during adolescence and emerging/early adulthood: Socialization, selection, and developmental transitions. In K. Sher (Ed.), *Handbook of substance use disorders.* New York: Oxford University Press.

Perkins, H. W. (2002). Surveying the damage: A review of research on consequences of alcohol misuse in college populations. *Journal of Studies on Alcohol* (Suppl. 14), 91–100.

Rutter, M. (1996). Transitions and turning points in developmental psychopathology: As applied to the age span between childhood and mid-adulthood. *International Journal of Behavioral Development, 19,* 603–626.

Schulenberg, J., Bachman, J. G., Johnston, L. D., & O'Malley, P. M. (1995). American adolescents' views on family and work: Historical trends from 1976–1992. In P. Noack, M. Hofer, & J. Youniss (Eds.), *Psychological responses to social change: Human development in changing environments* (pp. 37–64). Berlin: Walter de Gruyter.

Schulenberg, J. E., & Maggs, J. L. (2002). A developmental perspective on alcohol use and heavy drinking during adolescence and the transition to young adulthood. *Journal of Studies on Alcohol* (Suppl. 14), 54–70.

Schulenberg, J. E., Merline, A. C., Johnston, L. D., O'Malley, P. M., Bachman, J. G., & Laetz, V. B. (2005). Trajectories of marijuana use during the transition to adulthood: The big picture based on national panel data. *Journal of Drug Issues, 35,* 255–279.

Schulenberg, J. E., Wadsworth, K. N., O'Malley, P. M., Bachman, J. G., & Johnston, L. D. (1996). Adolescent risk factors for binge drinking during the transition to young adulthood: Variable- and pattern-centered approaches to change. *Developmental Psychology, 32,* 659–674.

Schulenberg, J. E., & Zarrett, N. R. (2006). Mental health during emerging adulthood: Continuity and discontinuity in courses, causes, and functions. In J. J. Arnett & J. L. Tanner (Eds.), *Emerging adults in America: Coming of age in the 21st century* (pp. 135–172). Washington, DC: American Psychological Association.

Shanahan, M. J. (2000). Pathways to adulthood in changing societies: Variability and mechanisms in life course perspective. *Annual Review of Sociology, 26,* 667–692.

Staff, J., Schulenberg, J. E., Maslowsky, J., Bachman, J. G., O'Malley, P. M., Maggs, J. L., et al. (2010). Substance use changes and social role transitions: Proximal developmental effects on ongoing trajectories from late adolescence through early adulthood. *Development and Psychopathology, 22,* 917–932.

Wechsler, H., Dowdall, G. W., Davenport, A., & Rimm, E. B. (1995). A gender-specific measure of binge drinking among college students. *American Journal of Public Health, 85,* 982–985.

White, H. R., Fleming, C. B., Kim, M. J., Catalano, R. F., & McMorris, B. J. (2008). Identifying two potential mechanisms for changes in alcohol use among college-attending and non-college-attending emerging adults. *Developmental Psychology, 44,* 1625–1639.

White, H. R., Labouvie, E. W., & Papadaratsakis, V. (2005). Changes in substance use during the transition to adulthood: A comparison of college students and their noncollege age peers. *Journal of Drug Issues, 22,* 281–306.

Williams, J., Powell, L. M., & Wechsler, H. (2002). *Does alcohol consumption reduce human capital accumulation?: Evidence from the College Alcohol Study* (ImpacTeen Working Paper Series, 18). Chicago: University of Illinois at Chicago.

Zucker, R. A. (2006). Alcohol use and the alcohol use disorders: A developmental-biopsychosocial systems formulation covering the life course. In D. Cicchetti & D. J. Cohen (Eds.), *Developmental psychopathology* (2nd ed): Vol. 3. *Risk, disorder, and adaptation* (pp. 620–656). Hoboken, NJ: Wiley.

CHAPTER 2

Use, Misuse, and Diversion of Scheduled Prescription Medications by College Students

Sean Esteban McCabe, James A. Cranford,
Christian J. Teter, David L. Rabiner, *and* Carol J. Boyd

Over the past 15 years there has been an increase in the medical use and nonmedical use of scheduled prescription medications, including stimulants, opioids, sedatives/anxiolytics, and sleeping medications, among children, adolescents, and young adults in the United States (Fortuna, Rabbins, Caiola, Joynt, & Halterman, 2010; Johnston, O'Malley, Bachman, & Schulenberg, 2007; McCabe, West, & Wechsler, 2007c; Olfson, Gameroff, Marcus, & Jensen, 2003; Thomas, Conrad, Casler, & Goodman, 2006; Zacny et al., 2003; Zito et al., 2003). Indeed, the prescribing rates for scheduled medications among adolescents and young adults have nearly doubled since 1994 (Fortuna et al., 2010). Scheduled prescription medications are considered medically sound and efficacious for treating a wide range of childhood and adolescent disorders but one consequence of increases in medical use may be a concomitant increase in nonmedical use—possibly due to greater availability.

Young adults 18 to 25 years old have the highest rates of nonmedical use, abuse, and dependence on scheduled medications compared to other age groups (Johnston et al., 2007; McCabe, Cranford, & Boyd, 2006a; Substance Abuse and Mental Health Services Administration [SAMHSA], 2009a), and nonmedical use of prescription medications among U.S. college students is now at its highest level in the past two decades (Johnston et al., 2007; McCabe, Cranford, Boyd, & Teter, 2007a). Given these high rates, the objective of this chapter is to describe the use, misuse, and diversion of four scheduled prescription medication classes (stimulants, pain/opioids, sedatives/anxiolytics, and sleeping medications) among college students in the United States. The chapter is not intended to be a systematic review of the literature; instead, the chapter summarizes several important prescription medication use behaviors, primarily from our own studies. In the following sections, we first describe the prevalence of prescription medication use, prescription medication misuse, prescription medication diversion, and nonmedical use of scheduled medications. Subsequent sections focus on four particularly important aspects of non-medical use of prescription medications, including (1) routes of administration of prescription medications; (2) co-ingestion of prescription medications and other drugs; (3) motivations associated with nonmedical use of prescription medications; and (4) symptoms of attention-deficit/hyperactivity disorder (ADHD) and nonmedical use of prescription stimulants. We then examine some of the consequences associated with nonmedical use of prescription medications. We conclude by considering subtypes of nonmedical prescription medication misuse.

Prescription medication use, misuse, and diversion among U.S. college students is an emerging research area albeit with several methodological limitations. First, many studies, including our own work, are limited by a focus on a specific geographic region, a narrow population (e.g., excluding community colleges), and/or by the use of a convenience sample (e.g., one institution). A second limitation is that several national college health studies do not include detailed measures regarding prescription medications or include measures that combine illicitly produced or "street" versions of drugs with scheduled prescription medications (Boyd & McCabe, 2008). A third limitation is that many studies do not distinguish among individuals who: (1) nonmedically use someone else's prescription medication(s) to self-treat a health condition; (2) nonmedically use someone else's prescription medication(s) to get high; (3) use their own medications more often than prescribed or at higher than prescribed doses to self-treat a health condition; and (4) misuse their own medications to get high (Boyd & McCabe, 2008; McCabe et al., 2007a). A fourth limitation is that previous studies focusing on nonmedical use of prescription medication among college students have been largely descriptive and atheoretical. A final limitation of existing research is that terms such as *nonmedical use, medical misuse, diversion, abuse,* and *dependence* have often been used inconsistently and/or without clear definitions (Compton & Volkow, 2006).

Related to the issue of language and for the purposes of this chapter, *nonmedical use* refers to the nonprescribed use of a scheduled psychotherapeutic medication, whereas *medical misuse* refers to the use of a scheduled psychotherapeutic medication by a patient with a legal prescription where the patient uses the medication in a manner not intended by the prescribing clinician (e.g., using higher or more frequent doses, using to get high). *Diversion* is defined as the exchange of scheduled medication that leads to the use of these drugs by people other than those whom the prescribing clinician intended. Finally, *abuse* and *dependence* are defined by DSM-IV criteria for diagnosis of substance abuse or dependence.

PRESCRIPTION MEDICATION USE

Scheduled medications are critical for the treatment of conditions and disorders such as ADHD, sleep disorders, anxiety disorders, and the treatment and management of pain in adolescents and young adults (Augustin, 2001; Greenhill et al., 2002; Savage, 2003; Zacny et al., 2003). Yet, despite the increases in the medical use of scheduled medications over the past 15 years, few studies have examined their medical use among college students.

One study that focused on medical use among college students was conducted at a single college (McCabe, 2008). The lifetime prescription medication use behaviors for four classes of scheduled medications (opioid, sedative/anxiety, sleeping, and stimulant medications) were examined at a large midwestern 4-year university in the United States, and the final random sample included 3,639 full-time undergraduate college students. The lifetime use of scheduled medications was as follows: 40% of undergraduate students did not use prescription medications; 40% used prescription medications prescribed by their doctors; 16% used both prescription medications as prescribed by their doctors as well as prescription medications that were not prescribed to them; and 4% used only prescription medication that was not prescribed to them (McCabe, 2008). Unfortunately, there are currently no data regarding the national prevalence of medical use of scheduled prescription medications among U.S. college students.

PRESCRIPTION MEDICATION MISUSE

Although the majority of legitimate medical users of scheduled medications use their medications appropriately (Fleming, Balousek, Klessig, Mundt, & Brown, 2007; Wilens, Gignac, Swezey, Monuteaux, & Biederman, 2006), case reports (Barrett & Pihl, 2002; Garland, 1998; Jaffe, 1991), poison center reports (Klein-Schwartz, 2003; Foley, Mrvos, &

Krenzelok, 2000), clinical studies (Wilens et al., 2006), and epidemiological studies (Arria et al., 2008; Upadhyaya, Rose, Wang, & Brady, 2005) indicate that individuals have used their own prescription medications for reasons other than those intended by the prescribing clinician. To date, existing studies regarding prescription medication misuse among college students focus primarily on the medical misuse of stimulant medications for ADHD. At least four studies have examined medical misuse among prescribed users of stimulant medications for ADHD in college student samples (Arria et al., 2008; Rabiner et al., 2009a; Upadhyaya et al., 2005; Sepulveda et al., 2008). Sepulveda and colleagues (2008) examined medical misuse among college students who were prescribed stimulant medications by a physician to treat their ADHD in the past 12 months. Of the 55 college students using stimulant medication for ADHD, approximately 36% reported using too much (e.g., higher doses, more frequent doses), 19% reported concomitant use with alcohol and other drugs, and 10% intentionally got high on their stimulant medication in the past 12 months. Arria and colleagues (2008) investigated various behaviors among 45 students who medically used a prescription stimulant for ADHD. They found that approximately 27% (n = 12) had overused their own prescription stimulants in their lifetime. Next, Rabiner and colleagues (2009a) reported that of 115 respondents who had received stimulant medications for ADHD 31% had misused their stimulant medications in the past 6 months (Rabiner et al., 2009a). Finally, Upadhyaya and colleagues (2005) found that approximately 25% of those students prescribed stimulants for ADHD reported ever using their medication to get high. Although these studies focus exclusively on stimulant medications at individual colleges, the results serve as evidence that more research is needed to examine misuse of scheduled medications among college students and to identify characteristics of misusers.

PRESCRIPTION MEDICATION DIVERSION

The diversion sources of nonmedical use of opioid, sedative/anxiety, sleeping, and stimulant medications have been examined in a few recent college-based studies (Garnier et al., 2010; McCabe & Boyd, 2005; McCabe, Teter, & Boyd, 2006c; McCabe et al., 2007a). Among nonmedical users who reported their source(s) of diversion, prescription stimulant, pain, sedative/anxiolytic, and sleeping medications were most likely to come from *peer* sources (McCabe & Boyd, 2005). Notably, one study found there were about twice as many of nonmedical users of stimulants in the past year who obtained these medications from peer sources on a college campus than medical users of prescription stimulant medications for ADHD who were prescribed these medications by a doctor (McCabe, Teter, & Boyd, 2006c). *Family* sources were the second leading source of diversion for each of the prescription medication classes (McCabe & Boyd, 2005). Drugs obtained from drug dealers and while traveling abroad made up less than 3% of reported sources of diversion. Interestingly, no students obtained their nonmedical prescription medications directly from the Internet. Arria and colleagues (2008) also found that college students who reported nonmedical use of prescription stimulants were most likely to obtain these medications from friends with prescriptions, and over 70% obtained them for free.

The sources for obtaining abusable prescription medications for nonmedical use can differ significantly by gender (McCabe & Boyd, 2005; McCabe et al., 2007a). For example, college women were more likely than men to obtain prescription sedative/anxiolytic, sleeping, and pain medications from *family* sources (McCabe & Boyd, 2005; McCabe et al., 2007a).

Approximately 27% of students who were prescribed any of the four classes of medications in the past year were approached to divert (e.g., sell, trade, or give away) their medications. Undergraduate students who were prescribed stimulant medications for ADHD were the most likely to be approached to divert their medications (54%), followed by those who were prescribed pain medications (26%), sedatives/anxiolytics (19%), and sleeping medications (14%).

Three recent studies examined the prevalence of diversion among college students who were prescribed stimulant medication for ADHD and found the prevalence of diversion by prescribed stimulant medication users was 26% in the previous 6 months (Rabiner et al., 2009a), 35% in the previous 12 months (Sepulveda et al., 2008), and 62% in their lifetime (Garnier et al., 2010). Taken together, these results suggest that careful therapeutic monitoring could contribute to reductions in the diversion and nonmedical use of prescription medications.

NONMEDICAL USE OF SCHEDULED MEDICATIONS

There have been well-documented increases in the nonmedical use of prescription drugs such as stimulants, sedatives/anxiolytics, sleeping medications, and prescription opioids, and this form of drug use is second only to marijuana use among adolescent and young adult substance users (Johnston et al., 2007; McCabe et al., 2007c; SAMHSA, 2009a). The past-year nonmedical use and abuse/dependence of scheduled prescription medications is most prevalent among individuals 18 to 25 years old (Johnston, O'Malley, Bachman, & Schulenberg, 2009; Kroutil et al., 2006; McCabe et al., 2006a; SAMHSA, 2009a).

Three large-scale national studies serve as the most comprehensive sources of data on nonmedical use of prescription medications among college students in the United States. The Monitoring the Future (MTF) Study data show that the past-year nonmedical use of prescription medications (i.e., stimulants, opioids, sedatives, tranquilizers) increased steadily among U.S. college students from 7% in 1992 to 15% in 2006 (Johnston et al., 2007).

The National Survey on Drug Use and Health (NSDUH) found that the nonmedical use of prescription stimulant medications such as Adderall is more prevalent among U.S. college students ages 18–25 than among their same-age peers not in college (Herman-Stahl, Krebs, Kroutil, & Heller, 2007; SAMHSA, 2009b). In contrast, college students tend to report lower rates of nonmedical use of prescription opioids such as Vicodin and OxyContin and prescription sedatives/anxiolytics than their same-age peers not attending college (Johnston et al., 2009; SAMHSA, 2005).

A secondary analysis using the College Alcohol Study (CAS) data on samples of randomly selected college students from a nationally representative sample of 119 colleges in 1993, 1997, 1999, and 2001 found that the past-year prevalence rates of nonmedical use increased between 1993 and 2001, while the illicit use of drugs other than marijuana increased significantly in prevalence between 1993 and 1997, followed by slight decreases in 1999 and 2001 (McCabe et al., 2007c). Notably, the past-year prevalence rates for nonmedical use of prescription medications in 2001 ranged from 0% at the lowest-use schools to 31% at the highest-use school (see Figure 2.1). Interestingly, nonmedical use of prescription stimulants was more prevalent at U.S. colleges with more competitive admission standards and at colleges located in the northeastern region of the U.S. (McCabe, Teter, Boyd, Knight, & Wechsler, 2005a). In addition, no students from the three historically black colleges and universities reported nonmedical use of prescription stimulants. Taken together, these findings highlight the variation in nonmedical use of prescription medications among U.S. colleges.

Nationally, the lifetime prevalence of nonmedical use of prescription opioids (e.g., Vicodin, Percocet, Percodan, Darvocet) was 12% and the past-year prevalence was 7% among U.S. college students (McCabe, Teter, Boyd, Knight, & Wechsler, 2005c). Among college students who reported nonmedical use of prescription opioids in their lifetime, the majority began nonmedical use *before* starting college (McCabe et al., 2007a). Among college students who reported nonmedical use of prescription opioids in

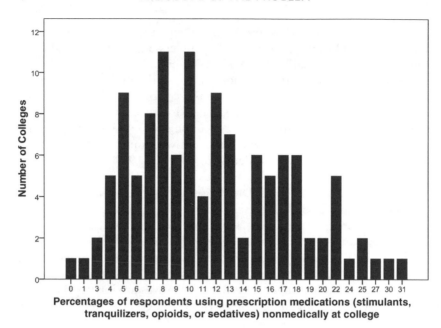

FIGURE 2.1. Distribution of past-year nonmedical use of scheduled prescription medications (stimulants, tranquilizers, opioids, sedatives) across 119 U.S. colleges. Data from McCabe (unpublished).

the past year, 63% used on one or two occasions, and 37% used on three or more occasions (McCabe, Teter, & Boyd, 2005b). McCabe and colleagues (2007b) examined the most commonly misused prescription opioids by past-year nonmedical users; these included hydrocodone (50%), codeine (38%), oxycodone (14%), and propoxyphene (10%).

Nationally, the lifetime prevalence of nonmedical use of prescription stimulants (Ritalin, Adderall, and Dexedrine) was 7%, and the past-year prevalence was 4% among U.S. college students (McCabe, Knight, Teter, & Wechsler, 2005a). Teter, McCabe, LaGrange, Cranford, and Boyd (2006) found that among college students who reported nonmedical use of prescription stimulants in their lifetime, the majority began nonmedical use *after* starting college. Approximately 48% of students who reported nonmedical use of prescription stimulants in the past year used on one or two occasions, and 52% used on three or more occasions (McCabe et al., 2006b). Teter and colleagues (2006) found that 76% of past-year nonmedical users of prescription stimulants reported using an amphetamine-dextroamphetamine combination agent (e.g., Adderall), while 25% reported using methylphenidate (e.g., Ritalin, Concerta, Metadate, Methylin).

ROUTES OF ADMINISTRATION
OF PRESCRIPTION MEDICATIONS

Despite the possible deleterious effects associated with nonmedical use of prescription medications, few studies have examined routes of administration associated with nonmedical use among adolescents (Compton & Volkow, 2006; Zacny et al., 2003). The use of prescription opioids via intranasal and other nonoral routes of administration is an extremely dangerous drug use behavior that has been linked to a number of adverse physical consequences (Jewers et al., 2005; Watson et al., 2004; Yewell, Haydon, Archer, & Manaligod, 2002). Additionally, the rate of delivery of drugs to the brain directly correlates to the abuse potential of the drug, and intranasal as well as other nonoral routes of administration are expected to deliver a drug to the brain at a much faster rate than oral administration (Kollins, MacDonald, & Rush, 2001; Roset et al., 2001; Volkow & Swanson, 2003).

Existing research on college students has shown that the two leading routes of administration associated with nonmedical use of prescription stimulants and opioids are oral and intranasal administration (Barrett, Darredeua, Bordy, & Pihl, 2005; McCabe et al., 2007a; McCabe & Teter, 2007; White, Becker-Blease, & Grace-Bishop, 2006). Among past-year nonmedical users of prescription stimulants (n = 212), approximately 58.5% reported an oral-only route of administration of prescription stimulants, 34.9% reported intranasal and oral administration, and 6.6% reported other routes of administration (McCabe & Teter, 2007). In addition, among lifetime nonmedical users of prescription opioids (n = 640), approximately 84.4% reported an oral-only route, 10.9% reported intranasal and oral administration, and 4.7% reported other routes of administration (McCabe et al., 2007a). Approximately 7 in every 10 intranasal users of prescription opioids or stimulants had positive drug abuse screens on the DAST-10 in the past year (McCabe et al., 2007a; McCabe & Teter, 2007). The route and rate of administration have important implications for the addictive potential of prescription medications; therefore, nonoral routes of administration should be assessed and monitored closely when considering risks associated with nonmedical use.

CO-INGESTION OF PRESCRIPTION
MEDICATIONS AND OTHER DRUGS

There is growing evidence that nonmedical use of prescription stimulants, tranquilizers, and opioids is highly correlated with other drug use behaviors such as cigarette smoking, heavy drinking, and illicit drug use (Arria et al., 2008; Barrett et al., 2005; McCabe, 2008; McCabe et al., 2005a, 2005b). National surveillance data, epidemiological studies, and several anecdotal case reports document the adverse consequences that can occur as a result of simultaneous use (i.e., co-ingestion) of prescription medications and other drugs (e.g., Cone et al., 2004; McCabe, Cranford, Morales, & Young, 2006c; SAMHSA, 2004; Watson et al., 2004). While marijuana and alcohol are the most common drugs used simultaneously, adolescents and young adults have particularly high rates of simultaneous use involving prescription medications. At least one study of college students found that the past-year prevalence of polydrug use involving alcohol and at least one prescription medication class (i.e., pain medication, stimulant medication, sedative medication, and sleeping medication) was 12.1% (McCabe et al., 2006b). Remarkably, the majority of nonmedical users of pain medication, stimulant medication, and sedative medication reported co-ingestion with alcohol (McCabe et al., 2006c). Simultaneous co-ingestion of prescription medications and alcohol was associated with more drug problems than nonmedical use not involving co-ingestion with alcohol. There is limited information available regarding the co-ingestion of prescription medications and substances other than alcohol among college students.

MOTIVATIONS FOR NONMEDICAL USE OF SCHEDULED MEDICATIONS

In order to fully comprehend the risks associated with nonmedical use of prescription medications, it is necessary to understand the motives for nonmedical use. McCabe and colleagues (2007a) found that college students were most likely to report "because it relieves pain" as a reason for using prescription opioids not prescribed to them by a doctor (63% of all lifetime nonmedical users). Other common motives were "because it gives me a high" (31.9%) and "because of experimentation" (26.8%). Forty percent of lifetime nonmedical users reported using prescription opioids *only* to relieve pain; for these 40%, their odds for drug abuse did not differ from those of students who did not report nonmedical use of prescription opioids (see Figure 2.2). By contrast, the odds for drug abuse were over 15 times greater among undergraduate students who reported "other motives" for nonmedical use compared to students who did not report nonmedical use of prescription opioids (McCabe et al., 2007a).

Several previous studies have examined the motives associated with nonmedical use of prescription stimulants among college students (Arria et al., 2008; Rabiner et al., 2009b; Teter, McCabe, Cranford, Boyd, &

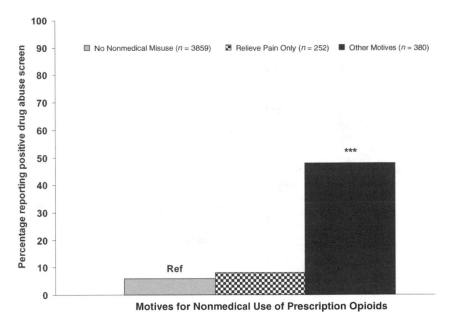

FIGURE 2.2. Motives for nonmedical use of prescription opioids and drug abuse. Data from McCabe et al. (2007a). The reference group for logistic regression analysis was composed of respondents who did not report nonmedical use of prescription opioids in their lifetime. Odds ratios were adjusted for gender, race/ethnicity, class year, and living arrangement. A cutpoint score of 3 or more was used for the Drug Abuse Screening Test, Short Form (DAST-10). *** $p < .001$ based on logistic regression results.

Guthrie, 2005; Teter et al., 2006). Teter and colleagues (2006) found the most prevalent motives among nonmedical users were to: (1) help with concentration (65%); (2) help study (60%); (3) increase alertness (48%); (4) get high (31%); and (5) experiment (30%). Previous work found that the motive "to get high" was strongly associated with other substance use; over one-third of those who endorsed the motive "to get high" had used cocaine in the past year compared to fewer than 2% of those who did not report nonmedical use of prescription stimulants (Teter et al., 2005). Teter and colleagues (2006) found that motives for nonmedical use of prescription stimulants were associated with age of initiation (see Figure 2.3). Compared with students who started before college, students who started during college were more likely to report the motives of improving concentration and helping to study. In contrast, precollege nonmedical users of prescription stimulants were more likely

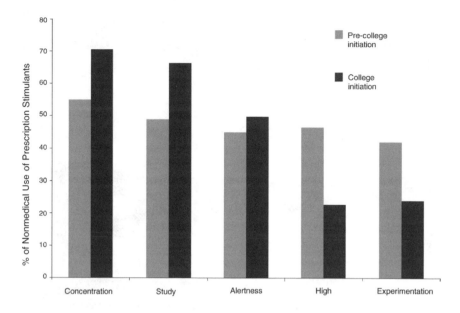

FIGURE 2.3. Motives for nonmedical use of prescription stimulants and age of initiation ($n = 382$, $p < .01$). Data from Teter et al. (2006).

than their counterparts to report using to get high, to lose weight, and to experiment.

While these studies were some of the first systematic attempts to investigate the motives for nonmedical use of prescription medications among college students, important gaps in our knowledge remain. Further longitudinal work is needed to examine the hypothesis that motives for nonmedical use of prescription medications can be used to identify individuals at higher risk for adverse health outcomes including, but not limited to, substance abuse.

ADHD SYMPTOMS AND NONMEDICAL USE OF PRESCRIPTION STIMULANTS

Attention problems adversely effect students' academic performance (Blasé et al., 2009), and students reporting nonmedical use of ADHD drugs also report greater concerns about their academic performance, (Rabiner et al., 2009b). Thus, some students may initiate nonmedical ADHD medication misuse to "treat" problems with attention—or possibly untreated ADHD—that they experience as undermining their academic success.

To investigate this possibility, Rabiner and colleagues (2009b) examined nonmedical use in relation to students' ratings of ADHD symptoms. High levels of inattentive symptoms, but not hyperactive–impulsive symptoms, were associated with nonmedical use of ADHD drugs, and nearly 25% of nonmedical users rated themselves as having attention difficulties at or above the median level reported by students who had been diagnosed with ADHD.

In related work, Peterkin, Crone, Sheridan, and Wise (2010) examined the association between screening positive for ADHD and nonmedical use of ADHD medications in a convenience sample of 184 college students. Twenty-five percent reported nonmedical use, and 71% of these students had screened positive for ADHD. Nonmedical users of ADHD medications were nearly seven times as likely to report high levels of ADHD symptoms than other students. Finally, Arria and colleagues (2010) compared self-reported ADHD symptoms among three groups of students enrolled in a 4-year longitudinal study: (1) persistent nonmedical users of prescription stimulants (i.e., students reporting nonmedical use during the past 12 months in three consecutive annual surveys); (2) persistent marijuana users who did not use prescription stimulants; and (3) students using neither ADHD medication or marijuana. After adjusting for race/ethnicity, sex, socioeconomic status, and other illicit drug use, scoring above the clinical cutoff on the ADHD scale nearly tripled the odds of being in the stimulant group compared to the nonuser group, and more than doubled the odds of being in the nonmedical use group compared to the marijuana group. Consistent with findings from Rabiner et al. (2009a), it was self-reported inattentive and not hyperactive–impulsive symptoms that predicted being in the nonmedical use group.

In a second longitudinal study, Rabiner, Anastopoulos, Costello, Hoyle, and Swartzwelder (2010) surveyed more than 800 students about nonmedical use during their first semester in college, and again during the spring semester of their sophomore year, to identify factors that predicted the onset of nonmedical use. After controlling for gender, race, and social fraternity/sorority status, students' reports of attention problems and substance use both predicted the initiation of nonmedical use of ADHD medications. Furthermore, although substance use predicted the nonmedical use of other prescription medications, the effect of attention problems was restricted to ADHD medication alone.

Collectively, these studies strongly suggest that a subset of students who take ADHD medications without a prescription do so to address attention difficulties that they experience as undermining their academic success. Some of these students may have undiagnosed ADHD, although problems with attention may occur for a wide variety of reasons. In either case, self-treating by using ADHD medications is highly problematic, and students should be educated about the importance of pursuing an appropriate evaluation of such attention difficulties.

CONSEQUENCES ASSOCIATED WITH NONMEDICAL USE OF PRESCRIPTION MEDICATIONS

There have only been a few studies linking adverse consequences directly to the nonmedical use of prescription medications. One of the main challenges to examining consequences associated with nonmedical use of prescription medications is the high rate of polydrug use involving prescription medications and other substances. For example, previous research has found that almost all nonmedical users also reported using other drugs, and the majority of nonmedical users of pain medication, stimulant medication, and sedative medication co-ingest prescription medications with alcohol and/or other drugs (McCabe et al., 2005a, 2005b; McCabe & Teter, 2007). More than 90% of past-year nonmedical users of prescription stimulants also reported using other drugs (not including alcohol) in the past year (McCabe & Teter, 2007). Nevertheless, Rabiner and colleagues (2009b) found that students who reported nonmedical use of ADHD medication in the past 6 months reported the following adverse effects from ADHD medications: sleep difficulties (72%), irritability (62%), feeling dizzy/lightheaded (35%), headaches (33%), stomachaches (33%), and sadness (25%). This last finding by Rabiner and colleagues (i.e., that one-quarter of nonmedical users of ADHD medication reported "sadness") is consistent with recent data demonstrating that *frequency* of nonmedical prescription stimulant use and *nonoral routes* of prescription stimulant administration are associated with depressed mood (Teter, Falone, Cranford, Boyd, & McCabe, 2010). Approximately 50% of frequent nonmedical prescription stimulant users or those reporting nonoral administration of prescription stimulants reported depressed mood. Despite the apparent high rates of adverse effects associated with nonmedical use of prescription stimulants, over 70% of students reporting nonmedical use rated the overall impact on them as positive, and very few students felt they had been negatively affected (Rabiner et al., 2009b).

Reports in the popular press have documented several deaths of undergraduate college students as a result of co-ingestion of alcohol and scheduled prescription medications (e.g., Leinwand, 2005; Petrillo & Cantlupe, 2005). There are potential serious risks to individuals who obtain prescription medications from nonclinician sources. For example, they do not benefit from a thorough clinical assessment, and they do not receive important medical information that accompanies a prescription for scheduled medications. The nonmedical user is likely to be unaware of the medication's potential for interaction with other substances or the medication's documented contraindications and precautions. For example, the death of a 19-year-old male was directly attributed to co-ingestion of methylphenidate and alcohol. The patient developed hyperpyrexia and tachycardia, as well as cardiac lesions—signs and symptoms consistent with amphetamine toxicity (Massello & Carpenter, 1999).

Substance abuse and dependence is another potential consequence of nonmedical use of prescription medications (Griffiths & Weerts, 1997; Kollins et al., 2001; McCabe, West, Morales, Cranford, & Boyd, 2007b; Zacny et al., 2003). Relative to advances made in the study of the prevalence of nonmedical use, there is very little information regarding the prevalence and risk factors for the nonmedical abuse or dependence on prescription medications among college students. There is evidence that a considerable proportion of nonmedical users of prescription medications in the U.S. population meet criteria for abuse or dependence (Kroutil et al., 2006; McCabe et al., 2007b; Zacny et al., 2003). Among lifetime nonmedical users, an estimated 21–31% go on to develop abuse, while 6–13% go on to develop dependence during their lifetime (McCabe et al., 2007b).

In a Web-based survey, McCabe (2008) found that the past-year prevalence of a positive screen for drug abuse (on the DAST-10) was 3.2% for lifetime nonusers, 5.5% for lifetime medical users only, 29.2% for lifetime medical users and nonmedical users, and 35.3% for lifetime nonmedical users only. The higher rates of a positive screen for drug abuse among lifetime nonmedical users of prescription medications held steady across each of the four classes of prescription medications (see Figure 2.4).

These findings provide evidence that nonmedical users of each prescription medication class are at substantially higher risk of a positive screening for drug abuse (on the DAST-10). In contrast, medical users without any history of nonmedical use were at considerably lower risk of screening positive for drug abuse. Furthermore, the odds of a positive screen for drug abuse did not differ significantly between individuals who reported medical use only and those who reported no use of prescription medications. The elevated substance use rates found among those reporting any nonmedical use suggest that this behavior is part of a "multi-problem" behavior pattern (Biglan, Brennan, Foster, & Holder, 2004). Thus, screening instruments that cover a wide range of drugs are most appropriate for nonmedical users of prescription medications. Based on the lacuna in knowledge at the national level, more research is needed at U.S. colleges to better understand the consequences associated with the nonmedical use of scheduled medications.

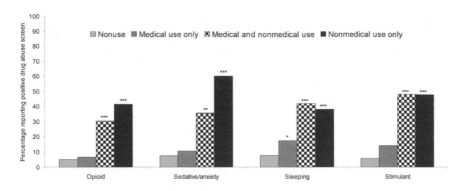

FIGURE 2.4. Past-year drug abuse as a function of lifetime medical use and nonmedical use of four classes of prescription medications. Data from McCabe (2008). The reference group for logistic regression analysis was nonusers. Odds ratios were adjusted for gender, race/ethnicity, class year, family income, living arrangement, fraternity or sorority membership, and age at onset for use of alcohol, nicotine, and marijuana. A cutpoint score of 3 or more was used for the DAST-10. * $p < .05$; ** $p < .01$; *** $p < .001$ based on logistic regression results.

SUBTYPES OF NONMEDICAL USE
OF PRESCRIPTION MEDICATIONS

There appear to be different subtypes of nonmedical use of prescription medications. A recent study used three characteristics associated with the nonmedical use of prescription medications (i.e., motive, route of administration, and co-ingestion) across four separate scheduled medication classes (i.e., pain, sedative/anxiety, sleeping, and stimulant medications) to examine nonmedical subtypes and drug-related problems (McCabe, Boyd, & Teter, 2009). Self-treatment subtypes were characterized by motives consistent with the prescription medication's pharmaceutical main indication, oral-only routes of administration, and no co-ingestion with alcohol. Recreational subtypes were characterized by recreational motives, oral or nonoral routes, and/or co-ingestion. Mixed subtypes consisted of other combinations of motives, routes, and co-ingestion. Among those who reported any nonmedical use of prescription medications, approximately 13% were classified into the recreational subtype, while 39% were in the self-treatment subtype, and 48% were in the mixed subtype. Approximately 50% of those in subtypes other than self-treatment screened positive for drug abuse (on the DAST-10). We found that nonmedical users in the mixed subtypes resembled nonmedical users in the recreational subtypes, but differed significantly from nonmedical users in the self-treatment subtypes. Most notably, the odds of a positive drug abuse screen were generally lower among self-treatment subtypes than other subtypes (see Figure 2.5).

POLICY, CLINICAL, PREVENTION, AND INTERVENTION IMPLICATIONS

The key developmental transition to college marks a time of growth but also of increased vulnerability. Most notably, college students often become fully responsible for their own medication management for the first time in their lives and are presented with more opportunities for—and a higher expectation of—substance use. Thus, prescription medication use, misuse, and diversion respresents an important college health topic, and existing research in this area suggests several implications for policy, prevention, and intervention. Given the therapeutic efficacy of scheduled prescription medications for treating a wide range of health conditions and disorders, institutions of higher education must balance the medical necessity of these medications and the risk for nonmedical use and diversion among college students.

There are steps that can be taken by colleges and universities to understand the scope of prescription medication use, misuse, and diversion on their campuses:

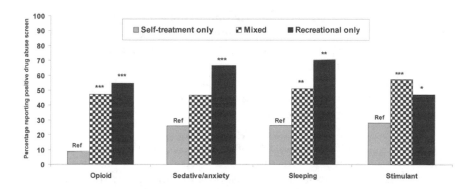

FIGURE 2.5. Past-year drug abuse as a function of nonmedical prescription medication use subtypes. Data from McCabe et al. (2009). The reference group for logistic regression analysis was self-treatment only. Odds ratios were adjusted for gender, race/ethnicity, class year, and living arrangement. A cutpoint score of 3 or more was used for the DAST-10. * $p < .05$; ** $p < .01$; *** $p < .001$ based on logistic regression results.

• Colleges and universities are encouraged to assess their own campuses because prevalence rates of medication use, nonmedical use, and diversion of prescription medications can vary considerably across schools.

• Colleges and universities are encouraged to revise their codes of student conduct policies and add language regarding the diversion and nonmedical use of prescription medications. It should be made clear to students that these behaviors are considered school violations because many policies exclude such language.

• Colleges and universities are encouraged to provide locked storage units in residence halls and other living arrangements for students with prescribed scheduled medications to safely store these medicines, especially since college students often become fully responsible for their own medication management for the first time in their lives.

• Physicians should instruct all patients who require scheduled medications about the abuse potential of these medications and the need to store their prescription in a secure location.

• Colleges and universities should take steps to educate students about the potential dangers associated with the nonmedical use of prescription medications. For example, because scheduled medications are so widely prescribed, and generally safe, many students may be unaware of the potentially serious adverse health consequences, especially when these drugs are used in conjunction with alcohol and other substances. Students may also be unaware that they can develop problems of abuse and dependence with these compounds.

Clinicians must balance the risks and benefits of medications with abuse potential when assessing, treating, and monitoring their patients. Psychotropic medications such as opioids, stimulants, sedatives, and anxiolytics demonstrate a long-standing history of effectiveness when used appropriately; however, they can be misused for a variety of purposes. There are steps that can be taken by clinicians to help minimize the misuse of these beneficial medications:

• Periodic screening and assessment can lead to the identification of those at risk for the nonmedical use of prescription medications. Screening and assessment scales may be useful tools in this regard. Knowing who is at risk for nonmedical use is a key step to the safe and effective use of abusable prescription medications. Additionally, differentiating subtypes of nonmedical prescription medication users could help identify individuals who are untreated (or inadequately treated) for a legitimate health condition and/or those who need a more comprehensive substance use assessment.

• Given that many individuals obtain diverted prescription medications for nonmedical use from friends, peers, and family members, clinicians prescribing these medications should exercise caution and periodically monitor their patients' behavior over the course of treatment. They may consider limiting both the quantity of medication prescribed and well as the number of refills, which in turn requires more frequent clinician–patient interactions and therapeutic monitoring. These steps could result in both a reduction in the overall supply of controlled substances available for diversion and nonmedical use, and improved treatment of target symptoms for which the medications were initially prescribed.

• Clinicians should be continually educated about the benefits and risks of abusable prescription medications. It has even been suggested that this type of education should be mandatory. For example, take the following statement by expert Steven D. Passik, MD: "Doctors and other professionals involved in pain management should be required to have continuing medical education credits in the pain addiction interface upon licensing renewal" (Passik, 2010). This is a clear endorsement of mandatory education and could be applied to the treatment of ADHD, anxiety, and insomnia as well.

• Clinicians should be familiar with effective medication alternatives that carry less risk for abuse. Medications that carry less risk for abuse based on their pharmacological profile are available for many conditions. For example, the Food and Drug Administration approved atomoxetine, a nonstimulant norepinephrine reuptake inhibitor (lacking stimulant-like abuse potential) for the treatment of ADHD.

• The use of pharmaceutical delivery systems that are not easily manipulated for alternate routes of administration (e.g., injection, snorting) might help limit the abuse of some prescription medications. As technology improves, more and more delivery systems will become available that make it difficult to alter each medication's pharmacokinetic profile (e.g., absorption rate), which is key to reducing its abuse potential.

• Furthermore, the use of additional aides to help safely and effectively prescribe and monitor medications, such as prescription drug monitoring programs (PDMPs), is appropriate. Centralized prescription databases such as PDMPs, which are available in over 30 states, allow clinicians to access patients' prescription records. Although these programs vary by state, they may (*if used properly*) help curb the misuse of prescription medications. For example, they could enhance monitoring and detection of drug-seeking behaviors, such as doctor shopping or the use of multiple pharmacies to obtain controlled substances.

CONCLUSIONS

While previous research has provided valuable information regarding nonmedical use of prescription medications, much remains to be learned about medical use, misuse, abuse, and diversion of prescription medications among U.S. college students. Through the research detailed in this chapter, we have established the following:

• More than half of college students reported ever having a prescription for at least one of the following four scheduled medication classes: stimulant, opioid, sedative/anxiolytic, and sleeping medication. The majority of college students who are prescribed scheduled medications appear to use their medications appropriately.

• More than one in every four college students—with their own legal prescriptions—also engaged in nonmedical use and/or were approached to divert their scheduled medications. More than one in every seven college students engages in nonmedical use of scheduled medications each year. The prevalence of nonmedical use of scheduled medications ranges greatly across colleges, from 0% at the lowest-use schools to over 30% at the highest-use schools.

• Motivations and routes of administration associated with nonmedical use of scheduled prescription medications vary and are differentially associated with drug-use-related problems. Nearly all nonmedical users of scheduled prescription medications have misused other substances, and the majority of nonmedical users have co-ingested scheduled prescription medications with alcohol. Thus, screening instruments that cover a wide range of drugs are most appropriate for nonmedical users of prescription medications.

• Medical misuse, diversion, and nonmedical use of scheduled prescription medications all represent risk behaviors that can be directly associated with drug abuse and adverse health outcomes in college students.

There are different subtypes of nonmedical use but we do not know nearly enough about these subtypes, and future work needs to consider subtypes over time. We are just beginning to know how many college students misuse their own medications or divert their medications across the four classes of abusable medications. It is necessary to expand beyond single-college campus studies and examine individual-level and college-level characteristics associated with the use, misuse, abuse, and diversion of prescription medications in a national study of college students. Finally, it is essential to move away from examining nonmedical use of prescription medications with only a cross-sectional lens, and begin to examine trajectories of nonmedical use, medical misuse, and diversion.

ACKNOWLEDGMENTS

The development of this chapter was supported by Research Grant Nos. R01DA024678, R01DA031160, R03DA018239, and R03DA019492 from the National Institute on Drug Abuse, National Institutes of Health.

REFERENCES

Arria, A. M., Caldeira, K. M., O'Grady, K. E., Vincent, K. B., Johnson, E. P., & Wish, E. D. (2008). Nonmedical use of prescription stimulants among college students: Associations with attention-deficit-hyperactivity disorder and polydrug use. *Pharmacotherapy, 28*, 156–169.

Arria, A. M., Garnier-Dykstra, L. M., Caldeira, K. M., Vincent, K. B., O'Grady, K. E., & Wish, E. D. (2011). Persistent nonmedical use of prescription stimulants among college students: Possible association with ADHD symptoms [Electronic version ahead of print]. *Journal of Attention Disorders, 15(5)*, 347–356.

Augustin, S. G. (2001). Anxiety Disorders. In M. A. Koda-Kimble, L. Y. Young, W. A. Kradjan, & B. J. Guglielmo (Eds.), *Applied therapeutics: The clinical use of drugs* (pp. 74.1–74.48). Philadelphia: Lippincott Williams & Wilkins.

Barrett, S. P., & Pihl, R. O. (2002). Oral methylphenidate-alcohol co-abuse. *Journal of Clinical Psychopharmacology, 22*, 633–634.

Barrett, S. P., Darredeua, C., Bordy, L. E., & Pihl, R. O. (2005). Characteristics of methylphenidate misuse in a university student sample. *Canadian Journal of Psychiatry, 50*, 457–461.

Biglan, A., Brennan, P. A., Foster, S. L., & Holder, H. D. (2004). *Helping adolescents at risk: Prevention of multiple problem behaviors.* New York: Guilford Press.

Boyd, C. J., & McCabe, S. E. (2008). Coming to terms with the nonmedical use of prescription medications. *Substance Abuse Treatment, Prevention and Policy, 3*, 22.

Compton, W. M., & Volkow, N. D. (June 2006). Abuse of prescription drugs and the risk of addiction. *Drug and Alcohol Dependence, 1*, 4–7.

Cone, E. J., Fant, R. V., Rohay, J. M., Caplan, Y. H., Ballina, M., Reder, R. F., & Haddox, J. D. (2004). Oxycodone involvement in drug abuse deaths. II. Evidence for toxic multiple drug-drug interactions. *Journal of Analytical Toxicology, 28*, 616–624.

Fleming, M. F., Balousek, S. L., Klessig, C. L., Mundt, M. P., & Brown, D. D. (2007). Substance use disorders in a primary care sample receiving daily opioid therapy. *The Journal of Pain, 8*, 573–582.

Foley, R., Mrvos, R., & Krenzelok, E. P. (2000). A profile of methylphenidate exposures. *Journal of Clinical Toxicology, 38*, 625–30.

Garland, E. J. (1998). Intranasal abuse of prescribed methylphenidate. *Journal of the American Academy of Child and Adolescent Psychiatry, 37*, 573–574.

Garnier, L. M., Arria, A. M., Caldeira, K. M., Vincent, K. B., O'Grady, K. E., & Wish, E. D. (2010). Sharing and selling of prescription medications in a college student sample. *Journal of Clinical Psychiatry, 71*, 262–269.

Greenhill, L. L., Pliszka, S., Dulcan, M. K., Bernet, W., Arnold, V., Beitchman, J., Benson, R. S., Bukstein, O., Kinlan, J., McClellan, J., Rue, D., Shaw, J. A., & Stock, S. (2002). Practice parameter for the use of stimulant medications in the treatment of children, adolescents, and adults. *Journal of the American Academy of Child and Adolescent Psychiatry, 41*, 26S–49S.

Griffiths, R. R., & Weerts, E. M. (1997). Benzodiazepine self-administration in humans and laboratory animals—implications for problems of long-term use and abuse. *Psychopharmacology, 134*, 1–37.

Herman-Stahl, M. A., Krebs, C. P., Kroutil, L. A., & Heller, D. C. (2007). Risk and protective factors for methamphetamine use and nonmedical use of prescription stimulants among young adults aged 18 to 25. *Addictive Behaviors, 32*, 1003, 1015.

Jaffe, S. L. (1991). Intranasal abuse of prescribed methylphenidate by an alcohol and drug abusing adolescent with ADHD. *Journal of the American Academy of Child and Adolescent Psychiatry, 30*, 773–775.

Jewers, W. M., Rawal, Y. B., Allen, C. M., Kalmar, J. R., Fox, E., Chacon, G. E., et al. (2005). Palatal perforation associated with intranasal prescription narcotic abuse. *Oral Surgery, Oral Medicine, Oral Pathology, Oral Radiology, Endodontology, 99*, 594–597.

Johnston, L. D., O'Malley, P. M., Bachman, J. G., & Schulenberg, J. E. (2007). *Monitoring the Future national survey results on drug use, 1975–2006: Vol. II. College students and adults ages 19–45* (NIH Publication No. 07-6206). Bethesda, MD: National Institute on Drug Abuse.

Johnston, L. D., O'Malley, P. M., Bachman, J. G., & Schulenberg, J. E. (2009). *Monitoring the Future National Survey Results on Drug Use, 1975–2008: Vol. II. College students and adults ages 19–50* (NIH Publication No. 09-7403). Bethesda, MD: National Institute on Drug Abuse.

Klein-Schwartz, W. (2003). Pediatric methylphenidate exposures: 7-year experience of poison centers in the United States. *Clinical Pediatrics, 42*, 159–164.

Kollins, S. H., MacDonald, E. K., & Rush, C. R. (2001). Assessing the abuse potential of methylphenidate in nonhuman and human subjects: A review. *Pharmacology, Biochemistry, and Behavior, 68*, 611–627.

Kroutil, L. A., Van Brunt, D. L., Herman-Stahl, M. A., Heller, D. C., Bray, R. M., & Penne, M. A. (2006). Nonmedical use of prescription stimulants in the United States. *Drug and Alcohol Dependence, 84*, 135–143.

Leinwand, D. (2005, May 25). Prescription drug users not just after a high. *USA Today.* Retrieved from *www.usatoday.com/news/health/2005-05-25-drugs_x.htm.*

Massello, W., & Carpenter, D. A. (1999). A fatality due to the intranasal abuse of methylphenidate (Ritalin). *Journal of Forensic Sciences, 44*, 220–221.

McCabe, S. E. (2008). Screening for drug abuse among medical and nonmedical users of prescription drugs in a probability sample of college students. *Archives of Pediatrics and Adolescent Medicine, 162*, 225–231.

McCabe, S. E., & Boyd, C. J. (2005). Sources of prescription drugs for illicit use. *Addictive Behaviors, 30*(7), 1342–1350.

McCabe, S. E., Boyd, C. J., & Teter, C. J. (2009). Subtypes of nonmedical prescription drug misuse. *Drug and Alcohol Dependence, 102*, 63–70.

McCabe, S. E., Cranford, J. A., & Boyd, C. J. (2006a). The relationship between past-year drinking behaviors and nonmedical use of prescription drugs: Prevalence of co-occurrence in a national sample. *Drug and Alcohol Dependence, 84*, 281–288.

McCabe, S. E., Cranford, J. A., Boyd, C. J., & Teter, C. J. (2007a). Motives, diversion and routes of administration associated with nonmedical use of prescription opioids. *Addictive Behaviors, 32*, 562–575.

McCabe, S. E., Cranford, J. A., Morales, M., & Young, A. (2006b). Simultaneous and concurrent poly-drug use of alcohol and prescription drugs: Prevalence, correlates and consequences. *Journal of Studies on Alcohol, 67*, 529–537.

McCabe, S. E., Knight, J. R., Teter, C. J., & Wechsler, H. (2005a). Nonmedical use of prescription stimulants among U. S. college students: Prevalence and correlates from a national survey. *Addiction, 100*, 96–106.

McCabe, S. E., & Teter, C. J. (2007). Drug use related problems among nonmedical users of prescription stimulants: A web-based survey of college students from a Midwestern university. *Drug and Alcohol Dependence, 91*, 69–76.

McCabe, S. E., Teter, C. J., & Boyd, C. J. (2005b). Illicit use of prescription pain medication among college students. *Drug and Alcohol Dependence, 71*(1), 37–47.

McCabe, S. E., Teter, C. J., & Boyd, C. J. (2006c). Medical use, illicit use and diversion of prescription stimulant medication. *Journal of Psychoactive Drugs, 38*, 43–56.

McCabe, S. E., Teter, C. J., Boyd, C. J., Knight, J. R., & Wechsler, H. (2005c). Nonmedical use of prescription opioids among U. S. college students: Prevalence and correlates from a national survey. *Addictive Behaviors, 30*(4),789–805.

McCabe, S. E., West, B. T., Morales, M., Cranford, J. A., & Boyd, C. J. (2007b). Does early onset of non-medical use predict prescription drug abuse and dependence?: Results from a national study. *Addiction, 102*, 1920–1930.

McCabe, S. E., West, B. T., & Wechsler, H. (2007c). Trends and college-level characteristics associated with the nonmedical use of prescription drugs among U. S. college students from 1993 to 2001. *Addiction, 102*, 455–465.

Olfson, M., Gameroff, M. J., Marcus, S. C., & Jensen, P. S. (2003). National trends in the treatment of attention deficit hyperactivity disorder. *American Journal of Psychiatry, 160*, 1071–1077.

Passik, S. D. (2010, July 22). REMS for opioids. FDA as a stakeholder in problems of pain and addiction: Enter risk evaluation and mitigation strategies (REMS). *Medscape.* Retrieved from *www.medscape.com/viewarticle/725505_2.*

Peterkin, A. L., Crone, C. C., Sheridan, M. J., & Wise, T. N. (2010, April 21). Cognitive performance enhancement: Misuse or self-treatment [Electronic version ahead of print]? *Journal of Attention Disorders, 15*(4), 263–268.

Petrillo, L., & Cantlupe, J. (2005, February 19). Painkiller linked to 3 local deaths. *San Diego Union Tribune.* Retrieved from *www.signonsandiego. com/uniontrib/20050219/news_7m19drug.html.*

Rabiner, D. L., Anastopoulos, A. D., Costello, E. J., Hoyle, R. H., McCabe, S. E., & Swartzwelder, H. S. (2009a). The misuse and diversion of prescribed ADHD medications by college students. *Journal of Attention Disorders, 13,* 144–153.

Rabiner, D. L., Anastopoulos, A. D., Costello, E. J., Hoyle, R. H., McCabe, S. E., & Swartzwelder, H. S. (2009b). Motives and perceived consequences of nonmedical ADHD medication use by college students: Are students treating themselves for attention problems? *Journal of Attention Disorders, 13,* 259–270.

Rabiner, D. L., Anastopoulos, A. D., Costello, E. J., Hoyle, R. H., & Swartzwelder, H. S. (2010). Predictors of nonmedical ADHD medication use by college students. *Journal of Attention Disorders, 13,* 640–648.

Roset, P. N., Farre, M., de la Torre, R., Mas, M., Menoyo, E., & Hernandez, C. (2001). Modulation of rate of onset and intensity of drug effects reduces abuse potential in healthy males. *Drug and Alcohol Dependence, 64,* 285–298.

Savage S. R. (2003). Opioid medications in the management of pain. In A. W. Graham, T. K. Schultz, M. F. Mayo-Smith, R. K. Ries, & B. B. Wilford (Eds.), *Principles of addiction medicine* (pp. 1452–1463). Chevy Chase, MD: American Society of Addiction Medicine.

Sepulveda, D. R., Thomas, L. M., McCabe, S. E., Boyd, C. J., Cranford, J. A., & Teter, C. J. (2008, June). *Misuse of prescribed stimulant medication for ADHD and associated patterns of substance use: A preliminary analysis among college students.* Presentation at the 70th annual meeting, College on Problems of Drug Dependence, San Juan, Puerto Rico.

Skinner, H. (1982). The Drug Abuse Screening Test. *Addictive Behaviors, 7,* 363–371.

Substance Abuse and Mental Health Services Administration (SAMHSA). (2004). *The DAWN Report: Oxycodone, hydrocodone, and polydrug use, 2002..* Rockville, MD: Author.

Substance Abuse and Mental Health Services Administration (SAMHSA). (2005). *College enrollment status and past year illicit drug use among young adults: 2002, 2003, and 2004..* Rockville, MD: Author.

Substance Abuse and Mental Health Services Administration (SAMHSA). (2009a). *Results from the 2008 National Survey on Drug Use and Health: Detailed tables.* Rockville, MD: Author.

Substance Abuse and Mental Health Services Administration (SAMHSA). (2009b). *Nonmedical use of Adderall® among full-time college students.* Rockville, MD: Author.

Teter, C. J., Falone, A. E., Cranford, J. A., Boyd, C. J., & McCabe, S. E. (2010). Nonmedical use of prescription stimulants and depressed mood among college students: Frequency and routes of administration. *Journal of American College Health, 53,* 253–262.

Teter, C. J., McCabe, S. E., Cranford, J. A., Boyd, C. J., & Guthrie, S. K. (2005). Prevalence and motivations for the illicit use of prescription stimulants in an undergraduate student sample. *Journal of American College Health, 53,* 253–262.

Teter, C. J., McCabe, S. E., LaGrange, K., Cranford, J. A., & Boyd, C. J. (2006). Illicit use of specific prescription stimulants among college students: Prevalence, motives, and routes of administration. *Pharmacotherapy, 26,* 1501–1510.

Thomas, C. P., Conrad, P., Casler, R., & Goodman, E. (2006). Trends in the use of psychotropic medications among adolescents, 1994 to 2001. *Psychiatric Services, 57,* 63–69.

Upadhyaya, H. P., Rose, K., Wang, W., & Brady, K. T. (2005). Attention-deficit/hyperactivity disorder, medication treatment, and substance use patterns among adolescents and young adults. *Journal of Child and Adolescent Psychopharmacology, 15,* 799–809.

Volkow, N. D., & Swanson, J. M. (2003). Variables that affect the clinical use and abuse of methylphenidate in the treatment of ADHD. *American Journal of Psychiatry, 160,* 1909–1918.

Watson, W. A., Litovitz, T. L., Klein-Schwartz, W., Rodgers, G. C., Youniss, J., Reid, N., et al. (2004). 2003 annual report of the American Association of Poison Control Centers Toxic Exposure Surveillance System. *American Journal of Emergency Medicine, 22,* 335–404.

White, B. P., Becker-Blease, K. A., & Grace-Bishop, K. (2006). Stimulant medication use, misuse, and abuse in an undergraduate and graduate student sample. *Journal of American College Health, 54,* 261–268.

Wilens, T. E., Gignac, M., Swezey, A., Monuteaux, M. C., & Biederman, J. (2006). Characteristics of adolescents and young adults with ADHD who divert or misuse their prescribed medications. *Journal of American Academy of Child and Adolescent Psychiatry, 45,* 408–414.

Yewell, J., Haydon, R., Archer, S., & Manaligod, J. M. (2002). Complications of intranasal prescription narcotic abuse. *Annals of Otology, Rhinology and Laryngology, 111,* 174–177.

Zacny, J., Bigelow, G., Compton, P., Foley, K., Iguchi, M., & Sannerud, C. (2003). College on Problems of Drug Dependence taskforce on prescription opioid nonmedical use and abuse: Position statement. *Drug and Alcohol Dependence, 69,* 215–232.

Zito, J. M., Safer, D. J., dosReis, S., Gardner, J. F., Magder, L., Soeken, K., et al. (2003). Psychotropic practice patterns for youth: A 10-year perspective. *Archives of Pediatric and Adolescent Medicine, 157,* 17–25.

PART II

BIOLOGICAL AND NEUROPSYCHOLOGICAL ASPECTS OF SUBSTANCE USE

CHAPTER 3

Chronic Effects of Heavy Alcohol and Marijuana Use on the Brain and Cognition in Adolescents and Young Adults

Krista M. Lisdahl *and* Susan Tapert

Alcohol continues to be the most popular drug among teens and young adults, with almost a third of 12th graders and 40% of college students reporting recent binge drinking (Johnston, O'Malley, Bachman, & Schulenberg, 2010; Johnston, O'Malley, Bachman, & Schulenberg, 2009). Furthermore, 58% of teen drinkers also use marijuana (Martin, Kaczynski, Maisto, & Tarter, 1996), contributing to frequent comorbidity between alcohol and marijuana use disorders (Agosti, Nunes, & Levin, 2002). Indeed, marijuana is the most commonly used illicit drug, with 42% of 12th graders using marijuana in their lifetime (Johnston et al., 2010) (for further information on substance use rates, see Schulenberg & Patrick, Chapter 1, this volume). In this chapter, we provide an overview of the cognitive and brain changes associated with heavy alcohol and marijuana use in teens and young adults. Then, we explore potential clinical and public health implications of these findings.

ADOLESCENCE AND YOUNG ADULTHOOD: A SENSITIVE NEURODEVELOPMENTAL PERIOD?

Adolescence is an incredibly dynamic time that is, among other things, marked by increased risk-taking behaviors (Eaton et al., 2006; Gardener

& Steinberg, 2005), which coincide with significant neurodevelopmental changes in both gray matter and white matter. Gray matter contains neuron cell bodies, dendrites, synaptic connections, and support cells, while white matter is made up of bundles of myelinated axons that connect brain regions. Several brain regions associated with executive functioning (e.g., problem solving, planning, working memory, and emotional regulation), including the prefrontal cortex (PFC), parietal cortex, and cerebellum, continue to undergo gray matter synaptic pruning into the mid-20s (Giedd et al., 1996a; Gogtay et al., 2004; Lenroot & Giedd, 2006; Sowell et al., 2004; Sowell, Thompson, Holmes, Jernigan, & Toga, 1999; Sowell, Trauner, Gamst, & Jernigan, 2002). Maturation of white matter tracts appears to continue into the early 30s, yielding improvements in efficient neural conductivity (Barnea-Goraly et al., 2005; Giedd et al., 1999; Nagel et al., 2006; Jernigan & Gamst, 2005; Paus et al., 1999). Some scholars have emphasized that it is not the late maturation of the PFC (which regulates executive functioning) alone that is responsible for increased impulsivity and risk-taking behavior during adolescence, but rather it is due to the differing developmental trajectories of the PFC and the limbic system. The limbic system, including brain regions like the amygdala and hippocampus, has a role in emotion, sexual behaviors, motivation, and memory. During the teen years, the limbic system develops earlier than the PFC (Galvan et al., 2006; Giedd et al., 1996b; Casey, Getz, & Galvan, 2008). As the PFC undergoes neuronal maturation, greater top-down control of the limbic system results in improved inhibitory control and affective processing (Casey et al., 2008; Casey, Galvan, & Hare, 2005; Casey et al., 1997; Liston et al., 2006; Monk et al., 2003).

It should also be noted that boys and girls differ in the timing and rate of neurodevelopment (see Lenroot & Giedd, 2010, for review). More specifically, gray matter volumes peak earlier for females in executive centers (PFC, parietal and temporal cortices), indicating that females undergo synaptic pruning earlier, and there are greater age-related white matter increases in males; overall, this results in relatively larger brain volumes in boys compared to girls (Giedd et al., 1996b; Nagel et al., 2006; Lenroot et al., 2007; Lenroot & Giedd, 2010). Larger relative volumes in boys do not necessarily denote an advantage or disadvantage; rather, boys and girls may use different neuronal structures to complete tasks at a similar level. Delayed brain development may underlie risk for impulse-control-related psychiatric disorders, including drug and alcohol misuse. Further, chronic alcohol or marijuana exposure during the teen or young adult years may differentially impact the trajectory of brain development for boys and girls.

ALCOHOL USE DISORDERS
AND NEUROCOGNITION
IN ADOLESCENTS AND YOUNG ADULTS

Animal studies have suggested that compared to adults, teens may be particularly vulnerable to the neurotoxic effects of alcohol (see Barron et al., 2005; Monti et al., 2005; Spear, 2010). Converging lines of evidence suggest that teenage onset of alcohol abuse or dependence (alcohol use disorders, or AUDs) is associated with neurocognitive deficits, even though teens have substantially shorter periods of exposure compared to adults. Specifically, neuropsychological studies have found that AUDs during adolescence and young adulthood are associated with poorer verbal retrieval (Brown, Tapert, Granholm, & Delis, 2000; Hanson, Medina, Padula, Tapert, & Brown, 2011), attention (Tapert & Brown, 1999), visuospatial functioning (Hanson et al., 2011; Giancola, Mezzich, & Tarter, 1998; Sher, Martin, Wood, & Rutledge, 1997; Tapert, Granholm, Leedy, & Brown, 2002b), language (Moss, Kirisci, Gordon, & Tarter, 1994), and executive functioning (Hanson et al., 2011). Withdrawal symptoms seem to be particularly sensitive predictors of cognitive deficits, including poorer visuospatial functioning and memory retrieval (Brown et al., 2000; Brown & Tapert, 1999; Hanson et al., 2011; Tapert, Baratta, Abrantes, & Brown, 2002a).

Studies utilizing high-resolution magnetic resonance imaging (MRI) to measure brain structure have revealed abnormalities in teens with AUDs, including reduced hippocampal volume (De Bellis et al., 2000; Nagel, Schweinsburg, Phan, & Tapert, 2005; Medina, Schweinsburg, Cohen-Zion, Nagel, & Tapert, 2007c) and reduced volume in the PFC (De Bellis et al., 2005; Medina et al., 2008), suggesting that heavy alcohol exposure during adolescence can result in neuronal atrophy in brain regions underlying executive functioning and memory. Using functional MRI (fMRI) to assess blood flow changes during cognitive tasks, our group has shown that despite similar behavioral performance on a spatial working memory task, teens with AUDs have increased brain response in the parietal and reduced response in the occipital, PFC, and cerebellar regions (Tapert et al., 2004). Results indicate that the teen brain may compensate for alcohol-induced neuronal insult by relying on other areas (e.g., parietal cortex—which plays a role in working memory) to successfully complete tasks. Gender may also moderate these effects; Caldwell et al. (2005) found that, after controlling for typical blood alcohol concentrations (BACs), females with AUDs demonstrated reduced PFC response compared to female controls, while the males showed the opposite pattern. Overall, females demonstrated more alcohol-related abnormalities in the executive control brain region (PFC) than males, which was consistent with our brain structural findings (Medina et al., 2008). Further, young adult women with AUDs who underwent a similar fMRI spatial working memory task demonstrated overall reduced brain activation along with poorer behavioral performance (Tapert et al., 2001). Thus, young adult women with AUDs may no longer be able to compensate as effectively as teens, so we see further performance decrements with continued alcohol use.

BINGE ALCOHOL USE AND NEUROCOGNITION IN ADOLESCENTS AND YOUNG ADULTS

Given the alarming rates of binge drinking in both teenagers and young adults, especially college students (Johnston et al., 2009, 2010), it is important to determine whether binge drinking (defined as four standard alcohol drinks on an occasion in females and five drinks for males), even in the absence of an AUD, is associated with cognition and brain changes. This problematic drinking pattern has induced neuronal damage and long-lasting behavioral deficits in adolescent and adult animals (see Barron et al., 2005; Monti et al., 2005; Spear, 2010). However, there have been relatively few human studies to date that specifically examine the effects of intermittent binge drinking in adolescents and young adults. Thus far, studies have reported cognitive deficits associated with binge drinking in otherwise healthy young adults, including poorer sustained attention (Hartley, Elsabagh, & File, 2004), memory (Hartley et al., 2004; Scaife & Duka, 2009), spatial working memory (Townshend & Duka, 2005; Scaife & Duka, 2009), psychomotor speed (Hartley et al., 2004), and response inhibition and rule acquisition in females (Townshend & Duka, 2005; Scaife & Duka, 2009), although two studies actually found faster motor response during a visuospatial task (Townshend & Duka, 2005; Scaife & Duka, 2009). Given the high rates of binge drinking in college students, these results are of great concern. It is likely that these cognitive problems are in part to blame for the lower grades seen in students who are heavy drinkers.

Although this area has been less studied, preliminary evidence suggests underlying structural and functional brain changes associated with binge drinking in youth. In accord with its role connecting brain regions to each other, improved white matter is associated with increased connectivity and more efficient processing. Using diffusion tensor imaging (DTI), an MRI technique that quantifies white matter integrity, McQueeny et al. (2009) found that adolescent binge drinkers, compared to light drinkers, had significantly reduced white matter quality (as measured by lower fractional anisotropy, or FA) in several brain regions that connect the brain stem, motor areas, limbic regions, and cortex including the PFC (i.e., the corpus callosum, superior longitudinal fasciculus, corona radiata, internal and external capsules, and commissural, limbic, brain stem, and cortical projection fibers). Greater symptoms of hangover and increased estimated peak BAC (see Figure 3.1) estimates were significantly correlated with poorer white matter integrity in white matter tracts connecting the two hemispheres, frontal lobe, and cerebellar tracts. In a similar sample, our group (Schweinsburg, McQueeny, Nagel, Eyler, & Tapert, 2010) found that teenage binge drinkers had abnormal brain response during a verbal encoding task. Further, unlike the controls, the binge drinkers failed to engage the hippocampus during novel verbal encoding.

Taken together, these studies suggest that intermittent recent binge drinking, even without the presence of an AUD, can also result in significant cognitive, structural, and functional brain changes in both males and females. Given the fact that approximately 40% of college students engage in this drinking pattern, this is a major concern. This pattern of

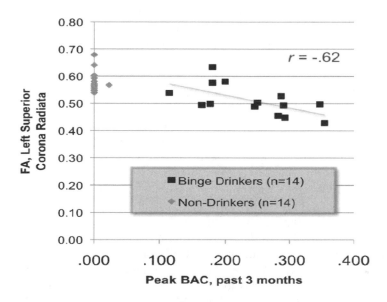

FIGURE 3.1. Reduced white matter integrity, shown by lower fractional anisotrophy (FA) in the corona radiata (a white matter tract connecting the cortex with the basal ganglia and spinal cord), is associated with increased estimated BAC in adolescent binge drinkers. Data from McQueeny et al. (2009).

brain findings suggests that recent binge drinking may lead to poorer learning of new information, reduced ability to hold new information in mind, and less efficient brain processing. Combined with other alcohol-related consequences (e.g., hangover, poor sleep, emotional stress), these cognitive problems may reduce performance in the classroom. Indeed, studies have found that problematic binge drinking has been predictive of a poorer end-of-semester grade point average (Read, Merrill, Kahler, & Strong, 2007).

HEAVY MARIJUANA USE AND NEUROCOGNITION IN ADOLESCENTS AND YOUNG ADULTS

Similar to alcohol findings, animal studies have found increased cellular changes associated with exposure to THC (delta-9-tetrahydrocannabi-nol, one of the major psychoactive compounds in marijuana) during adolescence compared to adulthood (e.g., Cha, White, Kuhn, Wilson, & Swartzwelder, 2006; Rubino et al., 2009; Schneider & Koch, 2003). Human findings suggest that earlier age of marijuana-use onset is associated with more severe cognitive consequences; marijuana users who started using during adolescence (before the age of 17) were more likely to demonstrate cognitive problems, including poorer attention, verbal memory, overall intelligence, and verbal fluency (Ehrenreich et al., 1999; Wilson et al., 2000). Despite the high prevalence of marijuana use in teens and animal studies suggesting adolescent vulnerability, there are relatively few studies examining the neurocognitive effects of heavy marijuana use in adolescents.

In a longitudinal study following adolescents with substance use disorders (SUDs) over time, Tapert and colleagues (2002b) found that greater cumulative marijuana use over an 8-year follow-up period was associated with poorer attention functioning. Thus far, studies conducted in adolescents with minimal psychiatric comorbidities have suggested subtle cognitive deficits associated with adolescent marijuana use, including processing speed (Fried, Watkinson, & Gray, 2005; Medina et al., 2007a), attention (Hanson et al., 2010; Harvey, Sellman, Porter, & Frampton, 2007; Medina et al., 2007a), memory (Fried et al., 2005; Hanson et al., 2010; Harvey et al., 2007; Medina et al., 2007a; Schwartz, Gruenewald, Klitzner, & Fedio, 1989), and executive functioning (Hanson et al., 2010; Harvey et al., 2007; Medina et al., 2007a). We (Medina et al., 2007a) compared neuropsychological functioning in a sample of demographically matched healthy controls and marijuana-using adolescents without comorbid psychiatric disorders who underwent a month of monitored abstinence. After controlling for alcohol exposure, compared to controls, marijuana users had deficits in complex attention, verbal story learning, sequencing ability, and slower psychomotor speed compared to controls (see Figure 3.2; Medina et al., 2007a). However, it can be difficult to determine whether these cognitive problems predated substance use, as these studies did not exclude for a family history of SUD or assess baseline cognitive functioning prior to the onset of marijuana use.

Few studies have utilized neuroimaging methods to assess the brain structural consequences of marijuana use in adolescents. Using high-resolution MRI, our laboratory has examined brain volumes in a subsample of aforementioned adolescent marijuana users (ages 16–19) and healthy controls. In one of our first analyses, we found that adolescent marijuana users (who were also heavy alcohol users) did not significantly differ from healthy controls in their hippocampal volumes, although correlations between hippocampal volumes and verbal memory were abnormal compared to the controls (Medina et al., 2007c). Given the sustained attention and sequencing problems observed in these marijuana-using teens, we measured PFC volumes in 16 marijuana users and 16 healthy controls without comorbid psychiatric disorders. We found marginal marijuana group-by-gender interactions in predicting PFC volume; female mari-

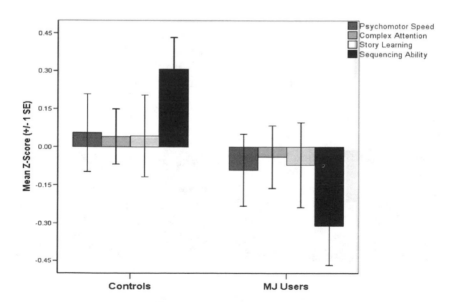

FIGURE 3.2. Deficits in mean z-score psychomotor speed, complex attention, verbal story learning, and sequencing ability were observed in teen marijuana users following 1 month of abstinence. Data from Medina et al. (2007a).

juana users demonstrated comparatively larger volumes, while male users had smaller volumes compared to same-gender controls (Medina et al., 2009). Marijuana group status and total PFC volume interacted in predicting executive functioning; among the marijuana users (especially the girls), larger PFC volumes were associated with *poorer* executive functioning, while the opposite pattern was seen among the controls, suggesting that larger PFC volumes in the marijuana users was detrimental. Most recently, we found increased posterior inferior cerebellar vermis (a brain region related to affective regulation) volumes in adolescent marijuana users compared to controls (Medina, Nagel, & Tapert, 2010). Again, these *larger* volumes were associated with *poorer* executive functioning. A similar brain structure finding was reported in marijuana-using teens with bipolar disorder (Jarvis et al., 2008).

Subtle white matter abnormalities have also been observed in adolescent and young adult marijuana users. Our group found that increased depressive symptoms in marijuana users were associated with smaller white matter volume (Medina, Nagel, McQueeny, Park, & Tapert, 2007b), suggesting that marijuana use during adolescence may disrupt white matter connections between areas involved in mood regulation. Using DTI, we found that marijuana users had significantly poorer white matter integrity, measured by lower FA in 10 brain regions, especially in regions underlying executive functioning and working memory (see Figure 3.3; Bava et al., 2009). Increased FA was also seen in regions underlying vision, suggesting possible overrecruitment of these brain regions in marijuana users compared to controls. With one exception (DeLisi et al., 2006), these results are consistent with other studies that have dem-

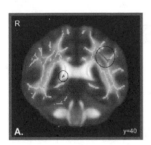 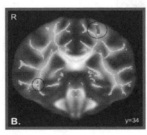 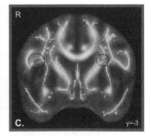

FIGURE 3.3. Fractional anisotropy (FA), or white matter integrity, in adolescent marijuana users and controls. Circled areas indicate lower FA, or poorer white matter integrity, in marijuana users ($p < .01$). (A) Left superior longitudinal fasciculus; (B) postcentral gyrus; (C) inferior frontal gyrus. Data from Bava et al. (2009).

onstrated reduced white matter integrity in young adult marijuana users who initiated use during adolescence (Arnone et al., 2008; Ashtari et al., 2009).

There is also evidence of inefficient brain activation patterns in young marijuana users. Young adults who initiated marijuana use early (younger than 16 years old) demonstrate greater brain functioning abnormalities compared to late-onset users (Becker, Wagner, Gouzoulis-Mayfrank, Spuentrup, & Daumann, 2010). Studies utilizing fMRI with adolescents have found abnormal PFC, limbic, and parietal activation patterns in marijuana users, compared to controls, in response to tasks involving cognitive inhibition (Tapert et al., 2007), verbal working memory (Jacobsen, Pugh, Constable, Westerveld, & Mencl, 2007; Jager, Block, Luijten, & Ramsey, 2010), and spatial working memory (Schweinsburg et al., 2008). Jager et al. (2010) recently reported that marijuana-using teenage boys (ages 13–19) demonstrated excessive activation in executive (PFC) regions during a verbal working memory task, especially during initial encoding, compared to nonusing healthy controls. Consistent with this finding, our laboratory (Tapert et al., 2007) found that after controlling for alcohol use, marijuana users demonstrated increased executive (right dorsolateral PFC, bilateral medial frontal), working memory (parietal), and visual (occipital) activation during inhibitory "no-go" trials (i.e., tests of impulse control), compared to normal controls, even though they had marginally poorer performance. Further, teen marijuana users with lighter use histories demonstrated the greatest brain activation in response to both the cognitive inhibition and spatial working memory tasks (Tapert et al., 2007; Schweinsburg et al., 2008), while teens with more intense use histories (earlier onset, longer duration, increased lifetime use) had lower activation than controls. This finding suggests that during *initial* marijuana exposure the brain may successfully compensate by recruiting additional neuronal resources, although this compensation may falter with more problematic and increased marijuana use patterns.

Taken together, the above studies suggest that heavy marijuana use during adolescence may lead to structural changes such as abnormal gray matter pruning or dendritic sprouting and reduced white matter myelination. These changes have been associated with poor neuronal efficiency and poorer cognitive functioning, especially psychomotor speed, executive functioning, emotional control, and learning and memory, even after a month of monitored abstinence. Given the high rates of marijuana use in teens and young adults, this may mean a large proportion of college students are experiencing cognitive difficulties that may negatively impact their performance. Indeed, we have found increased school difficulty and reduced grades in marijuana-using teens (Medina et al., 2007a).

POTENTIAL LIMITATIONS
OF THE EXISTING LITERATURE

It is important to note some limitations of the above research. Although several of the studies described above did control for family history of SUD and excluded subjects with Axis I comorbid psychiatric disorders, it is still difficult to determine whether the brain and cognitive abnormalities may have predated the onset of adolescent drug use. Risk factors associated with early drug experimentation (such as poor cognitive inhibition, attention problems, conduct disorder, and family history of SUD) are themselves related to subtle cognitive and brain abnormalities (Aronowitz et al., 1994; Hanson et al., 2010; Hill et al., 2007b; Hill et al., 2007a; Nigg et al., 2004; Ridenour et al., 2009; Schweinsburg et al., 2004; Spadoni, Norman, Schweinsburg, & Tapert, 2008; Tapert & Brown, 2000; Tapert, Barrata, Abrantes, & Brown, 2002a). Therefore, longitudinal research on teenagers prior to alcohol and marijuana exposure is needed to explore the influence of early drug use on adolescent neurodevelopment.

RECOVERY OF FUNCTION WITH ABSTINENCE?:
A MESSAGE OF HOPE

There is even less research available to help determine whether sustained abstinence from alcohol and marijuana results in recovery of cognitive functions, although findings thus far are hopeful. Our lab recently found that having greater days of abstinence from alcohol and drugs at a 10-year follow-up neuropsychological evaluation was associated with improved executive functioning, even after controlling for baseline executive functioning and education (Hanson et al., 2011). In teenagers, short-term memory impairments were mildly improved following 6 weeks of marijuana abstinence (Schwartz et al., 1989). Recently, our lab reported that adolescent marijuana users demonstrated significant improvements in verbal list learning and verbal working memory within the first 3 weeks of abstinence, although sustained attention problems persisted throughout 3 weeks of abstinence (Hanson et al., 2010; see Figure 3.4).

Another study found that adolescent marijuana users who abstained for a minimum of 3 months did not demonstrate any cognitive deficits compared to controls (Fried et al., 2005). Finally, in a cross-sectional study, recent marijuana users demonstrated increased activation in brain regions underlying executive control and attention, such as the insula and PFC, compared to abstinent ex-users (Schweinsburg et al., 2010). This preliminary evidence suggests that the inefficient brain response seen

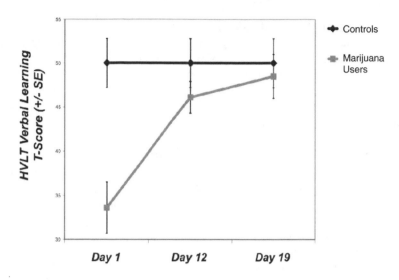

FIGURE 3.4. Immediate verbal learning (HVLT) *T*-scores significantly improve with approximately 2 weeks of abstinence from heavy marijuana use in adolescents. Data from Hanson et al. (2010).

in teenage marijuana users may begin to normalize after several weeks of abstinence. In sum, these results suggest there may be subtle recovery of cognitive functioning with increasing lengths of abstinence from marijuana and alcohol. It remains unclear whether complete recovery of neurocognitive functioning occurs in adolescents with greater lengths of abstinence; additional longitudinal studies are under way to help answer these questions. Still, these preliminary findings can be utilized to help increase motivation for abstinence in alcohol- and marijuana-using college students, as it is expected that with continued abstinence they will experience improvements in attention, verbal memory, and neuronal processing speed.

CONCLUSIONS: EFFECTS OF ALCOHOL AND MARIJUANA USE ON THE TEEN AND YOUNG ADULT BRAIN

Alarming numbers of teenagers and young adults regularly use marijuana and engage in binge drinking (Johnston et al., 2009, 2010). Animal and human research suggests that adolescence may be a vulnerable period for drug exposure due to critical neurodevelomental processes that peak during this period. Indeed, adolescents and young adults who use marijuana regularly or engage in binge drinking tend to show inferior cognitive skills compared to teens who abstain or use lightly. In the case of marijuana, these cognitive problems persist even following 1 month of abstinence, although there is evidence that sustained abstinence for at least 3 months may reverse these deficits. This chapter has outlined several studies that suggest AUDs, binge drinking, and chronic marijuana use during the teenage and early adult years result in gray matter and white matter structural abnormalities that are oftentimes correlated with cognitive deficits. Finally, evidence is mounting that heavy teenage alcohol and marijuana use may disrupt brain activation, leading to inefficient neuronal activation early on and diminished activation with continued heavy use into young adulthood.

Even subtle brain abnormalities and cognitive problems in teens and young adults may lead to important psychosocial consequences. The combined negative consequences of drug and alcohol use, such as hangovers, emotional stress), and drug-induced sleep deprivation (Cohen-Zion et al., 2009), and its chronic effects on brain structure may lead to even more pronounced cognitive problems in college students who are active users of alcohol and marijuana. Students may miss information presented in class due to poorer processing speed, initial learning, complex attention, and working memory. Indeed, researchers have found that drug-induced cognitive disadvantage may lead to lower-than-expected school performance, self-reported school problems, risky decision making, and poorer emotional regulation (Kloos, Weller, Chan, & Weller, 2009; Lynskey & Hall, 2000; Medina et al., 2007a).

Given these concerns, it is critical to disseminate these research findings to high school and college students, therapists, teachers, school administrators, general physicians, pediatricians, and parents to help prevent and reduce heavy alcohol and marijuana use. Fortunately, high-quality psychoeducational materials regarding the effects of alcohol and drugs on the brain, including colorful pamphlets made for teens and young adults, are available at no cost through the National Institute on Drug Abuse (NIDA) (*www.nida.nih.gov*) and the National Institute on Alcohol Abuse and Alcoholism (NIAAA) (*www.niaaa.nih.gov*). It is important to note, however, that giving more personalized feedback about the health effects of drugs and alcohol has been shown to be more effective in reducing use than simple psychoeducation (see Larimer & Cronce, 2007; see also Cronce & Larimer, Chapter 8, and Walters, Lee, & Walker, Chapter 9, this volume).

To date, however, no individualized feedback programs have integrated information regarding the effects of drugs on the brain and congnition. More global feedback focused on group or normative performance results could be integrated at this time. For example, after filling out an online survey, a student who engages in weekly marijuana use could be informed that "even with similar verbal intelligence and reading ability, marijuana users scored more than half a standard deviation lower on an executive functioning task, achieved a half-point lower GPA, and were more likely to demonstrate behavioral problems in school (26% vs. 0%) compared to peers who did not regularly use marijuana" (Medina et al., 2007a). A student who engaged in binge drinking within the past 3 months could be advised that "even with similar verbal intelligence, young adults who were recent binge drinkers remembered 7% fewer words following a delay compared to non-binging young adults" (Medina, Price, Hawkins, Budion, & McQueeny, 2011). This normative feedback could be developed further and disseminated more globally by college campus services aimed at health education and drug prevention. Therapists could also utilize this neurocognitive information during brief motivational interviewing sessions to help educate students about the negative effects of alcohol and marijuana use on the brain. Therapists could go even further by ordering neuropsychological testing and giving truly individualized feedback regarding the student's cognitive functioning.

In summary, heavy binge drinking or chronic marijuana use has been shown to negatively impact cognition and brain function in otherwise healthy teens and young adults. Given the high rates of binge drinking and marijuana use on college campuses, this is an important public health concern for universities worldwide. Normative feedback regarding effects of chronic drug use on thinking abilities and brain health needs to be integrated into current prevention, harm-reduction, and treatment programs. More globally, interventions proven effective in lowering alcohol and drug exposure in teens and young adults need to be implemented more aggressively on college campuses not only to reduce symptoms of drug abuse and dependence, but to prevent long-term neuronal damage and ensure optimal brain health and cognitive functioning in students.

ACKNOWLEDGMENTS

This chapter and much of the research presented within it were made possible through funding by the National Institute on Alcohol Abuse and Alcoholism Grant Nos. R01 AA13419 (Susan Tapert, Principal Investigator), R37 AA07033 (Sandra Brown, Principal Investigator), and T32 AA013525 (Susan Riley, Principle Investigator), and by National Institute on Drug Abuse Grant R01 DA021182 and 5P20 DA024194-0002 (Susan Tapert); F32 DA020206 (Krista M. Lisdahl, completed), R03 DA027457 (Krista M. Lisdahl, Principal Investigator); F32 DA024476 (Sunita Bava, Principal Investigator), and F31 DA026263 (Joanna

Jacobus, Principal Investigator). We would like to acknowledge the vast scientific contributions of our collaborators and graduate and undergraduate research assistants in the University of Wisconsin—Milwaukee Brain Imaging and Neuropsychology (BraIN) Laboratory and the University of California, San Diego, Adolescent Brain Imaging Project (ABIP).

REFERENCES

Agosti, V., Nunes, E., & Levin, F. (2002). Rates of psychiatric comorbidity among U.S. residents with lifetime cannabis dependence. *American Journal of Drug and Alcohol Abuse, 28*(4), 643–652.

Arnone, D., Barrick, T. R., Chengappa, S., Mackay, C. E., Clark, C. A., & Abou-Saleh, M. T. (2008). Corpus callosum damage in heavy marijuana use: Preliminary evidence from diffusion tensor tractography and tract-based spatial statistics. *NeuroImage, 41*(3), 1067–1074.

Aronowitz, B., Liebowitz, M. R., Hollander, E., Fazzini, E., Durlach-Misteli, C., Frenkel, M., Mosovich, S., et al. (1994). Neuropsychiatric and neuropsychological findings in conduct disorder and attention-deficit hyperactivity disorder. *Journal of Neuropsychiatry and Clinical Neurosciences, 6*, 245–249.

Ashtari, M., Cervellione, K., Cottone, J., Ardekani, B. A., Sevy, S., & Kumra, S. (2009). Diffusion abnormalities in adolescents and young adults with a history of heavy cannabis use. *Journal of Psychiatric Research, 43*(3), 189–204.

Barnea-Goraly, N., Menon, V., Eckert, M., Tamm, L., Bammer, R., Karchemskiy, A., et al. (2005). White matter development during childhood and adolescence: A cross-sectional diffusion tensor imaging study. *Cerebral Cortex, 15*(12), 1848–1854.

Barron, S., White, A., Swartzwelder, H. S., Bell, R. L., Rodd Z. A., Slawecki, C. J., et al. (2005). Adolescent vulnerabilities to chronic alcohol or nicotine exposure: Findings from rodent models. *Alcoholism: Clinical and Experimental Research, 29*(9), 1720–1725.

Bava, S., Frank, L. R., McQueeny, T., Schweinsburg, B. C., Schweinsburg, A. D., & Tapert, S. F. (2009). Altered white matter microstructure in adolescent substance users. *Psychiatry Research, 173*(3), 228–237.

Becker, B., Wagner, D., Gouzoulis-Mayfrank, E., Spuentrup, E., & Daumann, J. (2010). The impact of early-onset cannabis use on functional brain correlates of working memory. *Progress in Neuro-Psychopharmacology and Biological Psychiatry, 34*(6), 837–845.

Brown, S. A., & Tapert, S. F. (1999). Neuropsychological correlates of adolescent substance abuse: four-year outcomes. *Journal of the International Neuropsychological Society, 5*(6), 481–493.

Brown, S. A., Tapert, S. F., Granholm, E., & Delis, D. C. (2000). Neurocognitive functioning of adolescents: Effects of protracted alcohol use. *Alcoholism: Clinical and Experimental Research, 24*, 164–171.

Caldwell, L. C., Schweinsburg, A. D., Nagel, B. J., Barlett, V. C., Brown, S. A., &

Tapert, S. F. (2005). Gender and adolescent alcohol use disorders on BOLD (blood oxygen level dependent) response to spatial working memory. *Alcohol and Alcoholism, 40*(3), 194–200.

Casey, B. J., Getz, S., & Galvan, A. (2008). The adolescent brain. *Developmental Review, 28*(1), 62–77.

Casey, B. J., Galvan, A., & Hare, T. A. (2005). Changes in cerebral functional organization during cognitive development. *Current Opinion in Neurobiology, 15,* 239–244.

Casey, B. J., Trainor, R. J., Orendi, J. L., Schubert, A. B., Nystrom, L. E., Giedd, J. N., et al. (1997). A developmental functional MRI study of prefrontal activation during performance of a go-no-go task. *Journal of Cognitive Neuroscience, 9*(6), 835–847.

Cha, Y. M., White, A. M., Kuhn, C. M., Wilson, W. A., & Swartzwelder, H. S. (2006). Differential effects of delta(9)-THC on learning in adolescent and adult rats. *Pharmacology, Biochemistry and Behavior, 83*(3), 448–455.

Cohen-Zion, M., Drummond, S. P. A., Padula, C. B., Winward, J., Kanady, J., Medina, K. L., et al. (2009). Sleep architecture in adolescent marijuana and alcohol users during acute and extended abstinence. *Addictive Behaviors, 34*(11), 967–969.

De Bellis, M. D., Clark, D. B., Beers, S. R., Soloff, P. H., Boring, A. M., Hall, J., et al. (2000). Hippocampal volume in adolescent-onset alcohol use disorders. *American Journal of Psychiatry, 157*(5), 737–744.

De Bellis, M. D., Narasimhan, A., Thatcher, D. L., Keshavan, M. S., Soloff, P., & Clark, D. B. (2005). Prefrontal cortex, thalamus and cerebellar volumes in adolescents and young adults with adolescent onset alcohol use disorders and co-morbid mental disorders. *Alcoholism: Clinical and Experimental Research, 29*(9), 1590–1600.

DeLisi, L. E., Bertisch, H. C., Szulc, K. U., Majcher, M., Brown, K., Bappal, A., et al. (2006). A preliminary DTI study showing no brain structural change associated with adolescent cannabis use. *Harm Reduction Journal, 3,* 17.

Eaton, L. K., Kann, L., Kinchen, S., Ross, J., Hawkins, J., Harris, W. A., et al. (2006). Youth risk behavior surveillance United States, 2005. *Morbidity and Mortality Weekly Report, 55,* 1–108.

Ehrenreich, H., Rinn, T., Kunert, H. J., Moeller, M. R., Poser, W., Schilling, L., et al. (1999). Specific attentional dysfunction in adults following early start of marijuana use. *Psychopharmacology, 142*(3), 295–301.

Fried, P. A., Watkinson, B., & Gray, R. (2005). Neurocognitive consequences of marijuana: A comparison with pre-drug performance. *Neurotoxicology and Teratology, 27*(2), 231–239. Epub 2004 Dec 2009.

Galvan, A., Hare, T. A., Parra, C.E., Penn, J., Voss, H., Glover, G., & Casey, B. J. (2006). Earlier development of the accumbens relative to orbitofrontal cortex might underlie risk-taking behavior in adolescents. *Journal of Neuroscience, 26*(25), 6885–6892.

Gardener, M., & Steinberg, L. (2005). Peer influence on risk taking, risk preference, and risky decision making in adolescence and adulthood: An experimental study. *Developmental Psychology, 41,* 625–635.

Giancola, P. R., Mezzich, A. C., & Tarter, R. E. (1998). Disruptive, delinquent and aggressive behavior in female adolescents with a psychoactive substance use disorder: Relation to executive cognitive functioning. *Journal of Studies on Alcohol, 59*, 560–567.

Giedd, J. N., Blumenthal, J., Jeffries, N. O., Castellanos, F. X., Liu, H., Zijden-bos, A., et al. (1999). Brain development during childhood and adolescence: A longitudinal MRI study. *Nature Neuroscience, 2*, 861–863.

Giedd, J. N., Snell, J. W., Lange, N., Rajapakse, J. C., Casey, B. J., Kozuch, P. L., et al. (1996a). Quantitative magnetic resonance imaging of human brain development: Ages 4–18. *Cerebral Cortex, 6*(4), 551–560.

Giedd, J. N., Vaituzis, A. C., Hamburger, S. D., Lange, N., Rajapakse, J. C., Kaysen, D., et al. (1996b). Quantitative MRI of the temporal lobe, amygdala, and hippocampus in normal human development: Ages 4–18 years. *Journal of Comparative Neurology, 366*, 223–230.

Gogtay, N., Giedd, J. N., Lusk, L., Hayashi, K. M., Greenstein, D., Vaituzis, A. C., et al. (2004). Dynamic mapping of human cortical development during childhood through early adulthood. *Proceedings of the National Academy of Science, 101*(21), 8174–8179.

Hanson, K. L., Medina, K. L., Nagel, B. J., Spadoni, A. D., Gorlick, A., & Tapert, S. F. (2010). Hippocampal volumes in adolescents with and without a family history of alcoholism. *American Journal of Drug and Alcohol Abuse, 36*, 161–167.

Hanson, K. L., Medina, K. L., Padula, C. B., Tapert, S. F., & Brown, S. A. (2011). How does adolescent alcohol and drug use affect neuropsychological functioning in young adulthood?: 10-year outcomes. *Journal of Child and Adolescent Substance Abuse, 20*, 135–154.

Hanson, K. L., Winward, J. L., Schweinsburg, A. D., Medina, K. L., Brown, S. A., & Tapert, S. F. (2010). Longitudinal study of cognition among adolescent marijuana users over three weeks of abstinence. *Addictive Behaviors, 35*(11), 970–976.

Hartley, D. E., Elsabagh, S., & File, S. E. (2004). Binge drinking and sex: Effects on mood and cognitive function in healthy young volunteers. *Pharmacology, Biochemistry and Behavior, 78*(3), 611–619.

Harvey, M. A., Sellman, J. D., Porter, R. J., & Frampton, C. M. (2007). The relationship between non-acute adolescent marijuana use and cognition. *Drug and Alcohol Review, 26*(3), 309–319.

Hill, S. Y., Kostelnik, B., Holmes, B., Goradia, D., McDermott, M., Diwadkar, V., et al. (2007a). fMRI BOLD response to the eyes task in offspring from multiplex alcohol dependence families. *Alcoholism: Clinical and Experimental Research, 31*(12), 2028–2035.

Hill, S. Y., Muddasani, S., Prasad, K., Nutche, J., Steinhauer, S. R., Scanlon, J., et al. (2007b). Cerebellar volume in offspring from multiplex alcohol dependence families. *Biological Psychiatry, 61*(1), 41–47.

Jacobsen, L. K., Pugh, K. R., Constable, R. T., Westerveld, M., & Mencl, W. E. (2007). Functional correlates of verbal memory deficits emerging during nicotine withdrawal in abstinent adolescent marijuana users. *Biological Psychiatry, 61*(1), 31–40.

Jager, G., Block, R. I., Luijten, M., & Ramsey, N. F. (2010). Cannabis use and memory brain function in adolescent boys: A cross-sectional multicenter functional magnetic resonance imaging study. *Journal of the American Academy of Child and Adolescent Psychiatry, 49*(6), 561–572.

Jarvis, K., DelBello, M. P., Mills, N., Elman, I., Strakowski, S. M., & Adler, C. M. (2008). Neuroanatomic comparison of bipolar adolescents with and without cannabis use disorders. *Journal of Child and Adolescent Psychopharmacology, 18*(6), 557–563.

Jernigan, T., & Gamst, A. (2005). Changes in volume with age: Consistency and interpretation of observed effects. *Neurobiology of Aging, 26*(9), 1271–1274.

Johnston, L. D., O'Malley, P. M., Bachman, J. G., & Schulenberg, J. E. (2009). *Monitoring the Future national survey results on drug use, 1975–2008: Vol. II. College students and adults ages 19–50* (NIH Publication No. 09-7403). Bethesda, MD: National Institute on Drug Abuse.

Johnston, L. D., O'Malley, P. M., Bachman, J. G., & Schulenberg, J. E. (2010). *Monitoring the Future national results on adolescent drug use: Overview of key findings, 2009* (NIH Publication No. 10-7583). Bethesda, MD: National Institute on Drug Abuse.

Kloos, A., Weller, R. A., Chan, R., & Weller, E. B. (2009). Gender differences in adolescent substance abuse. *Current Psychiatry Reports, 11*(2), 120–126.

Larimer, M. E., & Cronce, J. M. (2007). Identification, prevention, and treatment revisited: Individual-focused college drinking prevention strategies 1999–2006. *Addictive Behaviors, 32*(11), 2439–2468.

Lenroot, R. K., & Giedd, J. N. (2006). Brain development in children and adolescents: Insights from anatomical magnetic resonance imaging. *Neuroscience and Biobehavioral Reviews, 30*, 718–729.

Lenroot, R. K., & Giedd, J. N. (2010). Sex differences in the adolescent brain. *Brain and Cognition, 72*(1), 46–55.

Lenroot, R. K., Gogtay, N., Greenstein, D. K., Wells, E. M., Wallace, G. L., Clasen, L. S., et al. (2007). Sexual dimorphism of brain developmental trajectories during childhood and adolescence. *Neuroimage, 36*(4), 1065–1073.

Liston, C., Watts, R., Tottenham, N., Davidson, M. C., Niogi, S., Ulug, A. M., et al. (2006). Frontostriatal microstructure modulates efficient recruitment of cognitive control. *Cerebral Cortex, 16*(4), 553–560.

Lynskey, M., & Hall, W. (2000). The effects of adolescent cannabis use on educational attainment: A review. *Addiction, 95*(11), 1621–1630.

Martin, C. S., Kaczynski, N. A., Maisto, S. A., & Tarter, R. E. (1996). Polydrug use in adolescent drinkers with and without DSM-IV alcohol abuse and dependence. *Alcoholism: Clinical and Experimental Research, 20*(6), 1099–1108.

McQueeny, T., Schweinsburg, B. C., Schweinsburg, A. D., Jacobus, J., Bava, S., Frank, L. R., et al. (2009). Altered white matter integrity in adolescent binge drinkers. *Alcoholism: Clinical and Experimental Research, 33*(7), 1278–1285.

Medina, K. L., Hanson, K., Schweinsburg, A. D., Cohen-Zion, M., Nagel, B. J., & Tapert, S. F. (2007a). Neuropsychological functioning in adolescent marijuana users: Subtle deficits detectable after 30 days of abstinence. *Journal of the International Neuropsychological Society, 13*(5), 807–820.

Medina, K. L., Price, J., Hawkins, M., Budion, B., & McQueeny, T. M. (2011). *Binge drinking predicts poor verbal memory in young adults.* Manuscript submitted for publication.

Medina, K. L., McQueeny, T., Nagel, B. J., Hanson, K., Schweinsburg, A. D., & Tapert, S. F. (2008). Prefrontal cortex volumes in adolescents with alcohol use disorders: Unique gender effects. *Alcoholism: Clinical and Experimental Research, 32,* 386–394.

Medina, K. L., McQueeny, T., Nagel, B. J., Hanson, K. L., Yang, T., & Tapert, S. F. (2009). Prefrontal morphometry in abstinent adolescent marijuana users: Subtle gender effects. *Addiction Biology, 14*(4), 457–468.

Medina, K. L., Nagel, B. J., McQueeny, T., Park, A., & Tapert, S. F. (2007b). Depressive symptoms in adolescents: Associations with white matter volume and marijuana use. *Journal of Child Psychology and Psychiatry, 48*(6), 592–600.

Medina, K. L., Nagel, B. J., & Tapert, S. F. (2010). Cerebellar vermis abnormality in adolescent marijuana users. *Psychiatry Research: Neuroimaging, 182*(2), 152–159.

Medina, K. L., Schweinsburg, A. D., Cohen-Zion, M., Nagel, B. J., & Tapert, S. F. (2007c). Effects of alcohol and combined marijuana and alcohol use during adolescence on hippocampal asymmetry. *Neurotoxicology and Teratology, 29,* 141–152.

Monk, C. S., McClure, E. B., Nelson, E. E., Zarahn, E., Bilder, R. M., Leibenluft, E., et al. (2003). Adolescent immaturity in attention-related brain engagement to emotional facial expressions. *Neuroimage, 20*(1), 420–428.

Monti, P. M., Miranda, R., Nixon, K., Sher, K. J., Swartzwelder, H. S., Tapert, S. F., et al. (2005). Adolescence: Booze, brains, and behavior. *Alcoholism: Clinical and Experimental Research, 29*(2), 207–220.

Moss, H. B., Kirisci, L., Gordon, H. W., & Tarter, R. E. (1994). A neuropsychologic profile of adolescent alcoholics. *Alcoholism: Clinical and Experimental Research, 18,* 159–163.

Nagel, B. J., Medina, K. L., Yoshii, J., Schweinsburg, A. D., Moadab, I., & Tapert, S. F. (2006). Age-related changes in prefrontal white matter volume across adolescence. *NeuroReport, 17*(13), 1427–1431.

Nagel, B. J., Schweinsburg, A. D., Phan, V., & Tapert, S. F. (2005). Reduced hippocampal volume among adolescents with alcohol use disorders without psychiatric comorbidity. *Psychiatry Research, 139*(3), 181–190.

Nigg, J. T., Glass, J. M., Wong, M. M., Poon, E., Jester, J. M., Fitzgerald, H. E., et al. (2004). Neuropsychological executive functioning in children at elevated risk for alcoholism: Findings in early adolescence. *Journal of Abnormal Psychology, 113*(2), 302–314.

Paus, T., Zijdenbos, A., Worsley, K., Collins, D. L., Blumenthal, J., Giedd, J. N., et al. (1999). Structural maturation of neural pathways in children and adolescents: *In vivo* study. *Science, 283*(5409), 1908–1911.

Read, J. P., Merrill, J. E, Kahler, C. W., & Strong, D. R. (2007). Predicting functional outcomes among college drinkers: Reliability and predictive validity of the Young Adult Alcohol Consequences Questionnaire. *Addictive Behaviors, 32*(11), 2597–2610.

Ridenour, T. A., Tarter, R. E., Reynolds, M., Mezzich, A., Kirisci, L., & Vanyukov, M. (2009). Neurobehavior disinhibition, parental substance use disorder, neighborhood quality and development of cannabis use disorder in boys. *Drug and Alcohol Dependence, 102*(1–3), 71–77.

Rubino, T., Realini, N., Braida, D., Guidi, S., Capurro, V., Viganò, D., et al. (2009). Changes in hippocampal morphology and neuroplasticity induced by adolescent THC treatment are associated with cognitive impairment in adulthood. *Hippocampus, 19*(8), 763–772.

Scaife, J. C., & Duka, T. (2009). Behavioural measures of frontal lobe function in a population of young social drinkers with binge drinking pattern. *Pharmacology, Biochemistry and Behavior, 93*(3), 354–362.

Schneider, M., & Koch, M. (2003). Chronic pubertal but not adult chronic cannabinoid treatment impairs sensorimotor gating, recognition memory and performance in a progressive ratio task in adult rats. *Neuropsychopharmacology, 28*, 1760–1790.

Schwartz, R. H., Gruenewald, P. J., Klitzner, M., & Fedio, P. (1989). Short-term memory impairment in cannabis-dependent adolescents. *American Journal of Diseases in Children, 143*(10), 1214–1219.

Schweinsburg, A. D., McQueeny, T., Nagel, B. J., Eyler, L. T., & Tapert, S. F. (2010). A preliminary study of functional magnetic resonance imaging response during verbal encoding among adolescent binge drinkers. *Alcohol, 44*(1), 111–117.

Schweinsburg, A. D., Nagel, B. J., Schweinsburg, B. C., Park, A., Theilmann, R. J., & Tapert, S. F. (2008). Abstinent adolescent marijuana users show altered fMRI response during spatial working memory. *Psychiatry Research, 163*(1), 40–51.

Schweinsburg, A. D., Paulus, M. P., Barlett, V. C., Killeen, L. A., Caldwell, L. C., Pulido, C., et al. (2004). An fMRI study of response inhibition in youths with a family history of alcoholism. *Annals of the New York Academy of Sciences, 1021*, 391–394.

Schweinsburg, A. D., Schweinsburg, B. C., Medina, K. L., McQueeny, T., Brown, S. A., & Tapert, S. F. (2010). The influence of recency of use on fMRI response during spatial working memory in adolescent marijuana users. *Journal of Psychoactive Drugs, 42*(3), 401–412.

Sher, K. J., Martin, E. D., Wood, P. K., & Rutledge, P. C. (1997). Alcohol use disorders and neuropsychological functioning in first-year undergraduates. *Experimental and Clinical Psychopharmacology, 5*(3), 304–315.

Sowell, E. R., Thompson, P. M., Holmes, C. J., Jernigan, T. L., & Toga, A. W. (1999). In vivo evidence for post adolescent brain maturation in frontal and striatal regions. *Nature Neuroscience, 2*(10), 859–861.

Sowell, E. R., Thompson, P., Leonard, C. M., Welcome, S. E., Kan, E., & Toga, A. W. (2004). Longitudinal mapping of cortical thickness and brain growth in normal children. *Journal of Neuroscience, 24*(38), 8223–8231.

Sowell, E. R., Trauner, D. A., Gamst, A., & Jernigan, T. L. (2002). Development of cortical and subcortical brain structures in childhood and adolescence: A structural MRI study. *Developmental Medicine and Child Neurology, 44*(1), 4–16.

Spadoni, A. D., Norman, A. L., Schweinsburg, A. D., & Tapert, S. F. (2008). Effects of family history of alcohol use disorders on spatial working memory BOLD response in adolescents. *Alcoholism: Clinical and Experimental Research, 32*(7), 1135–1145.

Spear, L. P. (2010). The behavioral neuroscience of adolescence. *Neuroscience and Biobehavioral Reviews, 24*, 417–463.

Tapert, S. F., Baratta, M. V., Abrantes, A. M., & Brown, S. A. (2002a). Attention dysfunction predicts substance involvement in community youths. *Journal of the American Academy of Child and Adolescent Psychiatry, 41*(6), 680–686.

Tapert, S. F., & Brown, S. A. (1999). Neuropsychological correlates of adolescent substance abuse: Four year outcomes. *Journal of the International Neuropsychological Society, 5*(6), 481–493

Tapert, S. F., & Brown, S. A. (2000). Substance dependence, family history of alcohol dependence, and neuropsychological functioning in adolescence. *Addiction, 95*, 1043–1053.

Tapert, S. F., Brown, G. G., Kindermann, S. S., Cheung, E. H., Frank, L. R., & Brown, S. A. (2001). fMRI measurement of brain dysfunction in alcohol-dependent young women. *Alcoholism: Clinical and Experimental Research, 25*(2), 236–245.

Tapert, S. F., Granholm, E., Leedy, N. G., & Brown, S. A. (2002b). Substance use and withdrawal: Neuropsychological functioning over 8 years in youth. *Journal of the International Neuropsychological Society, 8*(7), 873–883.

Tapert, S. F., Schweinsburg, A. D., Barlett, V. C., Brown, S. A., Frank, L. R., Brown, G. G., et al. (2004). Blood oxygen level dependent response and spatial working memory in adolescents with alcohol use disorders. *Alcoholism: Clinical and Experimental Research, 28*(10), 1577–1586.

Tapert, S. F., Schweinsburg, A. D., Drummond, S. P., Paulus, M. P., Brown, S. A., Yang, T. T., et al. (2007). Functional MRI of inhibitory processing in abstinent adolescent marijuana users. *Psychopharmacology (Berlin), 194*, 173–183.

Townshend, J. M., & Duka, T. (2005). Binge drinking, cognitive performance and mood in a population of young social drinkers. *Alcoholism: Clinical and Experimental Research, 29*(3), 317–325.

Wilson, W., Mathew, R., Turkington, T., Hawk, T., Coleman, R. E., & Provenzale, J. (2000). Brain morphological changes and early marijuana use: A magnetic resonance and positron emission tomography study. *Journal of Addictive Diseases, 19*(1), 1–22.

CHAPTER 4

Emotional Dysregulation in the Moment

Why Some College Students May Not Mature Out of Hazardous Alcohol and Drug Use

Marsha E. Bates *and* Jennifer F. Buckman

... and I came to favor Edna St. Vincent Millay whom I read in college always while drinking two beers to help me feel her extreme emotions.

—JIM HARRISON, *The English Major*

THE COLLEGE DRINKING PROBLEM: IMPLICATIONS OF HETEROGENEITY FOR INTERVENTION

Late adolescence is a developmental stage of peak alcohol use (Chen, Dufour, & Yi, 2004). College populations, in particular, show a high prevalence of binge drinking (Carter, Brandon, & Goldman, 2010). Curtailing high-risk substance use behaviors, and thus preventing the immediate negative consequences of harmful alcohol and drug use, has been the emphasis of college prevention and intervention programs (e.g., Larimer, Cronce, Lee, & Kilmer, 2004; White, 2006). Such work is of substantial importance as hazardous college-age drinking and drug use often lead to poor scholastic performance, high-risk sexual behaviors, driving while intoxicated, legal problems, alcohol poisoning, and other negative health consequences, all of which can have immediate as well as future implications.

In this chapter, we discuss the importance of examining sources of heterogeneity, beyond levels of substance use, to better identify students on hazardous alcohol use trajectories. We posit that individual differences in students' biological propensity to use alcohol and drugs to regulate emotion may be an important dimension of this heterogeneity. From this perspective, those who have relatively greater difficulty regulating emotional arousal may be at heightened risk for persistent substance use aimed at modifying their emotional experiences. We suggest that this increased risk likely existed before, and may well persist beyond the college years.

An important observation that comes from longitudinal studies examining alcohol use in college students is that the majority of college binge drinkers and drug users mature out of health-compromising substance use behaviors as they leave college and assume adult roles such as work and marriage (Bachman, Wadsworth, O'Malley, Johnston, & Schulenberg, 1997). A significant minority, however, do not follow this normative trend, but rather continue or escalate substance use behaviors. Students with more long-standing or complex risk profiles may need more or different intervention strategies beyond those aimed primarily at reducing the immediate negative consequences of use in college populations. An individual's psychological and physiological makeup, for example, may interact with potentially hazardous though relatively common substance use patterns such as weekend binge drinking to increase the risk of substance use difficulties. Basic alcohol-related research about mechanisms of emotional regulation may present novel opportunities for intervention.

The 2010 Duke University conference "College Student Drinking and Drug Use: Multiple Perspectives on a Complex Problem" provided a forum to foster new ideas about translating basic human experimental research into intervention development, and to identify knowledge gaps in current treatment approaches for college drinking and drug use. This chapter describes new findings from laboratory-based studies that examine real-time, moment-to-moment changes in integrated central (CNS) and autonomic (ANS) nervous system self-regulation. We characterize how heart rate variability (HRV), a physiological index of adaptable emotional regulation, is affected by acute alcohol intoxication and varies with motivations for substance use. The results emphasize heterogeneity in students' physiological modulation of emotional arousal and provide new insight into the subset of young adults who may be at risk for hazardous substance use due to ineffective emotional self-regulation. We conclude the chapter by discussing the possible intervention implications of these findings.

EMOTIONAL REGULATION AND SUBSTANCE USE

Emotional regulation is a primary function of alcohol and other drug use (Cox & Klinger, 1988; Pandina, Johnson, & Labouvie, 1992). The desire to enhance positive affect and reduce negative affect is an important motivation for substance use in both adolescents and adults (e.g., Wills, Sandy, Shinar, & Yaeger, 1999). The influence of alcohol on emotion is affected by learned outcome expectancies whose motivational components drive future drinking behaviors and consequences across the life span (e.g., Fromme & D'Amico, 2000; Stacy, Newcomb, & Bentler, 1991; Zucker & Fitzgerald, 1991; see also Reich & Goldman, Chapter 5, this volume). Outcome expectancies for other drugs (e.g., marijuana, stimulants) appear to function similarly (Giacomuzzi, 1998). For some individuals, such as those with high sensation-seeking tendencies, alcohol and other psychoactive drugs are used as conduits for enhancing positive emotional experience (Comeau, Stewart, & Loba, 2001). For other individuals, such as those with depression and anxiety, alcohol is used as a means to combat intrusive emotional states (Grant, Stewart, & Mohr, 2009).

The inability to effectively adapt to negative emotional challenges, in particular, is thought to be central to the development and persistence of alcohol and other drug use disorders (Baker, Piper, McCarthy, Majeskie, & Fiore, 2004). There has been considerable interest in impaired affective regulation in contributing to late-stage addiction (Koob, 2009; Koob & Le Moal, 1997), yet relatively little attention has been directed at understanding its role in creating vulnerability for the use of alcohol and other drugs to modulate emotions prior to the development of addiction. It is likely, however, that decreased regulatory flexibility in neurophysiological subsystems that modulate emotional arousal is a vulnerability process in the initiation and maintenance of unhealthy substance use behaviors at earlier developmental stages.

Problems associated with the inability to effectively modulate emotional arousal are present across the life span. Temperament researchers document individual differences in infants' reactivity to novel stimuli and whether they are easy or difficult to soothe (Field, 1981; Hernandez-Reif, Field, Diego, & Ruddock, 2006). These very early variations in arousal modulation predict later development of externalizing and internalizing problems (Pitzer, Esser, Schmidt, & Laucht, 2009). Dysregulation of physiological arousal correlates with, and predicts, social competence problems in childhood (El-Sheikh, 2001). Conversely, heightened ANS self-regulation can serve a protective function in moderating the negative effects of family stressors on children's adjustment, and on academic and health outcomes (El-Sheikh, 2001; Katz & Gottman, 1997).

Individuals who modulate emotional arousal less efficiently in response to internal and environmental changes will be further challenged during episodes of acute intoxication. There is strong, multilevel evidence that emotional self-regulation is diminished in the moment by acute alcohol intoxication, and that this impaired regulation persists across time with chronic, heavy alcohol use. For example, acute intoxication (e.g., Curtin & Lang, 2007; Gilman, Ramchandani, Davis, Bjork, & Hommer, 2008) and chronic alcohol use (e.g., Bates, Bowden, & Barry, 2002; Fitzpatrick, Jackson, & Crowe, 2008; Johnson-Greene, Adams, Gilman, & Junck, 2002) change brain functions that support emotional regulation and impair the cognitive control of emotional experience and behavior. Thus, individual differences in the efficiency of psychological and physiological systems that modulate emotional arousal may make some individuals more susceptible to the use of alcohol and other drugs to regulate emotions. And, in turn, alcohol use both immediately and chronically interferes with the individual's ability to self-regulate emotions at multiple physiological and cognitive levels.

HRV AS A BIOMARKER
OF EMOTIONAL SELF-REGULATION

At any given moment, decisions to use drugs and alcohol are influenced by interrelated *changes* in internal states (e.g., effortful and automatic cognitive processes, bodily sensations of arousal, moods) and the environment (e.g., visual, auditory, and olfactory cues; behavior of other persons). Thus, understanding how people change on short, "moment-to-moment" time scales may be pivotal to better understanding and intervening in substance use behaviors (Shiffman, Stone, & Hufford, 2008). In our research, we use a dynamic systems perspective to define self-regulation as a process by which individuals continuously modify their behavior in a systematic way by using information about changes in internal states and in the environment (Boker, 2001). This definition has three important tenets: (1) Self-regulation is a moving target because it continuously unfolds in real time; (2) the need for self-regulation is instigated by change; and (3) the source of change can be internal (e.g., cognitions, memories, a racing heart) or external (e.g., a person, sight of a drink, the smell of tobacco or marijuana) to the individual. We focus on the functional regulatory aspects of emotion within this dynamic systems perspective of self-regulation (Thayer & Lane, 2000). Our working definition of emotion is an organismic response to events that involves the interrelated actions of multiple systems and subsystems (e.g., neural, autonomic, behavioral) to facilitate the rapid mobilization for action and flexible adaptation to change (Hagemann, Waldstein, & Thayer, 2003).

Questionnaire methods are useful for probing emotional regulation styles and coping strategies of which the individual is aware. These instruments aggregate individuals' characteristic modes of cognitive and behavioral response to challenges over time. Other methods are needed to assess self-regulation mechanisms that may not be accessible to conscious awareness, and to provide information about moment-to-moment changes in emotional arousal and its modulation. ANS functions react to emotionally salient information received from the outside world, as well as to internal changes, and are capable of altering arousal states, attention allocation, and energy mobilization (Iversen, Kupfermann, & Kandel, 2000). *Variability* in ANS functions, such as heart rate, occur outside of conscious awareness, yet have a profound effect on behavior (Thayer & Lane, 2000). HRV, for example, is a neurophysiological function that responds flexibly and rapidly to emotional triggers and can be quantified precisely as changes in the system unfold. Importantly, HRV is not merely a "peripheral" event, but rather is a component of an integrated ANS–CNS system that controls emotional arousal (Benarroch, 1997; Goldstein, 2001). This chapter discusses how HRV is related to substance use and can add to our understanding of emotional self-regulation.

HRV, or changes in the time interval between heartbeats, is a powerful measure of adaptive neurophysiological regulation (Porges, 2007). In healthy people, the interval between heartbeats changes continuously, reacting to and modulating arousal in response to internal and external stimuli (Berntson et al., 1997). A large number of HRV indices[1] have been developed and validated as indicators of cardiovascular system efficiency that predict both physical and mental health (e.g., Appelhans & Luecken, 2006). Lower levels of resting-state HRV prospectively predict lower levels of physical health, psychological resiliency, and social competence in childhood (Katz & Gottman, 1997), increased vulnerability to stress (Giardino, Lehrer, & Feldman, 2000), somatic and emotional illness (Friedman & Thayer, 1998), and less active coping skills (Fabes & Eisenberg, 1997). Further, resting state HRV is decreased by acute and chronic stressors in healthy adults (Giardino et al., 2000), dampened during alcohol intoxication (e.g., Koskinen, Virolainen, & Kupari,

---

[1]A description of indices is outside the scope of this chapter; the reader is referred to (Task Force, 1996).

1994), and chronically depressed in persons with alcohol use disorders (e.g., Ingjaldsson, Laberg, & Thayer, 2003). These studies imply that a high resting-state level of HRV is a robust biomarker of physical and emotional well-being.

In addition to resting-state HRV, dynamic *changes* in HRV can also be examined in response to real-time environmental challenges (e.g., Gray, Rylander, Harrison, Wallin, & Critchley, 2009; Newlin, 1992; Reed, Porges, & Newlin, 1999) to capture moment-to-moment self-regulation of ANS arousal. Unlike background or resting-state HRV levels, increases in HRV in response to emotional or substance-related stimuli can provide information about whether individuals, in the moment, are over- or underreactive to challenges from their internal or external environment. Here we describe the results of initial studies that examined *changes in* HRV when college students were exposed to emotional and substance-related picture cues, how acute alcohol intoxication affected these changes, and differences between subtypes of college drinkers in how they responded to emotional and alcohol- and drug-related picture cues. These studies address how students' HRV changes in response to emotional perturbations, and thus may be informative about their use of alcohol to alter emotion in the moment.

Alcohol Effects and Changes in HRV to Provocative Picture Cues

Below are selected highlights from several studies (Vaschillo et al., 2008; Mun, von Eye, Bates, & Vaschillo, 2008; Udo et al., 2009) that included data from 20 male and 16 female college students (mean age = 21.8) who were healthy, moderate to heavy (nondependent) drinkers without psychiatric diagnosis. Regular users of other drugs were excluded. Each student was randomly assigned to an alcohol, placebo, or control beverage group ($n = 12$ per group). The target blood alcohol concentration (BAC) in the alcohol group was 90 mg/dl, a typical BAC of college students following an evening of drinking (Kraus et al., 2005). The alcohol and placebo groups were told they would receive some amount of alcohol; the control group was told they were not receiving alcohol. Sensors were attached to collect electrocardiogram (ECG) and other physiological data. Participants first completed an initial low-demand baseline task (B1). They next consumed a beverage selected based on their group assignment and completed the same baseline task again (B2). Participants then viewed blocks of sequentially presented picture cues that were emotionally negative, emotionally positive, emotionally neutral, alcohol related, marijuana related or polydrug related. The presentation order of blocks, and pictures within blocks, was randomized. Cues were from the International

Affective Picture System (Lang, Bradley, & Cuthbert, 2001), the Normative Appetitive Picture System (Stritzke, Breiner, Curtin, & Lang, 2004), Tapert et al. (2003), and our lab. Participants self-reported standardized liking and arousal ratings for each picture (Lang et al., 2001).

Because prior research focused mainly on resting-state HRV, we developed a methodology to evaluate HRV changes in response to emotional stimulation and compared its ability to detect changes in emotional regulation to other traditional HRV indices (Vaschillo et al., 2008). Emotionally salient and alcohol-related picture cues were presented to participants at the rate of one cue per 10 seconds (i.e., a 0.1-Hz presentation frequency), and the power (amplitude) of the HRV spectral density function at 0.1 Hz was measured. The 0.1-Hz frequency is a resonance frequency of the cardiovascular system (Angelone & Coulter, 1964). Stimulation and response at this frequency provide an evaluation of moment-to-moment ANS reaction to external stimulation (Nickel & Nachreiner, 2003), as well as insight into the baroreflex mechanism that controls how the time interval between heartbeats varies in response to perturbation (Cevese, Gulli, Polati, Gottin, & Grasso, 2001), and how the level of arousal is modulated. We found that increases in several HRV indices during cue exposure were dampened by alcohol to varying extents, but only pNN50, an HRV index of large beat-to-beat changes in heart period that may reflect the compensatory neural processes that are engaged following activation (Ewing, Neilson, & Travis, 1984), and the 0.1-Hz index showed differentiated response to emotionally arousing cues compared to emotionally neutral cues (Vaschillo et al., 2008). Moreover, the 0.1-Hz HRV index was most sensitive to changes in response to negative picture cues and uniquely sensitive to expectancy effects of alcohol (placebo condition) compared to all other HRV indices.

Figure 4.1 shows the total HRV spectrum in response to the negative emotional picture cues averaged across participants in the control (top panel), placebo (middle panel), and alcohol (bottom panel) beverage groups. The high-amplitude 0.1-Hz peak induced by the negative picture cues observed in the control condition was substantially dampened in both the alcohol and placebo beverage groups. A similar pattern of reactivity can be seen in response to alcohol-related cues (Figure 4.2). When assessed separately by gender, both genders showed similar placebo responses, but men showed greater alcohol-induced dampening of the 0.1-Hz HRV peak than women (Udo et al., 2009). In summary, acute alcohol intoxication substantially reduced HRV response to both emotional and substance-related picture cues, particularly in men, thereby reducing the cardiovascular system's ability to respond to, and modulate, arousal in response to emotional and substance-related cues. HRV response was also susceptible to the placebo condition, demonstrating the

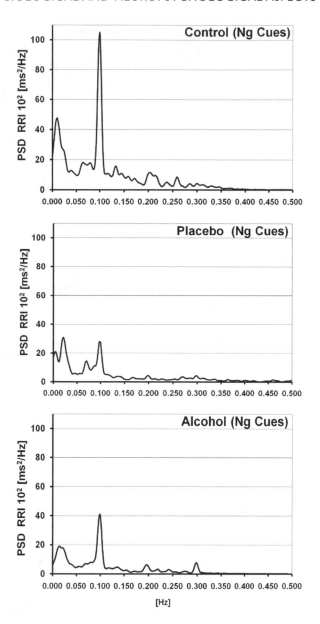

FIGURE 4.1. Average HRV spectra of the control (upper panel), placebo (middle panel), and alcohol (bottom panel) beverage groups in response to negative emotional (Ng) picture cues. PSD, power spectral density (power of the signal at each frequency); RRI, interval between normal heartbeats; Hz, Hertz (a unit of frequency).

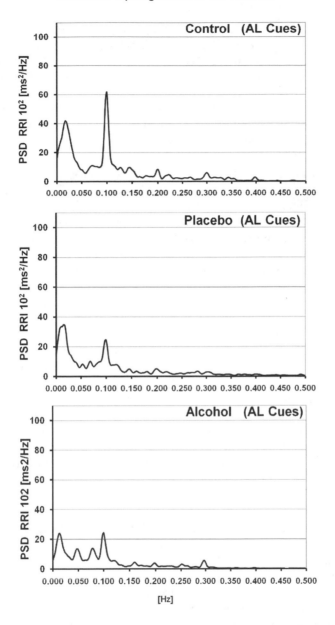

FIGURE 4.2. Average HRV spectra of the control (upper panel), placebo (middle panel), and alcohol (bottom panel) beverage groups in response to alcohol-related (AL) picture cues. PSD, power spectral density (power of the signal at each frequency); RRI, interval between normal heartbeats; Hz, Hertz (a unit of frequency).

comprehensive integration of behavioral, cognitive, and neurobiological systems that motivate behavior. Thus, a physiological cascade of events that influence emotional self-regulation ensues from alcohol drinking as well as the expectancy of drinking alcohol in experienced student drinkers.

In order to explore the existence of subtypes of college drinkers who display different constellations of drinking behavior, drinking motivations, and physiological profiles, we used model-based cluster analysis (Mun et al., 2008) to group participants by *baseline* (resting) levels of HR and 0.1-Hz HRV, typical alcohol use, and reasons for drinking (Labouvie & Bates, 2002). We identified a "High Alcohol Risk" cluster that had significantly higher alcohol use and more frequently identified disinhibition and emotional suppression as reasons for drinking than a second "Normative" cluster. The two clusters were then examined for differences in 0.1-Hz HRV *reactivity* to emotional, alcohol-related, and drug-related picture cues. The High Alcohol Risk group demonstrated significant and large effect size changes in 0.1-Hz HRV indices in response to all emotional and appetitive cues compared to response to neutral cues (Figure 4.3). The Normative group showed a significant change in HRV only in response to negative emotional cues.

The distinctively high patterns of arousal in response to emotional and substance-related cues in the High Alcohol Risk group emphasize the difference between high resting HRV levels (which, as previously noted, are associated with better physical and emotional health) and high levels of real-time changes in HRV in response to environmental cues, which may reflect the heightened salience of the cues and/or increased need for modulatory actions of the baroreflex to return arousal levels to baseline. In addition, the former group also reported using alcohol to suppress emotions and disinhibit behaviors more than the Normative group, perhaps suggesting that drinking had become an important tool for self-regulation in the High Alcohol Risk group. Finally, the observation that the High Alcohol Risk group showed high reactivity to drug cues, even though they were not currently regular users of drugs, may suggest the potential value of 0.1-Hz HRV reactivity as an indicator of risk for escalation in drug use.

We next examined heterogeneity in physiological and self-reported measures of arousal among 43 students (51% female) who 2 years earlier had been mandated to a brief intervention for violating university policies about on-campus substance use (Buckman, White, & Bates, 2010). We compared students who were involved in relatively minor alcohol-related violations (e.g., being present in a dormitory room where drinking was taking place, $n = 30$) to those who experienced more serious consequences such as emergency medical service ($n = 13$). Physiological data were col-

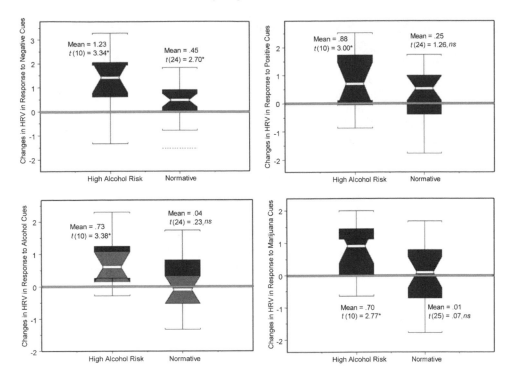

FIGURE 4.3. Box plots of within-individual changes in 0.1-Hz HRV indices in response to emotional and appetitive picture cues compared to response to neutral cues. Data from Mun, von Eye, Bates, and Vaschillo (2008). Copyright 2008 by the American Psychological Association.

lected, but there was no beverage administration. We found a consistent pattern of higher 0.1-Hz HRV *reactivity* and lower self-reported ratings of the arousal value of stimulus cues across all picture cue types (Figure 4.4) in the minor infraction group compared to the serious infraction group. The minor infraction group also reported significant increases in quantity and frequency of alcohol consumption from the baseline assessment (around the time of the infraction and mandated intervention) to 2 years later, whereas the serious infraction group did not. Thus, the group that showed an escalating pattern of alcohol use also showed a greater dissociation between physiological reactivity (which operates largely outside of conscious awareness) and subjectively reported ratings of arousal, compared to the serious infraction group. Taken at face value, it would seem that students with more serious and life-threatening alcohol use infractions would be at greater risk for future problematic alcohol use; however, the data suggest that the students who experienced less serious consequences from alcohol use were, in fact, at greater risk based on increased alcohol consumption and poorer emotional self-regulation. Future studies are needed to clarify the significance of this finding.

Taken together, these data demonstrate that dynamic changes in HRV that occur in response to provocative visual cues can serve as a method for evaluating how college students react to and modulate their arousal when confronted with environmental triggers that affect them emotionally or engage them in alcohol and drug use behaviors. A future goal is to determine the value of HRV in predicting and treating those students who are at high risk for persistent substance use problems due to emotional regulatory difficulties.

SUMMARY AND APPLICATIONS TO PREVENTION AND INTERVENTION IN COLLEGE SUBSTANCE USE

The English major (see opening quotation) drank beer in college while reading poetry so that he could feel the extreme emotions of the author. The findings reviewed in this chapter show that alcohol in fact dampens emotional arousal and its regulation in response to positive as well as negative emotional cues through its actions on the baroreflex. This highlights the potential incongruity between subjective beliefs about alcohol effects on emotional experience and physiological indices of emotional responding during episodes of acute alcohol intoxication.

Emotional experience, of course, comes about through the integrated functioning of many different cognitive and physiological systems. Given that alcohol simultaneously acts on all these systems, it is likely that the complex subjective experiences of alcohol intoxication and emotions reported by an individual are the output of many interrelated dynamic systems, which include but are not limited to the cardiovascular system. This reinforces the need to consider the individual as a complex adaptive system that, at any given moment, assimilates multiple sources of internal and external information to guide emotional responding. The findings presented here suggest that assessing HRV reactivity is valuable for identifying a basic source of heterogeneity among college students who may be on differing trajectories of substance use as they mature past the college years. That is, students with high alcohol use and either reduced resting HRV or heightened 0.1-Hz HRV index response to provocative cues may be at greater risk because they are physiologically less able to adapt to emotional challenges. Future studies should also assess other physiological systems to capture additional sources of heterogeneity.

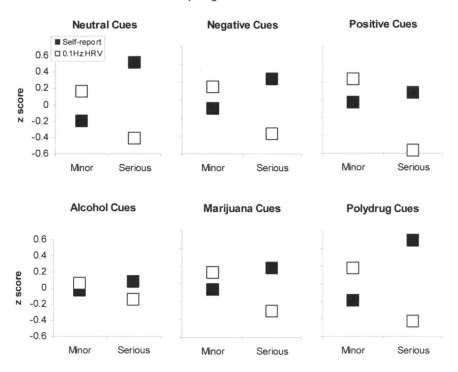

FIGURE 4.4. Self-reported versus physiologically measured arousal. Z-score transformed arousal ratings and 0.1-Hz HRV in response to emotional-, alcohol-, or drug-related picture cues in students mandated to a university substance use intervention program following a minor or serious incident.

Prior studies have shown that alcohol suppresses multiple indicators of ANS response to a variety of stressors and negative emotional stimuli (e.g., Greeley & Oei, 1999). Our assessment of HRV reactivity to emotional picture cues during an acute alcohol challenge showed that alcohol generally dampened increases in HRV response to all cue types, regardless of emotional valence. Thus, our results not only support "stress-response dampening" (Levenson, Sher, Grossman, Newman, & Newlin, 1980), but further suggest that alcohol intoxication diminishes the extent to which the baroreflex can react to all environmental perturbations, regardless of emotional content. This suggests that the route through which alcohol enhances the perception of increased positive emotion is not through a "tuning up" of the ANS arousal modulation system, as would be suggested by self-reported emotional experiences such as that of the English major.

Clinical Implications

These preliminary findings suggest that an individual's capacity to change neurophysiologically in response to challenges in their environment may be potentially valuable biomarkers of risk for persistent, harmful substance use behaviors. Further understanding of the heterogeneity in physiological reactions to environmental challenges may add to the ability to identify different subgroups of college students who may persist or escalate in maladaptive substance use behaviors beyond the college years. For example, one subtype was defined in our studies by heavy alcohol use and the use of alcohol to suppress negative emotions and become disinhibited. This subgroup showed heightened reactivity (and/or less modulation of reactivity) to emotional and substance-related stimulus cues relative to other student drinkers.

A final consideration is how interventions can address emotional regulatory difficulties in college drinkers. Existing cognitive-behavioral interventions for substance use rely on information processing that is, for the most part, voluntary, explicit, controlled, and "non-automatic." Within this context, a student who drinks heavily to modify emotional experience might be taught cognitive reappraisal strategies (i.e., to change how a situation is construed in order to decrease its emotional impact, Gross, 2002). Because cognitive emotional systems work together with neurophysiological systems to modulate arousal, multilevel intervention targeting both the voluntary (e.g., cognitive emotional) and involuntary (e.g., baroreflex) mechanisms that control emotion and arousal could be useful with students who drink heavily, and whose reasons for drinking are strongly linked to emotional suppression and behavioral disinhibition.

There is empirical support for behavioral interventions that remediate ANS dysfunction in arousal modulation. Resonance frequency breathing biofeedback (also known as HRV biofeedback), for example, increases modulation of arousal in normal as well as clinical samples. It increases baroreflex sensitivity, improves physical symptoms, reduces medication use, and decreases psychological distress in a variety of clinical samples (e.g., Karavidas et al., 2007; Lehrer & Vaschillo, 2004; Lehrer et al., 2003). This behavioral biofeedback technique, which is easily learned in the clinical setting, would be well suited to bolstering emotional resilience in persons who use psychoactive substances to modulate emotional experience. Thus far, however, HRV biofeedback has not been examined in populations engaging in hazardous alcohol or drug use. This is an important aim for future studies.

In conclusion, this chapter reviewed recent findings from laboratory-based studies that examined real-time, moment-to-moment changes in integrated CNS and ANS functioning. Although, in general, past substance use behavior is the best predictor of future behavior, and thus is an essential intervention target, this information alone has been insufficient to differentiate those who will mature out of high-risk substance use behaviors following college from those who will not. Our research program emphasizes the value of considering college-age substance users as a culmination of their internal milieu, their external environment, and the voluntary and involuntary mechanisms that act together to orient their attention, regulate their emotional responses, and guide their decision-making behavior. Further effort should be directed at developing methods that could allow treatment providers to assess physiological indicators of emotional self-regulation, in addition to considering prior substance use behavior. Vulnerable students might then be taught new biobehavioral techniques for handling the multitude of triggers, stressors, and difficulties that they encounter during and following the college years.

ACKNOWLEDGMENTS

This study was supported in part by grants and contracts from the National Institute on Alcohol Abuse on Alcoholism (Nos. R01 AA015248, K02 AA00325, K01AA017473 and HHSN275201000003C) and the National Institute on Drug Abuse (Nos. P20 DA017552 and 3P20 DA017552-05S1).

REFERENCES

Angelone, A., & Coulter, N. A., Jr. (1964). Respiratory sinus arrhythmia: A frequency dependent phenomenon. *Journal of Applied Physiology, 19*, 479–482.

Appelhans, B. M., & Luecken, L. J. (2006). Heart rate variability as an index of regulated emotional responding. *Review of General Psychology, 10*(3), 229–240.

Bachman, J. G., Wadsworth, K. N., O'Malley, P. M., Johnston, L. D., & Schulenberg, J. E. (1997). *Smoking, drinking, and drug use in young adulthood: The impacts of new freedoms and new responsibilities*. Mahwah, NJ: Erlbaum.

Baker, T. B., Piper, M. E., McCarthy, D. E., Majeskie, M. R., & Fiore, M. C. (2004). Addiction motivation reformulated: An affective processing model of negative reinforcement. *Psychological Review, 111*(1), 33–51.

Bates, M. E., Bowden, S. C., & Barry, D. (2002). Neurocognitive impairment associated with alcohol use disorders: Implications for treatment. *Experimental and Clinical Psychopharmacology, 10*(3), 193–212.

Benarroch, E. E. (1997). The central autonomic network. In P. A. Low (Ed.), *Clinical autonomic disorders* (2nd ed., pp. 17–23). Philadelphia: Lippincott-Raven.

Berntson, G. G., Bigger, J. T., Jr., Eckberg, D. L., Grossman, P., Kaufmann, P. G., Malik, M., et al. (1997). Heart rate variability: Origins, methods, and interpretive caveats. *Psychophysiology, 34*(6), 623–648.

Boker, S. M. (2001). Differential structural equation modeling of intraindividual variability. In L. M. Collins & A. G. Sayer (Eds.), *New methods for the analysis of behavior change* (pp. 5–27). Washington, DC: American Psychological Association.

Buckman, J. F., White, H. R., & Bates, M. E. (2010). Psychophysiological reactivity to emotional picture cues two years after college students were mandated for alcohol interventions. *Addictive Behaviors, 35*(8), 786–790.

Carter, A. C., Brandon, K. O., & Goldman, M. S. (2010). The college and noncollege experience: A review of the factors that influence drinking behavior in young adulthood. *Journal of Studies on Alcohol and Drugs, 71*, 742–750.

Cevese, A., Gulli, G., Polati, E., Gottin, L., & Grasso, R. (2001). Baroreflex and oscillation of heart period at 0.1 Hz studied by alpha-blockade and cross-spectral analysis in healthy humans. *Journal of Physiology, 531*, 235–244.

Chen, C. M., Dufour, M. C., & Yi, H. (2004). Alcohol consumption among young adults ages 18–24 in the United States: Results from the 2001–2002 NESARC survey. *Alcohol Research and Health, 28*, 94–10.

Comeau, N., Stewart, S. H., & Loba, P. (2001). The relations of trait anxiety, anxiety sensitivity, and sensation seeking to adolescents' motivations for alcohol, cigarette, and marijuana use. *Addictive Behaviors, 26*(6), 803–825.

Cox, W. M., & Klinger, E. (1988). A motivational model of alcohol use. *Journal of Abnormal Psychology, 97*(2), 168–180.

Curtin, J. J., & Lang, A. R. (2007). Alcohol and emotion: Insights and directives from affective science. In J. Rottenberg & S. Johnson (Eds.), *Emotion and psychopathology: Bridging affective and clinical science* (pp. 191–213). Washington, DC: American Psychological Association.

El-Sheikh, M. (2001). Parental drinking problems and children's adjustment: Vagal regulation and emotional reactivity as pathways and moderators of risk. *Journal of Abnormal Psychology, 110*, 499–515.

Ewing, D. J., Neilson, J. M. M., & Travis, P. (1984). New method for assessing cardiac parasympathetic activity using 24 hour electrocardiograms. *British Heart Journal, 52*, 396–402.

Fabes, R. A., & Eisenberg, N. (1997). Regulatory control and adults' stress-related responses to daily life events. *Journal of Personality and Social Psychology, 73*(5), 1107–1117.

Field, T. (1981). Infant arousal attention and affect during early interactions. *Advances in Infancy Research, 1*, 57–100.

Fitzpatrick, L. E., Jackson, M., & Crowe, S. F. (2008). The relationship between alcoholic cerebellar degeneration and cognitive and emotional functioning. *Neuroscience and Biobehavioral Review, 32*(3), 466–485.

Friedman, B. H., & Thayer, J. F. (1998). Autonomic balance revisited: Panic anxiety and heart rate variability. *Journal of Psychosomatic Research, 44*(1), 133–151.

Fromme, K., & D'Amico, E. J. (2000). Measuring adolescent alcohol outcome expectancies. *Psychology of Addictive Behaviors, 14*(2), 206–212.

Giacomuzzi, M. P. (1998). Early recollections of chemically dependent clients: Implications for relapse prevention treatment. *Dissertation Abstracts International, 58*(11-B), 6234. UMI No. AAM 9816320.

Giardino, N., Lehrer, P. M., & Feldman, J. (2000). The role of oscillations in self-regulation: Their contribution to homeostasis. In D. Kenney & F. J. McGuigan (Eds.), *Stress and health: Research and clinical applications* (pp. 27–52). London: Harwood.

Gilman, J. M., Ramchandani, V. A., Davis, M. B., Bjork, J. M., & Hommer, D. W. (2008). Why we like to drink: A functional magnetic resonance imaging study of the rewarding and anxiolytic effects of alcohol. *Journal of Neuroscience, 28*(18), 4583–4591.

Goldstein, D. S. (2001). *The autonomic nervous system in health and disease.* New York: Marcel Dekker.

Grant, V. V., Stewart, S. H., & Mohr, C. D. (2009). Coping-anxiety and coping-depression motives predict different daily mood-drinking relationships. *Psychology of Addictive Behavior, 23*(2), 226–237.

Gray, M. A., Rylander, K., Harrison, N. A., Wallin, B. G., & Critchley, H. D. (2009). Following one's heart: Cardiac rhythms gate central initiation of sympathetic reflexes. *Journal of Neuroscience, 29,* 1817–1825.

Greeley, J., & Oei, T. (1999). Alcohol and tension reduction. In K. E. Leonard & H. T. Howard (Eds.), *Psychological theories of drinking and alcoholism* (2nd ed., pp. 14–53). New York: Guilford Press.

Gross, J. J. (2002). Emotion regulation: Affective, cognitive, and social consequences. *Psychophysiology, 39*(3), 281–291.

Hagemann, D., Waldstein, S. R., & Thayer, J. F. (2003). Central and autonomic nervous system integration in emotion. *Brain and Cognition, 52*(1), 79–87.

Hernandez-Reif, M., Field, T., Diego, M., & Ruddock, M. (2006). Greater arousal and less attentiveness to face/voice stimuli by neonates of depressed mothers on the Brazelton Neonatal Behavioral Assessment Scale. *Infant Behavior and Development, 29*(4), 594–598.

Ingjaldsson, J. T., Laberg, J. C., & Thayer, J. F. (2003). Reduced heart rate variability in chronic alcohol abuse: Relationship with negative mood, chronic thought suppression, and compulsive drinking. *Biological Psychiatry, 54*(12), 1427–1436.

Iversen, S., Kupfermann, I., & Kandel, E. R. (2000). Emotional states and feelings. In E. R. Kandel, J. H. Schwartz, & T. M. Jessell (Eds.), *Principles of neural science* (4th ed., pp. 982–996). New York: McGraw-Hill.

Johnson-Greene, D., Adams, K. M., Gilman, S., & Junck, L. (2002). Relationship between neuropsychological and emotional functioning in severe chronic alcoholism. *Clinical Neuropsychologist, 16*(3), 300–309.

Karavidas, M. K., Lehrer, P. M., Vaschillo, E., Vaschillo, B., Marin, H., Buyske, S., et al. (2007). Preliminary results of an open label study of heart rate variability biofeedback for the treatment of major depression. *Applied Psychophysiology and Biofeedback, 32*(1), 19–30.

Katz, L. F., & Gottman, J. M. (1997). Buffering children from marital conflict and dissolution. *Journal of Clinical Child Psychology, 26*(2), 157–171.

Koob, G. F. (2009). Dynamics of neuronal circuits in addiction: Reward, anti-reward, and emotional memory. *Pharmacopsychiatry, 42*(Suppl. 1), S32–S41.

Koob, G. F., & Le Moal, M. (1997). Drug abuse: Hedonic homeostatic dysregulation. *Science, 278*(5335), 52–58.

Koskinen, P., Virolainen, J., & Kupari, M. (1994). Acute alcohol intake decreases short-term heart rate variability in healthy subjects. *Clinical Science, 87,* 225–230.

Kraus, C. L., Salazar, N. C., Mitchell, J. R., Florin, W. D., Guenther, B., Brady, D., et al. (2005). Inconsistencies between actual and estimated blood alcohol concentrations in a field study of college students: Do students really know how much they're drinking? *Alcoholism: Clinical and Experimental Research, 29,* 1672–1676.

Labouvie, E., & Bates, M. E. (2002). Reasons for alcohol use in young adulthood: Validation of a three-dimensional measure. *Journal of Studies on Alcohol, 63*(2), 145–155.

Lang, P. J., Bradley, M. M., & Cuthbert, B. N. (2001). *International Affective Picture System (IAPS): Instruction manual and affective ratings* (Tech. Rep. No. A-5). Gainesville: University of Florida, Center for Research in Psychophysiology.

Larimer, M. E., Cronce, J. M., Lee, C. M., & Kilmer, J. R. (2004). Brief intervention in college settings. *Alcohol Research and Health, 28,* 94–104.

Lehrer, P., & Vaschillo, E. (2004). Heart rate variability biofeedback: A new tool for improving autonomic homeostasis and treating emotional and psychosomatic diseases. *Japanese Journal of Biofeedback, 30,* 7–16.

Lehrer, P. M., Vaschillo, E., Vaschillo, B., Lu, S.-E., Eckberg, D. L., Edelberg, R., et al. (2003). Heart rate variability biofeedback increases baroreflex gain and peak expiratory flow. *Psychosomatic Medicine, 65,* 796–805.

Levenson, R. W., Sher, K. J., Grossman, L. M., Newman, J., & Newlin, D. B. (1980). Alcohol and stress response dampening: Pharmacological effects, expectancy, and tension reduction. *Journal of Abnormal Psychology, 89*(4), 528–538.

Mun, E. Y., von Eye, A., Bates, M. E., & Vaschillo, E. G. (2008). Finding groups using model-based cluster analysis: Heterogeneous emotional self-regulatory processes and heavy alcohol use risk. *Developmental Psychology, 44*(2), 481–495.

Newlin, D. B. (1992). A comparison of conditioning and craving for alcohol and cocaine. In M. Galanter (Ed.), *Recent developments in alcoholism: Vol. 10. Alcohol and cocaine: Similarities and differences* (pp. 147–164). New York: Plenum Press.

Nickel, P., & Nachreiner, F. (2003). Sensitivity and diagnosticity of the 0.1–Hz component of heart rate variability as an indicator of mental workload. *Human Factors, 45*(4), 575–590.

Pandina, R. J., Johnson, V., & Labouvie, E. W. (1992). Affectivity: A central mechanism in the development of drug dependence. In M. Glantz & R. Pickens (Eds.), *Vulnerability to drug abuse* (pp. 179–209). Washington, DC: American Psychological Association.

Pitzer, M., Esser, G., Schmidt, M. H., & Laucht, M. (2009). Temperamental predictors of externalizing problems among boys and girls: A longitudinal study in a high-risk sample from ages 3 months to 15 years. *European Archives of Psychiatry and Clinical Neuroscience, 259*(8), 445–458.

Porges, S. W. (2007). The polyvagal perspective. *Biological Psychology, 74*(2), 116–143.

Reed, S. F., Porges, S. W., & Newlin, D. B. (1999). Effect of alcohol on vagal regulation of cardiovascular function: Contributions of the polyvagal theory to the psychophysiology of alcohol. *Experimental and Clinical Psychopharmacology, 7*(4), 484–492.

Shiffman, S., Stone, A. A., & Hufford, M. R. (2008). Ecological momentary assessment. *Annual Review of Clinical Psychology, 4*, 1–32.

Stacy, A. W., Newcomb, M. D., & Bentler, P. M. (1991). Cognitive motivation and drug use: A 9-year longitudinal study. *Journal of Abnormal Psychology, 100*(4), 502–515.

Stritzke, W. G., Breiner, M. J., Curtin, J. J., & Lang, A. R. (2004). Assessment of substance cue reactivity: Advances in reliability, specificity, and validity. *Psychology of Addictive Behaviors, 18*, 148–159.

Tapert, S. F., Cheung, E. H., Brown, G. G., Frank, L. R., Paulus, M. P., Schweinsburg, A. D., et al. (2003). Neural responses to alcohol stimuli in adolescents with alcohol use disorder. *Archives of General Psychiatry, 60*, 727–735.

Task Force of the European Society of Cardiology and the American Society of Pacing and Electrophysiology. (1996). Heart rate variability: Standards of measurement, physiological interpretation, and clinical use. *Circulation, 93*, 1043–1065.

Thayer, J. F., & Lane, R. D. (2000). A model of neurovisceral integration in emotion regulation and dysregulation. *Journal of Affective Disorders, 61*(3), 201–216.

Udo, T., Bates, M. F., Mun, E. Y., Vaschillo, E. G., Vaschillo, B., Lehrer, P., et al. (2009). Gender differences in acute alcohol effects on self-regulation of arousal in response to emotional and alcohol-related picture cues. *Psychology of Addictive Behaviors, 23*, 196–204.

Vaschillo, E. G., Bates, M. E., Vaschillo, B., Lehrer, P., Udo, T., Mun, E. Y., et al. (2008). Heart rate variability response to alcohol, placebo, and emotional picture cue challenges: Effects of 0.1–Hz stimulation. *Psychophysiology, 45*, 847–858.

White, H. R. (2006). Reduction of alcohol-related harm on United States college campuses: The use of personal feedback interventions. *International Journal of Drug Policy, 17*, 310–319.

Wills, T. A., Sandy, J. M., Shinar, O., & Yaeger, A. (1999). Contributions of positive and negative affect to adolescent substance use: Test of a bidimensional model in a longitudinal study. *Psychology of Addictive Behaviors, 13*(4), 327–338.

Zucker, R. A., & Fitzgerald, H. E. (1991). Early developmental factors and risk for alcohol problems. *Alcohol Health and Research World, 15*(1), 18–24.

PART III

PSYCHOLOGICAL AND SOCIAL ASPECTS OF SUBSTANCE USE

CHAPTER 5

Drinking in College Students and Their Age Peers

The Role of Anticipatory Processes

Richard R. Reich *and* Mark S. Goldman

Because time always moves forward, behavioral processes are anticipatory in nature; that is, they produce behaviors geared toward accommodating events that have yet to occur (Goldman, 2002; Goldman, Darkes, Reich, & Brandon, 2010; Goldman, Reich, & Darkes, 2006). Anticipation clearly plays an influential role in human behavior, and work in a multitude of psychological areas has converged on this perspective (Goldman et al., 2006). Two recent reviews broadly illustrate this point: First, as a result of a vast amount of neuroscientific research, Holland and Gallagher (2004) described a shift in the conventional viewpoint on the function of human cognition: "The utility of learning and memory lies not in reminiscence about the past, but in allowing us to act in anticipation of future events" (p. 148). Second, and even more applicable to the material in this book, in summarizing the many theories on decision making with regard to addiction, Redish, Jensen, and Johnson (2008) identified a single common thread: "These literatures have converged on the concept that decisions are based on the *prediction* of value or expected utility of the decision" (p. 147). The purpose of this chapter is to show that developmental processes that occur in both college students and their same-age peers lead these young people to anticipate social and sexual benefits from using alcohol. These expectations may then consciously and unconsciously influence the decision to drink in this age group.

COLLEGE DRINKING
AS A DEVELOPMENTAL PROCESS

The recognition that college students consume considerable amounts of alcohol is so long-standing that it has become a truism in American culture. In the 1990s, however, a series of prominent newspaper reports of deaths due to excessive drinking among otherwise successful college students led the National Institute on Alcohol Abuse and Alcoholism (NIAAA) to create the Task Force on College Drinking in 1998. The report from this task force, issued in 2002 (Goldman, Boyd, & Faden, 2002), documented the excessive drinking seen in many college students, and the many deaths, injuries, and physical and sexual assaults that were associated with this drinking (an updated compilation of these statistics can be found in Hingson, Zha, & Weitzman, 2009).

In the context of the NIAAA completing its report on college student drinking, it was noted by the task force that many college students did not begin their drinking when they arrived at college but actually had extensive drinking histories prior to college entry. These observations, in conjunction with other reports and data sets, including various epidemiological findings, such as the National Research Council and Institute of Medicine's report on underage drinking) (Bonnie & O'Connell, 2004), led the NIAAA to generate a further initiative on underage drinking. The findings from this initiative informed *The Surgeon General's Call to Action to Prevent and Reduce Underage Drinking* (U.S. Department of Health and Human Services, 2007) and were directly reported in a special issue of the journal *Pediatrics* in 2008. This report placed the phenomenon of underage drinking within the increasingly understood developmental dynamics of adolescence and emerging adulthood. In particular, it was noted that the typical age of college attendance (around 18–22) overlaps extensively with lifetime peaks in heavy drinking episodes ("binges"). These peaks have been identified in a number of large epidemiological data sets including prevalence data from the National Survey on Drug Use and Health (Substance Abuse and Mental Health Services Administration, 2005).

Drinking data such as these raised the question of whether problematic drinking in college students was *caused* by the college experience, or was just coincidental with a specific developmental period of heavy drinking. To help address this question, two studies were recently completed in our laboratory: one, a review of published studies reporting on data sets that concurrently examined drinking in college students and noncollege same-age peers; and the second, a 5-year longitudinal study of young people in this age range that employed methods for close monitoring of drinking. This close monitoring approach (essentially capturing daily drinking) placed a kind of microscope on the consumption habits of young adults in this age range and obtained information on other variables previously identified as possibly related to drinking.

The review of college and non-college drinking examined 18 studies published over the past two decades (Carter, Brandon, & Goldman, 2010). Combining these studies was complicated because of variation in operational definitions of what constitutes a college student as well as variation in drinking outcomes. When we aggregated these metrics into the most global possible indices of quantity and frequency of consumption, however, this review indicated that college students indeed drank more frequently and in greater amounts than their nonstudent peers, but not dramatically so. Other factors also addressed in this review, however, suggested that it was not college attendance per se that could best be understood to play the determining role in elevating drinking. That is, it was unlikely that merely engaging in the academic aspects of college attendance increased drinking. Rather, concurrent factors such as living situation, age, full- versus part-time status, and type of college were more likely to have an influence on drinking behavior. For example, living in a fraternity house rather than at home with parents would likely portend greater drinking. Placed within the context of the developmental forces noted above, the review concluded that the overarching influences on alcohol consumption seemed to be best understood as a dense concentration of individuals in this developmental period within a single community (as might occur in a college environment as well as other contexts, e.g., the military), along with the availability of discretionary time. That is, many young people living in proximity to each other, with sufficient time to allocate to social functions (including drinking), seemed to be the recipe for extensive consumption.

Complementing the conclusions from this review, the second study longitudinally assessed daily drinking over 5 years beginning at ages 18–19 in college students and their same-age non-college peers. (All study participants had to be already drinking at recruitment; see study details for the reasoning behind this choice.) College students were defined as full-time status (= 9+ credit hours). Drinking was assessed both in terms of the usual quantity/frequency items (including frequency of getting "drunk"), and using 90-day timeline follow-back methods to obtain daily drinking practices. In one set of findings extracted from this data set (Goldman, Greenbaum, Darkes, Brandon, & Del Boca, 2011), we synchronized daily drinking records to an actual calendar year. During this calendar year (including summers), drinking levels varied considerably from ordinary weeks to "holiday" weeks (events such as Christmas, Thanksgiving, Fourth of July), as we have seen before in our earlier study of college students during the academic year (Del Boca, Darkes, Greenbaum, & Goldman, 2004). Remarkably, the second study showed that non-college individuals had consumption patterns similar to the college students. Not only did similar elevations occur across calendar events such as New Year's week, but even holidays specific to college, such as spring break, showed increased drinking in non-college students. That is, college and non-college students seemed relatively synchronized in their drinking, regardless of actual college attendance. In an extended analysis (over the full 5 years) of the same participants, quarterly data showed that the overlap observed in this selected chronological year continued through the entire 5-year study span, and the overlap seen in the time-line data also was seen for discrete item measures of drinking frequency, drinking quantity, and getting drunk. In sum, these data showed that for drinkers (recall that all participants in these studies were already drink-ers), consumption parameters during this age range did not appear be uniquely associated with college attendance.

RISK TAKING IN ANTICIPATION OF DEVELOPMENTALLY APPROPRIATE OUTCOMES

Because it is implausible that academic aspects of college attendance per se are the critical factors in escalating young adult drinking, and because drinking may increase wherever young people congregate in higher densi-ties with increased discretionary time, we must consider developmental processes common to all young people during this life period as most influ-ential. Although developmental processes are obviously highly complex and multifaceted, reviewers have recently highlighted two interrelated characteristics of this developmental period (Masten, Faden, Zucker, & Spear, 2008). One characteristic noted is the general increase in risk tak-ing that occurs across the entire population in this age group. Although considerable variation in risk taking occurs at any age, it appears that the entire distribution of risk taking shifts toward more riskiness at this time of life. For example, data from the Sensation Seeking Scale, a measure that includes risk taking as a component, has revealed increases through-out the teenage years, with a peak between 16 and 19, followed by slight decreases throughout the 20s (Zuckerman, Eysenck, & Eysenck, 1978). Although males typically show higher sensation-seeking scores than females, the late-teenage peak is common to both males and females. As just one example, risky driving may be a behavioral manifestation of this trait. Both males and females in their teens and 20s are more than twice as likely to be speeding in a fatal car accident as drivers above age 29 (Nell, 2002). This increased risk taking (as part of more general emotional dysregulation) may be responsible for the "paradox of adolescence": although adolescence is the healthiest and most resilient period of the lifespan, overall morbidity and mortality rates increase 200–300% between middle childhood and late adolescence/early adulthood (Dahl & Conway, 2009).

From an evolutionary perspective, the propensity of adolescents to tolerate more risk than they might at other times in their lives may offer advantages. Adolescence is the life phase in which the transition from adult oversight to independent living takes place; this transition requires risk tolerance because independent living is inherently risky, especially when the skills for such living are just coming online. Even more to the point, species survival through sexual reproduction necessitates mating. Although mating is an inherently social endeavor, it is also fundamentally risky, especially for males; the success or failure of mating attempts determines ones social standing and the likelihood of passing on one's genes. In the larger sense, this capacity has been called evolutionary fitness (Glimcher, 2002). Across many species, higher-status individuals get to mate with opposite-sex individuals who may produce more successful offspring; lower-status individuals may even be killed. That is, risk taking and mating may be synergistic. This dynamic is not unique to humans. Masten et al. (2008) note that risky behaviors geared toward social and/ or sexual goals "increase the probability of reproductive success for male individuals of a variety of species, including humans," and "facilitate ... emigration of sexually maturing adolescents away from genetic relatives" (p. S245).

How does alcohol enter into this dynamic? Alcohol is recognized as the perfect chemical facilitator of these activities for adolescents (socializing and risk taking). Adolescents have been shown to have greater sensitivity than adults to the social facilitative effects of alcohol, which thereby encourages the very behavior that seems fundamental to adolescence. At the same time, they have less sensitivity to aversive effects (e.g., sedation, hangover or ataxia; Masten at al., 2008), which thereby diminishes the discouragements that might accompany drinking for older individuals. And the nexus between alcohol use, socializing, and risk taking can be viewed from two perspectives. First, the act of drinking may be risky unto itself. The majority of those in this age group are underage and drinking illegally, and thus risk being caught. The acute toxicity of alcohol is also a risk that accompanies "drinking to get drunk." For people valuing risk, the display of intoxicated behavior, vomiting, or passing out can become a "badge of honor" signaling that a good time was had, thereby increasing social status. Second, and more to the purpose of this chapter, drinking can be viewed as a medium that enables risky but desired behaviors. Common expected drinking outcomes such as "reduced inhibitions" can lead to social and sexual activities that would be less likely to occur in the absence of an alcohol-induced state of stimulation (Reich & Gold-man, 2005). Other frequent expected outcomes include "bravery" and "confidence," which are viewed as being linked to both social status and alcohol consumption.

EXPECTED OUTCOMES: A BROADER PALETTE

An important distinction is worth making at this point about the reward-ing effects of alcohol. A very recent, comprehensive review of models of addiction (Redish at al., 2008) emphasizes expected outcomes as a key element in virtually all current animal and human models of addiction but focuses on expectations of pharmacological brain effects as the pen-ultimate motivation for substance consumption (including alcohol). In colloquial terms, these expectations would include the subjective experi-ence of getting "buzzed," "high," "wasted," "drunk," and so forth. It is possible, of course, that at the point of "addiction," psychopharma-cological effects are in fact primary. We should recognize, however, that the mixing of alcohol use, risk taking, and sociality occurs downstream of these psychopharmacological effects. That is, individuals drink to enhance their effectiveness in social situations that are often the context for drinking, and not just to experience internal, purely subjective effects that they might be able to experience in solitary drinking. Therefore, a truly comprehensive list of expected outcomes must include both direct neurophysiological effects and those effects that derive from the influence of alcohol on large organismic goals (i.e., evolutionary fitness). Research-ers are only just beginning to generate models, including animal models, of this more extensive list of sought-after outcomes (e.g., Varlinskaya & Spear, 2006).

LEARNING ANTICIPATED OUTCOMES WITHOUT DIRECT EXPERIENCE: VICARIOUS LEARNING

Humans do not require direct experience with alcohol to become knowl-edgeable about this full array of potentially desired outcomes. Humans are equipped with the powerful ability to learn through the experience of others, that is, vicariously. In recent years, a veritable explosion of information (especially information derived from the behavior of others) has been obtained about an array of neural mechanisms whose function seems to be to acquire information about the relationship among con-texts, behaviors, and outcomes (Mitchell, 2008). Through the discovery of biological mechanisms of vicarious learning such as mirror cells, along with brain regions sensitive to mentalizing (taking on the perspective of others), evidence is mounting that social information achieves privileged status in the brain. In other words, the human brain seems oriented to receive social information, relative to other types of information. This orientation allows for humans to make rapid and usually accurate inferences about others.

Obviously, vicarious learning provides an evolutionary advantage: it allows humans to make connections between behaviors and outcomes without requiring a "trial and error" approach to every minute behavior added to their repertoire, or having to engage in the possibly dangerous activities themselves. We know that much of what people learn about alcohol is vicarious. If learning about alcohol were a simple matter of direct experience, people would be like most animal species and choose to drink something that tastes better than the typical alcoholic drink. Yet children have learned a full array of expected alcohol effects before they have consumed their first sip (Christiansen, Smith, Roehling, & Goldman, 1989). Although young children seem more likely to associate aversive outcomes with alcohol use, research in our laboratory has shown that associations shift toward positive outcomes as children enter adolescence (Dunn & Goldman, 1996, 1998, 2000). As these expectations become more positive, they facilitate getting past the initial aversive taste and support the acceleration of drinking revealed in the epidemiological studies reviewed earlier. Parents, deviant peers, alcohol advertising, and adult-oriented television have all been implicated as sources for vicarious learning of alcohol's effects. For example, Donovan, Molina, and Kelly (2009) demonstrated that children have a tendency to adopt the alcohol expectancies of their parents, and that they are most likely to adopt consensual expectancies—those shared by both parents.

Some influences, however, may be more insidious than obvious factors such as parents or friends, and relate to the larger culture in which children are raised. For example, animated children's movies like *Pinocchio*, *The Rescuers*, and *Dumbo* depict characters consuming alcohol, and generally consumption is shown in connection with positive outcomes. Taking the latter as the quintessential example, after being cast as a "freak" because of his huge ears and having his mother taken away from him unjustly, Dumbo the elephant sinks into a deep depression. While being consoled by his mouse friend Timothy, Dumbo drinks from a water barrel inadvertently contaminated with alcohol. Dumbo then enters a state of intoxication unrivaled by even the most glorifying media image of alcohol, and seeming more like a psychedelic trip. As he emerges from this stupor in a tree, Dumbo's fortunes are transformed when he realizes how he got there: he flew with his oversized ears. He learned to fly while under the influence! The clear implication is that Dumbo would not likely have tried such a *risky* action without alcohol on board. Although Dumbo may be a bit obscure to children today, it may become less so soon as the 70th Anniversary Edition has been recently released on Blu-ray.

By watching parents, friends, or even Dumbo consume alcohol, people learn to anticipate alcohol's effects without ever having had a drop. These anticipated effects have been studied extensively in alcohol expectancy research.

ALCOHOL EXPECTANCY RESEARCH: EXPLICIT AND IMPLICIT

Expectancy theory originally was developed in the psychological domain to describe the performance of rodents in mazes that could not be explained by simple response–outcome relationships (Tolman, 1932). Most human alcohol expectancy research, however, has used conventional paper-and-pencil self-report measures. These measures, which have defined alcohol expectancies as the anticipated effects of alcohol use and yielded a great deal of information on drinking behavior, are described in recent reviews (Goldman, Darkes, & Del Boca, 1999; Goldman et al., 2006, 2010). Alcohol expectancies have been correlated with drinking, predicting up to 50% of drinking variance in error-attenuated models. As previously discussed, both cross-sectional and longitudinal developmental designs have shown alcohol expectancies to predict the onset of drinking in children. When studied concurrently with other known antecedents of drinking (e.g., family, peer, or cultural factors), alcohol expectancies have been shown to statistically mediate a portion of the relationship between these antecedents and drinking. Finally, when activated or diminished in controlled experiments, alcohol expectancies have caused increases and decreases in drinking, respectively. (For a more detailed summary of this research, see Goldman et al., 2006.)

To more comprehensively study expectancy theory and drinking behavior, our research group has embarked on multiple lines of research that have deviated from typical self-report measures. The intent of this more recent work has been to advance alcohol expectancy research beyond static psychometric (predictive) models, into theoretical models of expectancy operation. These advances took place in two stages. First, the foundation for operational models of alcohol expectancies was provided by construction of memory network models as used in cognitive science. These models have shown that expectancy memory networks may be understood as having two central dimensions: (1) valence (positive/negative); and (2) sedation (arousal/sedation). Interestingly, people tend to hold alcohol expectancies reflecting the full range of these dimensions. For example, alcohol's anticipated effects may simultaneously include sleepiness, euphoria, relaxation, and vomiting. In other words, the same person might have expectations for both happiness and sickness resulting from the same drinking episode. Research using approaches such as multidimensional scaling and free association to map out these memory networks has demonstrated that the alcohol expectancies people hold are not as important with regard to drinking (individuals with greater propensities to drink have more expectancies of *all* kinds), as the relative emphasis they put on each dimension (Rather & Goldman, 1994; Reich & Goldman, 2005). These and subsequent studies have repeatedly shown that heavier drinkers place a greater emphasis on positive and arousing alcohol expectancies than lighter drinkers.

These models of alcohol expectancy network structure provided the framework for the second line of research, which experimentally investigated expectancy operation; that is, the dependence of alcohol expectancy memory networks on context to activate anticipatory cognitions/affect that, in turn, influence behavioral outputs (both consumption and alcohol-related behaviors once consumption takes place). Practically speaking, alcohol expectancy memory networks may differ at a football game compared to dinner at a nice restaurant, and behavior should (and does) differ accordingly. A series of studies were conducted in our laboratory using tasks developed by cognitive psychologists to test memory activation following implicit primes. The term *implicit* simply means that participants were unaware of (not conscious of) the prime that influenced their performance on a subsequent task. Because initiation and pursuit of goals may be largely nonconscious (Custers & Aarts, 2010), approaches that tap these nonconscious processes are quite applicable to the investigation of alcohol-related goals. In addition, the use of implicit methods reduces demand characteristics by indirectly encouraging participants to provide the results that the experimenter "wants" to see, and thereby increases the validity of studies employing these approaches.

A final advantage of using implicit measures is their sensitivity to very subtle contextual shifts. For example, priming effects vastly differ with either slight or dramatic changes in stimuli; Reich, Noll, and Goldman (2005) demonstrated this sensitivity to slight modifications of the stimulti in an alcohol expectancy task by simply varying the first word of a list to be later recalled (beer versus milk). Other implicit priming studies in our lab have used alcohol words followed by the Stroop task (Kramer & Goldman, 2003), and in one simulated bar study the prime was followed by a false memory task (Reich, Goldman, & Noll, 2004). Each of these studies demonstrated that alcohol primes (all with comparison to alcohol-neutral primes) led to enhanced memory activation of positive and/or arousing alcohol expectancies. Not surprisingly, in each study this activation was contingent on the typical drinking of the participants. The greatest activation was found in the heaviest drinkers—those with the most drinking experience were the most sensitive to alcohol-specific contexts.

Showing that memory network activation was sensitive to context, although important, only provided support for a hypothetical mechanism that might influence drinking. To complete the picture, several studies conducted in our laboratory as well as in related laboratories also have shown that contextual priming can influence actual drinking. To this end, participants in these studies were exposed to primes in a procedure that was seemingly unrelated to a later "taste test" of an alcoholic beverage. These "unrelated experiment" studies have shown that exposure to television clips (Roehrich & Goldman, 1995), alcohol expectancy words (Stein, Goldman, & Del Boca, 2000), or a simulated bar (Lau-Barraco & Dunn, 2009) can lead to increases in actual drinking during the later taste test.

Beyond our immediate research group, many other investigators have used widely different implicit memory network measures (e.g., reaction time, recall, free associates) to study alcohol expectancies and related cognitions. To summarize this body of studies and to compare the predictive power of explicit and implicit measures, Reich, Below, and Goldman (2010) conducted a meta-analysis of studies that included both kinds of measures in one study. In 13 of the 16 studies that met this criterion, explicit measures accounted for more drinking variance than implicit measures (in 12 out of 13 studies accounting for unique variance), and the meta-analysis of the relative mean effect sizes confirmed the observed differences. Hence, these empirical findings indicated that implicit measurement was not somehow more central or fundamental to the prediction of behavior; that is, implicit measures were not supported as accessing more critical decision-making processes. At the same time, however, implicit measures did account for significant (incremental) drinking variance beyond that accounted for by explicit measures. This pattern of results supported the use of both explicit and implicit measures of alcohol expectancy and similar associative processes to predict drinking.

A very recent line of research in our laboratory has added one form of neuroimaging to open a new window on alcohol expectancy operation. To this end, Fishman, Goldman, and Donchin (2008) measured the P300 component of the event related potential (ERP) as an index of alcohol expectancy violation. Elevations in this component usually have been understood as indexing violations of preconceived expectancies; that is, individuals who strongly expected a particular outcome showed large

P300s if a different outcome appeared. After alcohol expectancies were assessed in college students using conventional paper-and-pencil measures, participants monitored using a dense array electroencephalogram (EEG) were presented with the sentence stem "On a Friday night, alcohol makes me ...," which was completed with an alcohol expectancy word (e.g., *happy*). The stem was repeated multiple times with different alcohol expectancy completions representing both positive and negative dimensions. For each of these presentations, participants either agreed or disagreed with the statement using a computer keyboard. Participants who more strongly endorsed positive alcohol expectancies on the paper-and-pencil measures had larger P300 EEG waves when presented with negative alcohol expectancy sentences. That is, expectancy violation was greatest for participants presented with expectancies incongruent with their own. These P300 results occurred too quickly (within 300 ms) to be contingent on conscious verbal if–then propositions, and suggested that decisions about alcohol outcomes were in process well before individuals might be aware of these decisions. This lack of awareness supports the idea that implicit processes are at least partially guiding drinking-related cognition.

THE SOCIAL NATURE
OF ALCOHOL EXPECTANCIES

Prior to reviewing alcohol expectancy studies, we described how adolescents and young adults take risks to obtain biologically meaningful rewards, and observed that these rewards were likely social in nature. We also argued that alcohol consumption may be understood as one risk taken to obtain such rewards, or as a facilitator of risk taking. What has yet to be explicitly tested using any type of alcohol expectancy measure is evidence that social alcohol expectancies are accorded the kind of "privileged" cognitive status that social neuroscientists have observed with other social information (Mitchell, 2008). In spite of the unavailability of studies that directly test this hypothesis, several lines of evidence point to this possibility.

First, in addition to the many anticipated effects already mentioned, which seem to reflect possible pharmacological effects of ethanol, social and sexual effects were often observed as alcohol expectancies. Among these effects, common expectancies reported in our research included sociability, talkativeness, attractiveness, and horniness (Reich & Goldman, 2005). Rarer, but repeatedly observed, expectancies included enhanced dancing and fighting. Second, we have found that social and sexual expectancies were always highly positively related to actual drinking. Reich and Goldman (2006) isolated social and sexual expectancies from other expectancies following a free-associating task where participants could give up to five responses to complete the phrase "Alcohol makes me _____." The more social and sexual responses each individual produced, the heavier his or her typical self-reported drinking tended to be.

Third, among other types of alcohol expectancies on standardized measures, social and sexual scales typically accounted for the greatest statistical prediction of drinking behavior (e.g., Goldman & Darkes, 2004). And fourth, effective expectancy challenge studies have had at their core the manipulation of social and sexual activities (e.g., Darkes & Goldman 1993, 1998). During these procedures participants were randomly assigned to receive drinks containing alcohol or placebo alcohol. Participants then interacted in social games with sexual content (rating the attractiveness of models in pictures) or without sexual content (Win, Lose, or Draw) to elicit expectancy-consistent behavior. Later, when asked to guess who had consumed alcohol based on their behaviors during these activities, participants were correct at about the level of a coin flip (chance). This level of accuracy, or more precisely, inaccuracy, occurred even when they were guessing about their own personal consumption. The expectancy challenge manipulation, which showed participants that many social and sexual effects of alcohol could be the result of placebo effects, has led to observable decreases in drinking in some college student samples. Variations in challenge strategies and findings across laboratories have yet to reveal a fully endorsable approach to reliable expectancy challenge.

CONCLUSIONS

Recent evidence suggests that college student drinking must be considered in light of the developmental characteristics of college-age people (including those who do not attend college). This chapter has highlighted two of these developmental characteristics: risk taking and elevated social motivation. We also have laid out a rationale for the role of alcohol expectancies, particularly social and sexual expectancies, as points of entry into fully appreciating how alcohol perfectly serves these developmental needs.

This body of research has some clear practical implications. First, context plays a role in (heavy) drinking behavior. Influential aspects of context are wide-ranging, encompassing temporal (e.g., calendar events), physical (e.g., a bar), media (e.g., movies), and social (e.g., presence of potential mates) factors. Not surprisingly, contexts where social or sexual outcomes are likely tend to be signals for heavier drinking. Knowledge of this contextual influence can help administrators anticipate when and where problematic drinking may occur. Also, identifying the most relevant expectancies with respect to decision making is critical for refining expectancy challenge programs, which represent one possible means of using expectancies to assist in the reduction of excessive drinking and its consequences in this age group. Social and sexual expectancies are already the point of focus in some expectancy challenge programs (Darkes & Goldman, 1993, 1998), which are designed to show the drinker that these effects are largely the result of placebo. Knowing that emerging adults are particularly tuned in to these effects may be helpful in improving such programs.

ACKNOWLEDGMENTS

This study was supported in part by National Institute on Alcohol and Alcoholism Grant Nos. R01 AA08333 and RO1 AA016091.

REFERENCES

Bonnie, R. J., & O'Connell. (Eds.). (2004). *Reducing underage drinking: A collective responsibility*. Washington, DC: National Academies Press.

Carter, A. C., Brandon, K. O., & Goldman, M. S. (2010). The college and noncollege experience: A review of factors that influence drinking behavior in young adulthood. *Journal of Studies on Alcohol and Drugs, 71*, 742–750.

Christiansen, B. A., Smith, G. T., Roehling, P. V., & Goldman, M. S. (1989). Using alcohol expectancies to predict adolescent drinking behavior at one year. *Journal of Consulting and Clinical Psychology, 57*, 93–99.

Custers, R., & Aarts, H. (2010). The unconscious will: How the pursuit of goals operates outside of conscious awareness. *Science, 329*, 47–50.

Dahl, R. E., & Conway, A. M. (2009). Self-regulation and the development of behavioral and emotional problems: Toward an integrative conceptual and translational research agenda. In S. Olson, & A. J. Sameroff (Eds.), *Biopsychosocial regulatory processes in the development of childhood behavioral problems* (pp. 290–318). New York: Cambridge University Press.

Darkes, J., & Goldman, M. S. (1993). Expectancy challenge and drinking reduction: Experimental evidence for a mediational process. *Journal of Consulting and Clinical Psychology, 61*, 344–353.

Darkes, J., & Goldman, M. S. (1998). Expectancy challenge and drinking reduction: Process and structure in the alcohol expectancy network. *Experimental and Clinical Psychopharmacology, 6*, 1–13.

Del Boca, F. K., Darkes, J., Greenbaum, P. E., & Goldman, M. S. (2004). Up close and personal: Temporal variability in the drinking of- individual college stu-

dents during their first year. *Journal of Consulting and Clinical Psychology,*
72, 155–164.

Donovan, J. E., Molina, B. S. G., & Kelly, T. M. (2009). Alcohol outcome expectancies as socially shared and socialized beliefs. *Psychology of Addictive
Behaviors, 23,* 248–259.

Dunn, M. E., & Goldman, M. S. (1996). Empirical modeling of an alcohol expectancy memory network in elementary school children as a function of grade.
Experimental and Clinical Psychopharmacology, 4, 209–217.

Dunn, M. E., & Goldman, M. S. (1998). Age and drinking-related differences
in the memory organization of alcohol expectancies in 3rd-, 6th-, 9th-, and
12th-grade children. *Journal of Consulting and Clinical Psychology, 66,*
579–585.

Dunn, M. E., & Goldman, M. S. (2000). Validation of multi-dimensional scal-
ing-based modeling of alcohol expectancies in memory: Age and drinking-
related differences in expectancies of children assessed as first associates.
Alcoholism: Clinical and Experimental Research, 24, 1639–1646.

Fishman, I., Goldman, M. S., & Donchin, E. (2008). The P300 as an electro-
physiological probe of alcohol expectancy. *Experimental and Clinical Psychopharmacology, 16,* 341–356.

Glimcher, P. W. (2002). Decisions, decisions, decisions: Choosing a biological science of choice. *Neuron, 36,* 323–332.

Goldman, M. S. (2002). Expectancy and risk for alcoholism: The unfortunate
exploitation of a fundamental characteristic of neurobehavioral adaptation.
Alcoholism: Clinical and Experimental Research, 26, 737–746.

Goldman, M. S., Boyd, G. M., & Faden, V. (Eds.). (2002). College drinking, what
it is, and what to do about it: A review of the state of the science [Special
issue]. *Journal of Studies on Alcohol, S14.*

Goldman, M. S., & Darkes, J. (2004). Alcohol expectancy multi-axial assessment
(A.E.Max): A memory network-based approach. *Psychological Assessment,*
16, 4–15.

Goldman, M. S., Darkes, J., & Del Boca, F. K. (1999). Expectancy mediation of
biopsychosocial risk for alcohol use and alcoholism. In I. Kirsch (Ed.), *How
expectancies shape experience.* Washington, DC: American Psychological
Association.

Goldman, M. S., Darkes, J., Reich, R. R., & Brandon, K. O. (2010). Anticipa-
tory processing as a transdisciplinary bridge in addiction. In D. Ross, H.
Kincaid, D. Spurrett, & P. Collins (Eds.), *What is addiction?* (pp. 291–334)
Cambridge, MA: MIT Press.

Goldman, M. S., Greenbaum, P. E., Darkes, J., Brandon, K. O., & Del Boca, F. K.
(2011). How many versus how much: 52 weeks of alcohol consumption in
emerging adults. *Psychology of Addictive Behaviors, 25,* 16–27.

Goldman, M. S., Reich, R. R., & Darkes, J. (2006). Expectancy as a unifying
construct in alcohol-related cognition. In R. W. Wiers & A. W. Stacy (Eds.),
Handbook of implicit cognition and addiction (pp. 105–121). Thousand
Oaks, CA: Sage.

Hingson, R. W., Zha, W., & Weitzman, E. R. (2009). Magnitude of and trends
in alcohol-related mortality and morbidity among U.S. college students

ages 18–24, 1998–2005. *Journal of Studies on Alcohol and Drugs, S16,* 12–20.

Holland, P. C., & Gallagher, M. (2004). Amygdala-frontal interactions and reward expectancy. *Current Opinion in Neurobiology, 14,* 148–155.

Kramer, D. A., & Goldman, M. S. (2003). Using a modified Stroop task to implicitly discern the cognitive organization of alcohol expectancies. *Journal of Abnormal Psychology, 112*(1), 171–175.

Lau-Barraco, C., & Dunn, M. E. (2009). Environmental context effects on alcohol cognitions and immediate alcohol consumption. *Addiction Research and Theory, 17,* 306–314.

Masten, A. S., Faden, V. B., Zucker, R. A., & Spear, L. P. (2008). Underage drinking: A developmental framework. *Pediatrics, 121*(Suppl. 4), S235–S251.

Mitchell, J. P. (2008). Contributions of functional neuroimaging to the study of social cognition. *Current Directions in Psychological Science, 17,* 142–146.

Nell, V. (2002). Why young men drive dangerously: Implications for injury prevention. *Current Directions in Psychological Science, 11,* 75–79.

Rather, B. C., & Goldman, M. S. (1994). Drinking-related differences in the memory organization of alcohol expectancies. *Experimental and Clinical Psychopharmacology, 2,* 167–183.

Redish, A. D., Jensen, S., & Johnson, A. (2008). A unified framework for addiction: Vulnerabilities in the decision process. *Behavioral and Brain Sciences, 31,* 415–487.

Reich, R. R., Below, M. C., & Goldman, M. S. (2010). Explicit and implicit measures of expectancy and related alcohol cognitions: A meta-analytic comparison. *Psychology of Addictive Behaviors, 24,* 13–25.

Reich, R. R., & Goldman, M. S. (2005). Exploring the alcohol expectancy memory network: The utility of free associates. *Psychology of Addictive Behaviors, 19,* 317–325.

Reich, R. R., & Goldman, M. S. (2006, June). *Dancing, sex, and violence: Effects of alcohol about which EtOH or rats haven't told us.* In D. McCarthy (Chair), Symposium conducted at the annual meeting of the Research Society on Alcoholism, Baltimore, MD.

Reich, R. R., Goldman, M. S., & Noll, J. A. (2004). Using the false memory paradigm to test two key elements of alcohol expectancy theory. *Experimental and Clinical Psychopharmacology, 12,* 102–110.

Reich, R. R., Noll, J. A., & Goldman, M. S. (2005). Cue patterns and alcohol expectancies: How slight differences in stimuli can measurably change cognition. *Experimental and Clinical Psychopharmacology, 13,* 65–71.

Roehrich, L., & Goldman, M. S. (1995). Implicit priming of alcohol expectancy memory processes and subsequent drinking behavior. *Experimental and Clinical Psychopharmacology, 3,* 402–410.

Stein, K. D., Goldman, M. S., & Del Boca, F. K. (2000). The influence of alcohol expectancy priming and mood manipulation on subsequent alcohol consumption. *Journal of Abnormal Psychology, 109,* 106–115.

Substance Abuse and Mental Health Services Administration. (2005). *Results from the 2005 National Survey on Drug Use and Health: National findings.*

Retrieved   from   *www.oas.samhsa.gov/NSDUH/2k5NSDUH/2k5results. htm#Ch3*.

Tolman, E. C. (1932). *Purposive behavior in animals and man*. New York: Appleton-Century-Crofts.

U.S. Department of Health and Human Services. (2007). *The Surgeon General's Call to Action to Prevent and Reduce Underage Drinking*. Retrieved from *www.surgeongeneral.gov/topics/underagedrinking/calltoaction.pdf*.

Varlinskaya, E. I., & Spear, L. P. (2006). Differences in the social consequences of ethanol emerge during the course of adolescence in rats: Social facilitation, social inhibition, and anxiolysis. *Developmental Psychobiology, 48*, 146–161.

Zuckerman, M., Eysenck, S. B., & Eysenck, H. J. (1978). Sensation seeking in England and America: Cross-cultural, age, and sex comparisons. *Journal of Consulting and Clinical Psychology, 46*, 139–149.

CHAPTER 6

The Effects of Alcohol on Other Behavioral Risks

Kim Fromme *and* Patrick D. Quinn

Over the past decade, public health concerns regarding alcohol use by college students have broadened beyond a primary focus on their amount of consumption to include the influence of alcohol on a variety of potentially hazardous behaviors. In addition to exhibiting the highest rates of alcohol consumption of all age groups (Johnston, O'Malley, Bachman, & Schulenberg, 2009), college students have high alcohol-related morbidity and mortality (Hingson, Zha, & Weitzman, 2009). Alcohol use may contribute to these statistics, as people appear to be more likely to take risks if they have been drinking (e.g., Neal & Fromme, 2007).

Fortunately, most students will mature out of heavy drinking patterns when they leave college and assume adult responsibilities (see Jochman & Fromme, 2010, for a review). However, the negative consequences that may result from behavioral risks during this developmentally limited period of excess could have permanent, detrimental effects. An unplanned pregnancy or arrest for driving under the influence (DUI) is likely to have long-lasting effects on the individual's future. Moreover, college students do not typically drink in isolation, and their alcohol use does not have exclusively personal consequences. Often it is the behaviors in which students engage with other people while they are drinking that create the most serious problems. Consequently, there is an urgent need to develop an understanding of the role alcohol actually plays in the behavioral risks frequently attributed to drinking. Aggression, risky sexual behaviors, sexual assault, and illicit drug use have all been associated with collegiate alcohol use, yet relatively little is known about whether alcohol plays a direct or moderated role in their occurrence. This chapter reviews the growing body of research that sheds light on this question.

THEORETICAL MODELS AND METHODS LINKING ALCOHOL AND BEHAVIORAL RISKS

Although cultural myth suggests that alcohol leads to behavioral risks, it is also possible that drinking simply covaries with a variety of behaviors, including drug use, sex, and aggression. From this perspective, third variables such as personality or opportunity might explain the co-occurrence of alcohol and other behavioral risks. Conversely, a hypothesized causal link has been explained by expectancy models that focus on beliefs about drinking (see Patel & Fromme, 2010, for a review) and by pharmacological models that focus on the effects of alcohol on cognitive processes (Steele & Josephs, 1990) or anxiety reduction (Ito, Miller, & Pollock, 1996). A key distinction between expectancy and pharmacological perspectives is whether drinking serves a motivational function, for example providing the drinker with an incentive or an excuse for engaging in risky behaviors (i.e., expectancy models), or whether the pharmacological properties of alcohol disrupt information processing or reduce fear that otherwise inhibits behavior. Below we summarize the three major theoretical models regarding the association between alcohol and behavioral risks.

General Deviance Models

General deviance or co-occurrence models (e.g., Jessor & Jessor, 1977) suggest that engagement in behavioral risks (also referred to as externalizing behaviors), including drinking, drug use, vandalism, aggression, and sexual risk taking, constitutes a syndrome of problem behavior, with personality traits such as impulsivity and sensation seeking leading some people to be drawn to these behaviors (Zuckerman, 1979). Indeed, the global associations among alcohol and other substance use, delinquency, and risky sexual behaviors support a general deviance syndrome and, to a large extent, reflect a common tendency toward these externalizing behaviors, in which impulsivity plays an important role (Cooper, Wood, Orcutt, & Albino, 2003). Also referred to as behavioral disinhibition or behavioral undercontrol, impulsivity represents an underlying genetic risk factor for both alcohol use and other externalizing behaviors (Young et al., 2009).

Additionally, shared contexts such as social activities, parties, and bars may also promote the co-occurrence of both drinking and other behavioral risks, without there being a causal link between them (Leigh & Stall, 1993). Bars, nightclubs, and house parties, for example, are common drinking environments for college students, and behavioral risks often occur within such environments (e.g., aggression; Parks, 2000).

Expectancy Models

According to expectancy theory, the relation between alcohol use and post-drinking behavior is caused by outcome expectancies, or beliefs about the effects of drinking alcohol (see Patel & Fromme, 2010, for a review). Expectancies about potential positive consequences of drinking may lead people to engage in certain behaviors when they drink. Expectancies may, for example, motivate people to combine alcohol with sexual behavior if they believe that alcohol makes sex more likely or enjoyable. Beliefs that one can "blame the bottle" may also provide post hoc justification for sexual indiscretion or unsafe sexual practices (Fromme, D'Amico, & Katz, 1999). These beliefs are learned, either through direct personal experience, vicarious observation, or sociocultural norms (e.g., Patel & Fromme, 2010).

Support for expectancy models comes primarily from research that has linked alcohol outcome expectancies with drinking patterns and problems (see Jones, Corbin, & Fromme, 2001, for a review). Extensions of the expectancy concept to substance use, sexual behavior, and a host of other behavioral risks have found consistent associations between expected outcomes and frequency of engaging in these behaviors (e.g., Fromme, Katz, & Rivet, 1997b). For example, expectations of sexual enhancement and disinhibition are associated with drinking to intoxication when combining alcohol with sex (Dermen & Cooper, 1994), and sex-related alcohol expectancies have been found to moderate the association between drinking and risky sexual practices during first and most recent intercourse (Dermen, Cooper, & Agocha, 1998). (For greater detail on expectancy research, see Reich & Goldman, Chapter 5, this volume.)

Pharmacological Models

One of the leading pharmacological explanations of the link between alcohol and behavioral risks is the attention allocation, or alcohol myopia, model (Giancola, Josephs, Parrott, & Duke, 2010; Steele & Josephs, 1990). This model posits that impaired attentional capacity and an inability to process and extract meaning from cues in the environment may lead the intoxicated individual to focus on immediate and salient cues without processing more peripheral ones. These cues include external factors (e.g., an attractive date) as well as internal factors (e.g., perceived risks). Alcohol may therefore contribute to behavioral risks by focusing drinkers' attention on immediate positive consequences (e.g., thrills or pleasure) and reducing their ability to effectively process potential negative consequences (e.g., getting hurt or arrested).

Support for pharmacological models is found in studies documenting alcohol's effects on attentional and memorial processes, specifically on the capacity to integrate previously learned information, retrieve information from memory, inhibit prepotent but inappropriate responses, and plan behavioral strategies (e.g., Casbon, Curtin, Lang, & Patrick, 2003; Curtin & Fairchild, 2003). Sexual arousal, for example, is thought to be a powerful internal cue that promotes desire for sex and, when combined with alcohol, leads to sexual risk taking (MacDonald, MacDonald, Zanna, & Fong, 2000). Consistent with an attention allocation model, alcohol intoxication has been found to interact with sexual arousal to lead to a greater reported likelihood of having unprotected sex (Ebel-Lam, MacDonald, Zanna, & Fong, 2009). In their review of alcohol myopia as an explanation for aggression and other behavioral risks, Giancola and colleagues (2010) offered several possible mechanisms through which alcohol-induced myopia may occur, including effects on negative affect, self-awareness, and empathy.

Expectancy-Mediated Pharmacological Models

Expectancy and pharmacological explanations for the association between alcohol and behavioral risks need not be mutually exclusive (e.g., Davis, Hendershot, George, Norris, & Heiman, 2007; Morris & Albery, 2001). For example, Davis et al. (2007) demonstrated the importance of examining predrinking beliefs about the risks and benefits of unprotected sex when testing alcohol myopia as an explanation for sexual decision making. Whereas intoxicated participants reported greater sexual risk intentions than sober participants, this effect was moderated by the individual's predrinking beliefs about the potential consequences of unprotected sex.

In a series of alcohol administration studies in our simulated bar laboratory, we tested the hypothesis that alcohol intoxication contributes to behavioral risks by altering people's expectations about the possible outcomes of engaging in those behaviors. In the first study, young adults who were moderate to heavy drinkers participated in two counterbalanced laboratory sessions in which they drank alcohol (average blood alcohol concentration [BAC] of .088%) or no alcohol (Fromme, Katz, & D'Amico, 1997a). After consuming their beverages, participants rated the likelihood of negative and positive outcomes of engaging in six types of behavioral risks (Illicit Drug Use, Aggressive/Illegal Acts, Risky Sex, Heavy Drinking, High Risk Sports, and Academic/Work Behaviors). Compared with ratings made when sober, intoxicated likelihood estimates of negative outcomes resulting from illicit drug use, risky sexual practices, and aggressive/illegal behaviors were significantly lower, and participants reported a greater likelihood of future drug use and risky sex. No effects of intoxication were found for expected positive outcomes, leading us to conclude that alcohol intoxication contributes to behavioral risks by reducing negative outcome expectancies.

To more closely approximate actual situations that involve intoxicated risk taking, we developed videotaped stimuli that depicted people engaging in a variety of risky activities (e.g., getting into a physical fight, sexual foreplay) but that ended before any outcomes of the behaviors were apparent (Fromme et al., 1997a). We found no differences between the no alcohol and placebo conditions in ratings of expected negative outcomes, but those receiving alcohol (average BAC = .081%) again provided lower ratings of expected negative outcomes for the behavioral risks. Similar to our first study, there were no differences in expected positive outcomes, but contrary to earlier findings, intoxicated participants reported no greater likelihood of engaging in the behavioral risks that were depicted in the videotaped stimuli. Differences between findings for behavioral intentions in these two studies likely related to the greater number and range of severity of the behavioral risks that were captured by the first study in comparison to those of the seven videotaped scenes.

Finally, in an effort to replicate and extend our findings to risky sexual behavior, we screened participants on the basis of their outcome expectancies about alcohol and sexual behavior (Fromme et al., 1999). For example, they were asked about their likelihood of being flirtatious or having sex without protection if they were drunk. High and low expectancy groups were randomly assigned to consume alcohol (target BAC of .08%), no alcohol, or placebo and then completed a revised version of the Cognitive Appraisal of Risky Events questionnaire (CARE-R) (Fromme, Katz, & Rivet, 1997b). The CARE-R measures expected positive and negative outcomes of four sexual practices (e.g., sex without protection against sexually transmitted diseases) with a "new" and a "regular" partner. Consistent with study hypotheses, participants who received alcohol provided lower ratings of potential negative outcomes with a new partner, but not with a regular partner. High-sex-expectancy participants provided higher ratings of potential positive outcomes and the likelihood of engaging in the risky sexual behaviors with a new (but not regular) partner, but we found no interaction between predrinking sex expectancies and beverage. Thus, for sex with a new partner, alcohol intoxication reduced negative expectancies, whereas predrinking expectancies were associated with more positive anticipated outcomes and a greater likelihood of engaging in risky sexual behaviors.

From our experimental studies, we concluded that alcohol intoxication reduced negative outcome expectancies and thereby contributed to greater risk-taking behavior when intoxicated than when sober. Because we found no evidence for an effect of placebo in any of these studies, we further concluded that alcohol-induced impairments in cognitive processing led to reductions in perceived personal vulnerability. Although our study was not designed to test the attention allocation model, we believe our findings are consistent with this model, as alcohol reduced expectations about potential negative, inhibitory outcomes but did not alter expectations about potential positive outcomes that may impel behavior (Steele & Josephs, 1990).

Methodologies to Assess Alcohol and Behavioral Risks

There are a variety of methodologies that can each uniquely inform our understanding of the relationship between alcohol use and behavioral risks. The preceding section illustrated the use of experimental studies manipulating beverage content to examine the effects of alcohol on beliefs and behavioral intentions. Although such experimental studies are ideal for establishing causal relations, survey methodologies, which can maximize external validity by capturing behaviors as they occur in the natural environment, are particularly valuable for understanding the relation between alcohol use and behavioral risks.

Survey methodologies can be divided into three relatively distinct categories (Leigh & Stahl, 1993). Global association studies correlate measures of overall alcohol use with frequencies of engaging in different behavioral risks. Situational association studies assess the frequency of specific behaviors that occur when alcohol is consumed. Although somewhat more precise than global association studies, situational assessments still fail to establish a temporal relation between alcohol use and behavioral risks. Finally, and perhaps most informatively for understanding temporal associations, event- or time-linked designs query respondents about specific events and whether (or how much) alcohol was consumed when that event occurred. Event-level methodologies range from retrospective reports of single events (e.g., a recent sexual encounter) to diary-based approaches in which participants provide information regarding alcohol use and behavioral risks each day over a set calendar period.

These three types of survey methodology provide varying levels of support for a link between alcohol and behavioral risks.

EVIDENCE FOR A LINK BETWEEN ALCOHOL AND BEHAVIORAL RISKS

Understanding the myriad of factors affecting behavioral risks and disentangling alcohol's effects from those of other influences is a daunting empirical task. Nevertheless, the potential mechanisms underlying the association between alcohol use and other behavioral risks have been subjected to increasing investigations. Below we provide a brief overview of the findings for alcohol use and aggression, risky sexual behavior, sexual assault, and illicit drug use.

Alcohol and Aggression

Global, event, and experimental studies provide compelling evidence that alcohol is associated with physical aggression. This association extends to general aggression (e.g., Swahn & Donovan, 2004), dating violence (Stappenbeck & Fromme, 2010), and aggression perpetration among married couples (Quigley & Leonard, 2000). From their comprehensive review and trajectory analysis of two cohorts of longitudinal samples, White and colleagues (White, Jackson, & Loeber, 2009) concluded that there is a strong and consistent association between substance use and violence.

Although it is widely accepted that alcohol intoxication, rather than expectancy, accounts for physical aggression (Bushman & Cooper, 1990; Chermack & Taylor, 1995), the precise mechanisms that underlie the alcohol–aggression link are debated. Impulsivity (Scott, Schafer, & Greenfield, 1999), cognitive abilities (Hoaken, Assaad, & Pihl, 1998a), executive cognitive functioning (Hoaken, Giancola, & Pihl, 1998b), provocation (Chermack & Taylor, 1995), and trait aggressivity (Parrott & Zeichner, 2002) all appear to moderate the effects of alcohol on aggression.

Alcohol and Risky Sexual Behavior

A substantial proportion of research on the association between alcohol and behavioral risks has focused on risky sexual behavior. These studies, however, have yielded conflicting findings (see Cooper, 2002). Global association studies have consistently documented a strong positive association between quantity and frequency indices of drinking, sexual frequency, and risky sexual behavior (e.g., Hingson, Strunin, Berlin, & Heeren, 1990), with heavier drinkers having more sexual experiences and being less likely to practice safe sex. Likewise, situational association studies have tended to support the co-occurrence of alcohol use and risky sexual behaviors (e.g., O'Leary, Goodhart, Jemmott, & Boccher-Lattimore, 1992).

With some exceptions (e.g., Leigh, 1993), event-level analyses have provided strong support for the link between alcohol use and the decision to have sex but have provided mixed support for an association between drinking and unsafe sexual practices (Cooper, 2002). For adolescents' first intercourse and first intercourse with most recent partner, Cooper, Peirce, and Huselid (1994) found that those who had been drinking prior to sex reported significantly more AIDS-related risk behaviors than those who had not been drinking. Yet, heterosexual, sexually active single adult women were no less likely to discuss sexually transmitted infection (STI) protection or use condoms when alcohol was consumed than when it was not (Testa & Collins, 1997).

Discrepancies among global, situational, and event-level findings for risky sex may be related to differences in samples (e.g., community versus college student) and level of measurement (e.g., global versus event). To help test the possibility that such differences might account for variability in the effects of alcohol on sexual behavior, Corbin and Fromme (2002) examined global, situational, and event-level associations between alcohol use and risky sexual behavior in a single sample of 576 college students. At the global level, and controlling for sexual frequency, we found no associations between alcohol and condom use for sex with either a new or regular partner. At the situational level, however, sexual intercourse with a new partner was more likely to involve both drinking and condom use, which was at least partially explained by high perceptions of risk for STIs with a new partner. Alcohol consumption was not an independent predictor of condom use with a regular partner.

In our event-level analysis, participants reported on first and most recent sex with the same partner. We found that first sex was associated with greater alcohol consumption and condom use, and less frequent use of oral contraceptives. On the other hand, most recent sex was unrelated to alcohol consumption and was less likely to involve condoms. From these global, situational, and event-level analyses, we concluded that it is important to consider contextual factors, such as characteristics of the sexual relationship, to understand the association between alcohol use and sexual practices. Other individual and situational factors, such as personality characteristics and the salience of environmental or internal cues, may also be helpful in determining the effect of alcohol on sexual risks (Cooper, 2006, 2010; Davis et al., 2007).

Alcohol and Sexual Assault

Of college men who acknowledged committing sexual assault on a date, 26% reported being intoxicated at the time of the assault, and another 29% reported being "mildly buzzed," for a total of 55% who were admittedly under the influence of alcohol at the time of the assault (Abbey, 1991). Of college women who experienced sexual assault, 21% reported being intoxicated and another 32% reported being "mildly buzzed", for a total of 53% who were under the influence of alcohol. Alcohol is thought to contribute to sexual assault through both beliefs about the effects of drinking and effects of alcohol on cognitive and motor skills (see Abbey, Zawacki, Buck, Clinton, & McAuslan, 2004; and Testa, 2002, for reviews).

Alcohol and Illicit Drug Use

National statistics indicate that 31.3% of heavy drinkers and 16.1% of binge drinkers used illicit drugs in the past month (Substance Abuse and Mental Health Services Administration, 2008). Trajectory analyses also find high correspondence between heavy drinking and marijuana use over time (Jackson, Sher, & Schulenberg, 2008), as well as between early onset of heavy drinking and other drug use (Chassin, Pitts, & Prost, 2002). Moreover, students who used marijuana in the past 30 days were more likely than others to engage in binge drinking (Mohler-Kuo, Lee, & Wechsler, (2003). Although these global associations are suggestive of a relation between alcohol use and illicit drug use, few studies have directly tested the possible causal role of alcohol intoxication. We are aware, for example, of no event-level studies demonstrating the co-occurrence of alcohol and drug use, which might help differentiate general deviance explanations from causal accounts.

In sum, efforts to elucidate the association between alcohol use and behavioral risks have yielded mixed findings. Inconsistencies are often a function of differences in populations, methodologies, and the failure to consider potential moderators. Focusing on data from a large, ethnically diverse longitudinal sample of emerging adults, the remainder of our chapter summarizes findings from event focused examinations of the association between alcohol and other behavioral risks.

EVENT-LEVEL ASSOCIATIONS BETWEEN ALCOHOL USE AND OTHER BEHAVIORAL RISKS

"The UT Experience!" (UTE) was a 6-year longitudinal study of the alcohol use and other behavioral risks of first-time college students (Fromme, Corbin, & Kruse, 2008). Unmarried high school graduates (N = 2,245) were recruited during the summer before they matriculated into The University of Texas at Austin. After providing informed consent (including parental consent for those under age 18), participants completed Web-based surveys during the summer following their senior year in high school, again each semester for years 1 through 3, and once annually during years 4 through 6. For each assessment, the surveys included detailed measures of participants' alcohol use and the other behavioral risks for the previous 3 months. In addition, once annually during years 1 through 4, the students completed 30 days of Web-based daily monitoring about their alcohol use and behavioral risks for the previous day and night. Lastly, smaller samples of students participated in lab-based assessments in each of the first 4 years.

Heavy Drinking Events and Behavioral Risks

In year 4 of the UTE, 150 students who were about to reach the legal drinking age of 21 were recruited to complete laboratory sessions that included a semistructured interview about their 21st birthday celebrations. Because the 21st birthday celebration often involves extreme alcohol consumption (Rutledge, Park, & Sher, 2008), it provides a unique opportunity to examine the association between high levels of intoxication and other behavioral risks. Trained interviewers helped reconstruct a detailed drink-by-time account of the type and amount of alcohol consumed during the individual's 21st birthday celebration. Taking into account the number of standard drinks consumed, the drinking duration, and the individual's weight and gender, we used standard methods to estimate each individual's blood alcohol concentration (eBAC; Mathews & Miller, 1979). At the end of their celebrations, participants reached an average eBAC of .22% (Wetherill & Fromme, 2009).

In addition, we assessed the occurrence of two categories of behaviors: Physical Consequences and Behavioral Risks. Achieving a higher celebration eBAC was associated with experiencing more physical consequences and engaging in more behavioral risks (Brister, Sher, & Fromme, in press). There was also a trend toward lighter drinkers experiencing fewer physical consequences at higher eBAC than heavier drinkers, but this was explained in part by their different types of 21st birthday celebrations. Lighter drinkers were more likely to celebrate in restaurants and with family members, whereas heavier drinkers more likely to celebrate in bars and with friends. Like many other single-event-focused studies, we found mixed evidence for the direct effects of alcohol on specific outcomes and findings further suggest the need to consider moderators (such as drinking history) in event-level analyses.

Daily Monitoring and Event-Level Associations between Alcohol Use and Behavioral Risks

The availability of daily reports allowed us to examine alcohol use and behavioral risks over 30-day periods annually from the first through the fourth years of college. In year 1 of the UTE, 1,654 participants were invited to monitor their drinking from September through May (i.e., not during the summer break). Of these individuals, 67% provided 14 or more days of data, including reports of their drinking and behavioral risks. This yielded a final sample size of 1,113 for a total of 30,224 days of daily monitoring data. Again, using the number of standard drinks consumed, the duration of the drinking event, and the student's gender and weight, we were able to estimate their BACs for each drinking day (Neal & Fromme, 2007). We calculated three measures of BAC: (1) average eBAC, which is the mean eBAC across the student's entire monitoring period; (2) daily eBAC, which reflected an individual's drinking on a given day, expressed as a function of the deviation from his or her average eBAC; and (3) an average eBAC × daily eBAC interaction, which took into account both an individual's average and daily eBAC. Average eBAC allowed us to assess whether heavier drinkers generally engaged in more behavioral risks; Daily eBAC addressed the question of whether drinking more during a given drinking episode increased the likelihood of engaging in behavioral risks; and the average × daily eBAC interaction allowed us to determine whether average consumption moderated the effects of daily drinking on the likelihood of engaging in behavioral risks. This interaction helped determine, for example, whether lighter drinkers were at greater risk than heavier drinkers when they drank more than their typical amount.

Results indicated that heavy drinkers were globally more likely to use drugs, drive after drinking, gamble, and have sex (Neal & Fromme, 2007). Consuming more alcohol put students at greater risk of having unsafe sex or engaging in aggressive behaviors on a given day. Specifically, a 0.01% increase in BAC was associated with a 4% increase in the odds of both unsafe sex and aggression. We also found that lighter drinkers who drank more than usual in an episode were more likely to engage in property crimes and to be either a victim or a perpetrator of sexual assault. Among lighter drinkers, a 0.01% increase in BAC was associated with a 12% increase in the odds of property crime, an 8% increase in sexual assault victimization, and a 10% (for women) or 16% (for men) increase in the odds of sexual assault perpetration. In contrast, that same increase in BAC was associated with smaller increases in the odds of property crime (4%), victimization (5%), and perpetration (5% for women, 12% for men) among heavier drinkers. These results indicated distinct effects of alcohol on different behavioral risks, with the most important findings related to the dangers associated with reaching higher BACs during a given episode, especially for lighter drinkers.

Subjective Response to Alcohol as a Risk Factor for Engaging in Other Behavioral Risks

In addition to the use of objective indices of intoxication, such as eBAC, there is increasing recognition that it is important to consider subjective measures of intoxication (Jackson, Sher, Gotham, & Wood, 2001). Alcohol response varies in the population in both magnitude and quality (Ray, MacKillop, & Monti, 2010), with some individuals subjectively experiencing the effects of alcohol more strongly than others. A lower acute response to alcohol, as measured by self-reported levels of intoxication, body sway, and other biological responses, has been shown to prospectively predict the development of alcohol-related problems (e.g., Schuckit & Smith, 1996). Although response to alcohol has traditionally been studied as a risk factor for the development of alcohol use disorders (see Morean & Corbin, 2010, for a review), recent research from our laboratory suggests that subjective alcohol response may also be another important factor in alcohol-induced behavioral risks.

Using four years of daily monitoring data from 1,867 participants in the UTE, we examined whether subjective response might contribute to behavioral risks at the event level (Quinn & Fromme, 2011). Our findings demonstrated that college students who, on average, experienced greater subjective response to the sedative effects of alcohol were more likely to use illicit drugs, have sex and unsafe sex, and act aggressively when they drank, even accounting for eBAC. Further, during episodes in which they experienced greater than their usual subjective intoxication, college students were more likely to use drugs, have sex, and have unsafe sex. That is, these findings indicate that students who tend to experience greater subjective intoxication relative to their peers (accounting for alcohol consumption as measured by eBAC) are more likely to engage in some behavioral risks, and this likelihood is greater during drinking episodes when students experience higher-than-usual subjective intoxication. Important questions remain, such as whether greater response to the stimulant effects of alcohol would produce similar results, and what drinking contexts produce greater-than-typical subjective response. Nevertheless, these findings suggest that alcohol-induced behavioral risks may be more likely among some students and in some specific contexts. In sum, behavioral risks may be a function not only of how much alcohol a student consumes, but also how strongly he or she responds to alcohol at the time.

CONCLUSIONS

In looking beyond simply how much students drink to the behaviors in which they engage while drinking, event-level research has provided new insights into the potential effect of alcohol on other behavioral risks. For example, our research (Neal & Fromme, 2007) has confirmed laboratory-based experimental findings suggesting that alcohol intoxication contributes to at least some behavioral risks. In particular, intoxicated students appear more likely to engage in aggression and risky sexual behavior, with results from both survey and laboratory methodologies providing support for the causal role of alcohol proposed by attention allocation theory. Further research is needed to determine alcohol's contribution to several other behavioral risks, particularly sexual assault and property crime, although our event-level studies suggest that intoxication may increase the likelihood of both, at least among less experienced drinkers. Finally, illicit drug use, and perhaps some other behavioral risks, appear more common among heavier drinkers, but perhaps not because of alcohol itself. The bulk of the evidence suggests that the use of alcohol and other substances may result in part from common underlying influences, such as impulsivity and other personality traits.

Importantly, however, our findings also suggest that merely examining event-level associations between objective indices of alcohol intoxication (i.e., BAC) and behavioral risks without considering the ways in which feelings of intoxication differ across students and across drinking events may underestimate the role of alcohol. For example, our recent event-level research on students' objective and subjective intoxication has found greater support for alcohol's association with property crime and substance use than have previous studies. Additional research, both event-level and laboratory-based, is needed to parse the unique and interactive effects of BAC and subjective response in helping establish a causal relation between these indices and behavioral risk taking, and to isolate the potential pharmacological or cognitive mechanisms underlying subjective response to alcohol.

IMPLICATIONS FOR COLLEGE PREVENTION

Findings summarized in this chapter have a number of implications for understanding and preventing alcohol-related behavioral risks by college students. Students are more likely to have risky sex (i.e., sex without protection against pregnancy and sexually transmitted infections) and act aggressively when they are intoxicated than when sober. Thus prevention efforts might focus on helping students make sexual decisions before they begin drinking—whether that decision is to have sex or not, or to ensure that proper protection is planned. Emotion-control strategies for managing feelings might also help diminish the occurrence of alcohol-related aggression. The additional association between alcohol intoxication and sexual assault indicates that prevention programs should incorporate alcohol use as a common risk factor for risky sex, aggression, and sexual assault.

Second, the primary focus of most college alcohol prevention programs tends to be on how much or how often students drink. Whereas frequency of binge drinking is clearly associated with a variety of negative outcomes (e.g. Wechsler, Dowdall, Maenner, Glendhill-Hoyt, & Lee, 1998), our findings also emphasize the importance of subjective feelings of intoxication in addition to absolute levels of alcohol use when attempting to intervene on alcohol-related behavioral risks. Regardless of how objectively intoxicated students may be (i.e., BAC level), their perceived level of impairment may be a critical determinant of their engagement in behavioral risks. Therefore both students' objective measures of drinking (i.e., how much and how frequently they drink) as well as their subjective feelings of intoxication should be addressed by college prevention programs.

Lastly, many college programs emphasize universal approaches to prevention, meaning that their programs are administered to groups of students regardless of the students' alcohol use patterns. For example, many programs are provided during new student orientation, or to all freshmen, student-athletes, or members of fraternities and sororities. These programs are often not prepared to deal with students who drink lightly. Unless an abstinence-only approach is taken, the students who drink lightly are already consuming alcohol at low, infrequent, and/or safer levels. In this case, teaching moderation skills would not seem relevant or appropriate. Findings we presented, however, indicate that these students who drink lightly face significant risks on the rare occasions when they exceed their typical levels of consumption. Consequently, universal prevention programs might incorporate models to educate light drinkers about the greater risks they experience (e.g., being a victim or perpetrator of sexual assault) whenever they reach higher levels of intoxication than they typically do.

In sum, college prevention programs might be expanded to address (1) alcohol use as a common risk factor for risky sex, aggression, and sexual assault; (2) both objective (i.e., amount and frequency of drinking) and subjective (i.e., feelings of intoxication) indices of drinking; and (3) the substantial risks that those who drink lightly might experience whenever they deviate from their otherwise safer patterns of consumption. By building upon empirically based findings about alcohol intoxication and subjective feelings of intoxication, prevention programs could be expanded to better address the association between drinking alcohol and experiencing other behavioral risks among college students.

REFERENCES

Abbey, A. (1991). Acquaintance rape and alcohol consumption on college campuses: How are they linked? *College Health, 39,* 165–169.

Abbey, A., Zawacki, T., Buck, P. O., Clinton, A. M., & McAuslan, P. (2004). Sexual assault and alcohol consumption: What do we know about their relationship and what types of research are still needed? *Aggression and Violent Behavior: A Review Journal, 9,* 271–303.

Brister, H. A., Sher, K. J., & Fromme, K. (in press). *21st birthday drinking and associated physical consequences and behavioral risks.*

Bushman, B. J., & Cooper, H. M. (1990). Effects of alcohol on human aggression: An integrative research review. *Psychological Bulletin, 107,* 341–354.

Casbon, T. S., Curtin, J. J., Lang, A. R., & Patrick, C. J. (2003). Deleterious effects of alcohol intoxication: Diminished cognitive control and its behavioral consequences. *Journal of Abnormal Psychology, 112,* 476–487.

Chassin, L., Pitts, S. C., & Prost, J. (2002). Binge drinking trajectories from adolescence to emerging adulthood in a high-risk sample: Predictors and substance abuse outcomes. *Journal of Consulting and Clinical Psychology, 70,* 67–78.

Chermack, S. T., & Taylor, S. P. (1995). Alcohol and human physical aggression: Pharmacological versus expectancy effects. *Journal of Studies on Alcohol, 56,* 449–456.

Cooper, M. L., (2002). Alcohol use and risky sexual behavior among college students and youth: Evaluating the evidence. *Journal of Studies on Alcohol*(Suppl. 14), 101–117.

Cooper, M. L. (2006). Does drinking promote risky sexual behavior? A complex answer to a simple question. *Current Directions in Psychological Science, 15,* 19–23.

Cooper, M. L. (2010). Toward a person x situation model of sexual risk-taking behaviors: Illuminating the conditional effects of traits across sexual situations and relationship contexts. *Journal of Personality and Social Psychology, 98,* 319–341.

Cooper, M. L., Peirce, R. S., & Huselid, R. F. (1994). Substance use and sexual risk-taking among black adolescents and white adolescents. *Health Psychology, 13,* 251–262.

Cooper, M. L., Wood, P. K., Orcutt, H. K., & Albino, A. (2003). Personality and the predisposition to engage in risky or problem behaviors during adolescence. *Journal of Personality and Social Psychology, 84,* 390–410.

Corbin, W. R., & Fromme, K. (2002). Alcohol use and serial monogamy as risk for sexually transmitted diseases in young adults. *Health Psychology, 21,* 229–236.

Curtin, J. J., & Fairchild, B. A. (2003). Alcohol and cognitive control: Implications for regulation of behavior during response conflict. *Journal of Abnormal Psychology, 112,* 424–436.

Davis, K. C., Hendershot, C. S., George, W. H., Norris, J., & Heiman, J. R. (2007). Alcohol's effects on sexual decision making: An integration of alcohol myopia and individual differences. *Journal of Studies on Alcohol and Drugs, 68,* 843–851.

Dermen, K. H., & Cooper, M. L. (1994). Sex-related alcohol expectancies among adolescents: II. Prediction of drinking in social and sexual situations. *Psychology of Addictive Behaviors, 8,* 161–168.

Dermen, K. H., Cooper, M. L., & Agocha, V.B . (1998). Sex-related alcohol expectancies and moderators of the relationship between alcohol use and risky sex in adolescents. *Journal of Studies on Alcohol, 59,* 71–77.

Ebel-Lam, A. P., MacDonald, T. K., Zanna, M. P., & Fong, G. T. (2009). An experimental investigation of the interactive effects of alcohol and sexual arousal on intentions to have unprotected sex. *Basic and Applied Social Psychology, 31,* 226–233.

Fromme, K., Corbin, W. R., & Kruse, M. I. (2008). Behavioral risks during the transition from high school to college. *Developmental Psychology, 44,* 1497–1504.

Fromme, K., D'Amico, E. J., & Katz, E. C. (1999). Intoxicated sexual risk-taking: An expectancy or cognitive impairment explanation? *Journal of Studies on Alcohol, 60,* 54–63.

Fromme, K., Katz, E., & D'Amico, E. J. (1997a). Effects of alcohol intoxication on the perceived consequences of risk taking. *Experimental and Clinical Psychopharmacology, 5,* 14–23.

Fromme, K., Katz, E., & Rivet, K. (1997b). Outcome expectancies and risk-taking behavior. *Cognitive Therapy and Research, 21,* 421–442.

Giancola, P. R., Josephs, R. A., Parrott, D. J., & Duke, A. A. (2010). Alcohol myopia revisited: Clarifying aggression and other acts of disinhibition through a distorted lens. *Perspectives on Psychological Science, 5,* 265–278.

Hingson, R. W., Strunin, L., Berlin, B. M., & Heeren, T. (1990). Beliefs about AIDS, use of alcohol and drugs, and unprotected sex among Massachusetts adolescents. *American Journal of Public Health, 80,* 295–299.

Hingson, R., Zha, W., & Weitzman, E. R. (2009). Magnitude of and trends in alcohol-related mortality and morbidity among U.S. college students ages 18–24, 1998–2005. *Journal of Studies on Alcohol and Drugs*(Suppl. 16), 12–20.

Hoaken, P. N. S., Assaad, J., & Pihl, R. O. (1998a). Cognitive functioning and the inhibition of alcohol-induced aggression. *Journal of Studies on Alcohol, 59*, 599–607.

Hoaken, P. N. S., Giancola, P. R., & Pihl, R. O. (1998b). Executive cognitive functions as mediators of alcohol-related aggression. *Alcohol & Alcoholism, 33*, 47–54.

Ito, T. A., Miller, N., & Pollock, V. E. (1996). Alcohol and aggression: A meta-analysis on the moderating effects of inhibitory cues, triggering events, and self-focused attention. *Psychological Bulletin, 120*, 60–82.

Jackson, K. M., Sher, K. J., Gotham, H. J, & Wood, P. K. (2001). Transitioning into and out of large-effect drinking in young adulthood. *Journal of Abnormal Psychology, 110*, 378–391.

Jackson, K. M., Sher, K. J., & Schulenberg, J. E. (2008). Conjoint developmental trajectories of young adult substance use. *Alcoholism: Clinical and Experimental Research, 32*, 723–737.

Jessor, R., & Jessor, S. L. (1977). *Problem behavior and psychosocial development.* New York: Academic Press.

Jochman, K. A., & Fromme, K. (2010). Maturing out of substance use: The other side of etiology. In L. M. Scheier (Ed.), *Handbook of drug use etiology* (pp. 565–578). Washington, DC: American Psychological Association.

Johnston, L. D., O'Malley, P. M., Bachman, J. G., & Schulenberg, J. (2009). *Monitoring the future national survey results on drug use, 1975–2008: Vol. 2. College students and adults ages 19–50* (NIIH Publication No. 09-7403). Bethesda, MD: National Institute on Drug Abuse.

Jones, B. T., Corbin, W., & Fromme, K. (2001). A review of expectancy theory and alcohol consumption. *Addiction, 96*, 57–72.

Leigh, B. C. (1993). Alcohol consumption and sexual activity as reported with a diary technique. *Journal of Abnormal Psychology, 102*, 490–493.

Leigh, B. C., & Stahl, R. (1993). Substance use and risky sexual behavior for exposure to HIV. *American Psychologist, 48*, 1035–1045.

MacDonald, T. K., MacDonald, G., Zanna, M. P., & Fong, G. T. (2000). Alcohol, sexual arousal, and intentions to use condoms in young men: Applying alcohol myopia theory to risky sexual behavior. *Health Psychology, 19*, 290–298.

Mathews, D. B., & Miller, W. R. (1979). Estimating blood alcohol concentration: Two computer programs and their applications in therapy and research. *Addictive Behaviors, 4*, 55–60.

Mohler-Kuo, M., Lee, J. E., & Wechsler, H. (2003). Trends in marijuana and other illicit drug use among college students: Results from 4 Harvard School of Public Health College Alcohol Study Surveys: 1993–2001. *Journal of American College Health, 52*, 17–24.

Morean, M. E., & Corbin, W. R. (2010). Subjective response to alcohol: A critical review of the literature. *Alcoholism: Clinical and Experimental Research, 34*, 385–395.

Morris, A. B., & Albery, I. P. (2001). Alcohol consumption and HIV risk behaviours: Integrating the theories of alcohol myopia and outcome expectancies. *Addiction Research and Theory, 9*, 73–86.

Neal, D. J., & Fromme, K. (2007). Event-level covariation of alcohol intoxication and behavioral risks during the first year of college. *Journal of Consulting and Clinical Psychology, 75,* 294–306.

O'Leary, A., Goodhart, F., Jemmott, L., & Boccher-Lattimore, D. (1992). Predictors of safer sex on the college campus: A social cognitive theory analysis. *Journal of American College Health, 40,* 254–263.

Parks, K. A. (2000). An event-based analysis of aggression women experience in bars. *Psychology of Addictive Behaviors, 14,* 102–110.

Parrott, D. J., & Zeichner, A. (2002). Effects of alcohol and trait anger on physical aggression in men. *Journal of Studies on Alcohol, 63,* 196–204.

Patel, A., & Fromme, K. (2010). Explicit outcome expectancies and substance use: Current research and future directions. In L. M. Scheier (Ed.), *Handbook of drug use etiology* (pp. 565–578). Washington, DC: American Psychological Association.

Quigley, B. M., & Leonard, K. E. (2000). Alcohol and the continuation of early marital aggression. *Alcoholism: Clinical and Experimental Research, 24,* 1003–1010.

Quinn, P. D., & Fromme, K. (2011). Predictors and outcomes of variability in subjective alcohol intoxication among college students: An event-level analysis across four years. *Alcoholism: Clinical and Experimental Research, 35,* 484–495.

Ray, L. A., MacKillop, J., & Monti, P. M. (2010). Subjective responses to alcohol consumption as endophenotypes: Advancing behavioral genetics in etiological and treatment models of alcoholism. *Substance Use and Misuse, 45,* 1742–1765.

Rutledge, P. C., Park, A., & Sher, K. J. (2008). 21st birthday drinking: Extremely extreme. *Journal of Consulting and Clinical Psychology, 76,* 511–516.

Schuckit, M. A., & Smith, T. L. (1996). An 8-year follow-up of 450 sons of alcoholic and control subjects. *Archives of General Psychiatry, 53,* 202–210.

Scott, K. D., Schafer, J., & Greenfield, T. K. (1999). The role of alcohol in physical assault perpetration and victimization. *Journal of Studies on Alcohol, 60*(4), 528–536.

Stappenbeck, C. A., & Fromme, K. (2010). A longitudinal investigation of heavy drinking and physical dating violence in men and women. *Addictive Behaviors, 35,* 479–485.

Steele, C. M., & Josephs, R. A. (1990). Alcohol myopia: Its prized and dangerous effects. *American Psychologist, 45,* 921–933.

Substance Abuse and Mental Health Services Administration. (2008). *Results from the 2007 National Survey on Drug Use and Health: National findings* (DHHS Publication No. SMA 08-4343). Rockville, MD: Author.

Swahn, M. H., & Donovan, J. E. (2004). Correlates and predictors of violent behavior among adolescent drinkers. *Journal of Adolescent Health, 34,* 480–492.

Testa, M. (2002). The impact of men's alcohol consumption on perpetration of sexual aggression. *Clinical Psychology Review, 22,* 1239–1263.

Testa, M., & Collins, R. L. (1997). Alcohol and risky sexual behavior: Event-based analyses among a sample of high-risk women. *Psychology of Addictive Behaviors, 11,* 190–201.

Wechsler, H., Dowdall, G. W., Maenner, G., Glendhill-Hoyt, J., & Lee, H. (1998). Changes in binge drinking and related problems among American college students between 1993 and 1997. *Journal of American College Health, 47,* 57–68.

Wetherill, R. R., & Fromme, K. (2009). Subjective responses to alcohol prime event-specific consumption and negative consequences. *Journal of Studies on Alcohol and Drugs, 70,* 593–600.

White, H. R., Jackson, K., & Loeber, R. (2009). Developmental sequences and comorbidity of substance use and violence. In M. D. Krohn, A. J. Lizotte, & G. P. Hall (Eds.), *Handbook on crime and deviance* (pp. 433–46). New York: Springer.

Young, S. E., Friedman, N. P., Miyake, A., Willcutt, E. G., Corley, R. P., Haberstick, B. C., et al. (2009). Behavioral disinhibition: Liability for externalizing spectrum disorders and its genetic and environmental relation to response inhibition across adolescence. *Journal of Abnormal Psychology, 118,* 117–130.

Zuckerman, M. (1979). Risk-taking activities. In C. E. Izard (Ed.), *Emotions in personality and psychopathology* (pp. 163–197). New York: Plenum Press.

CHAPTER 7

Personality and Contextual Factors in College Students' Drinking

Alvaro Vergés *and* Kenneth J. Sher

In the United States, the college years represent the period of life most strongly associated with heavy alcohol consumption and with alcohol use disorders (Dawson, Grant, Stinson, & Chou, 2004; Grant, 1997). While many high school students drink heavily prior to arriving on college campuses, a large proportion of collegiate binge drinkers initiate bingeing during college (Weitzman, Nelson, & Wechsler, 2003).

The most representative estimates of the prevalence of various college student drinking behaviors come from several studies conducted with national data sets in which the data were collected either specifically from college students (e.g., the College Alcohol Study [CAS; Wechsler, Davenport, Dowdall, Moeykens, & Castillo, 1994; Wechsler, Lee, Kuo, & Lee, 2000; Wechsler & Nelson, 2008]) or more generally from college-age young adults (e.g., Monitoring the Future [MTF; Johnston, O'Malley, & Bachman, 2002]). Numerous other studies have collected data at the individual institution level. Although the results of these studies are less generalizable, they often provide more extensive assessments of drinking and its correlates than national studies and thus remain valuable.

The present chapter provides an overview of the environmental and individual factors that increase the risk of heavy drinking during college. Data from the national studies are examined, along with our own data collected in two long-term longitudinal studies. The first one is the Alcohol, Health, and Behavior Project (AHB; see Sher, Walitzer, Wood, & Brent, 1991, for more details), a prospective study of 489 students (46% male, mean age = 18.2 years) who were freshmen in 1987. This sample consisted of roughly equal numbers of students who were either family history positive for paternal alcoholism (i.e., had alcoholic fathers) or family history negative (i.e., had no first- or second-degree relatives with alcoholism). Participants in the AHB study were assessed seven times over 16 years with a retention rate of 78% at year 16. The second study is the Intensive, Multivariate, Prospective Alcohol College-Transitions Study (IMPACTS; see Sher & Rutledge, 2007, for a detailed description). IMPACTS is a longitudinal study initiated in the summer prior to matriculation in the fall semester of 2002. Participants in IMPACTS included 3,720 first-time freshmen (88.0% of the original precollege sampling frame at a large midwestern university). In addition to a paper-and-pencil survey administered in the summer prior to their freshman year, all IMPACTS participants were invited to participate in semiannual Web-based surveys administered toward the end of the fall and spring semesters.

ENVIRONMENTAL FACTORS PREDICTING DRINKING

As Shore and colleagues (Shore, Rivers, & Berman, 1983) suggest, campus life may be so isolated from the "real world" that the campus environment is as important as (or more important than) personal background variables in predicting drinking. There are a number of environmental factors associated with college drinking that vary both across and within college campuses (Presley, Mcilman, & Leichliter, 2002). The CAS indicated that rates of heavy episodic drinking at 140 colleges ranged from 1% to 70% in 1993 (Wechsler et al., 1994), suggesting that campuses differ greatly from one another in terms of alcohol use, and likely differ in terms of risk factors for and consequences of heavy drinking. Not surprisingly, what constitutes a college environment is increasingly difficult to describe (Presley et al., 2002) because of heterogeneity both across campuses (intercampus differences) and within campuses (intracampus). Presley et al. (2002) suggest that colleges are part of a number of "supra" environments that are constantly changing. Note, however, that across four CAS reports from 1993 to 2001, the rates of binge drinking have remained relatively stable (Wechsler et al., 2002), and these findings are echoed in the MTF (Johnston, O'Malley, Bachman, & Schulenberg, 2009). This consistency has occurred despite the fact that there have been major changes in the profile of typical college attendees and campus environments, with more nontraditional and ethnically diverse students, more off-campus housing, and more influential local outlets adjacent to campus than in the past (Presley et al., 2002).

In this section, we address some of the environmental factors that lead to intercampus differences.

Type of College

Smaller institutions, as defined by the number of students, tend to have higher rates of weekly drinking than larger institutions (Presley et al., 2002). Further, greater social capital (e.g., social resources and volunteer services) in an institution has been associated with less alcohol use (Weitzman & Chen, 2005). Data from the CORE Institute (Presley, Meilman, & Cashin, 1996) show that schools with higher heavy drinking rates tend to have more fraternity housing and more students belonging to a fraternity or sorority, compared to schools with lower heavy drinking rates (Presley et al., 2002). In contrast, the difference in consumption between public and private campuses appears to be minimal (Wechsler et al., 2000).

In general, schools with higher rates of students living on campus have higher heavy drinking rates (Presley et al., 2002). Greater ethnic diversity is associated with lower binge-drinking rates among white students (Wechsler & Kuo, 2003). Consumption and heavy drinking at historically black institutions are lower than at predominately white institutions (Meilman, Presley, & Cashin, 1995), even when controlling for sex, proportion of students who are in Greek organizations, and proportion of students living on campus (Presley et al., 2002). Even white students at historically black schools had lower levels of alcohol consumption and heavy drinking than those in traditional university settings (Meilman et al., 1995), and Debro (1991) observed that black students at black institutions drank less than black students at traditional universities. In addition, Meilman et al. (1995) observed fewer alcohol-related consequences at the black institutions. It is unclear whether the protective influence of historically black colleges is due to aspects of the culture at those institutions (e.g., focus on spirituality, less disposable income, sense of purpose, pressure to succeed; Crowley, 1991) or whether those who choose to attend black colleges (including white students) are characteristically less heavy drinkers.

Presley et al. (2002) observed inconsistency in the relationship between consumption and attendance at women's colleges versus coeducational colleges, noting that the consumption rates for women at six women's colleges did not look very different than those for women attending coeducational institutions.

Class Schedule

Despite the increasing trend toward distance learning and technologies that reduce the reliance on traditional classroom instruction (National Center for Education Statistics, 2003), classroom instruction remains a key structural aspect of the college experience and there is considerable variation in class schedules across schools. In principle, class schedules could serve to either promote or inhibit college student drinking. It is often noted that the weekend begins on Thursday (the "thirsty Thursday" phenomenon) on many college campuses, adding another potential heavy drinking day to the drinking patterns of students. Wood, Sher, and Rutledge (2007) recently found that there was excessive drinking on Thursday, relative to other weekdays, and that this was, in fact, strongly moderated by Friday class schedule. Students with no Friday classes drank approximately twice as much on Thursdays as students with early Friday classes. Extensive analyses conducted over eight consecutive semesters of the IMPACTS study indicated that this effect could not be fully explained by selection (although heavier-drinking students did tend to avoid early Friday morning classes), suggesting that the absence of early classes is an environmental risk factor for drinking. Importantly, this potential risk factor is highly modifiable.

College Residence

The transition from living at home with parents to living in a student residence (e.g., dormitory; off-campus housing without parents) is characteristic of the passage from adolescence into young adulthood (Maggs, 1997) and is associated with an increase in alcohol use. As such, although this transition is a time of growth and opportunity, it is also a time of vulnerability to a high-risk environment (Maggs, 1997). According to a number of studies using national data, data from individual institutions, or community samples (e.g., Gfroerer, Greenblatt, & Wright, 1997; Harford & Muthen, 2001; Harford, Wechsler, & Muthen, 2002; O'Hare, 1990; White et al., 2006, but see Globetti, Stern, Marasco, & Haworth-Hoeppner, 1988), those students living on campus were more likely to drink and to report binge drinking and less likely to abstain than those living off campus with parents, even when the studies controlled for age, sex, and race (e.g., Gfroerer et al., 1997). Those living independently off campus tended to fall somewhere in between but frequently were not statistically different from those living on campus.

Harford and Muthen (2001) specifically examined change in drinking as a function of change in residence over a 3-year period using National Longitudinal Survey of Youth (NLSY) data. Students living in residence halls or in independent off-campus living arrangements showed elevations in heavy drinking, while those living off campus with their parents showed no such growth. In addition, a change to a dormitory or independent off-campus living arrangement from living off campus with parents was associated with an increase in subsequent drinking, indicating the powerful influence of the college environment. This finding is consistent with findings showing a clear increase in heavy drinking between high school and college (Baer, Kivlahan, & Marlatt, 1995; Johnston et al., 2009). Baer (1994) suggested that living situations during the first year in college may promote certain social processes; however, his study failed to identify differences in perceptions about drinking between students living in dormitory housing and those living off campus. (Perhaps this was because students living in independent off-campus housing were grouped with students who were living off campus with their parents.) Although the above work certainly is consistent with the idea of the college environment as a risk factor, Harford et al. (2002) also demonstrated that students who had been heavy drinkers in high school were more likely to live in coeducational residence halls or independently off campus, supporting a selection effect as well. However, Harford and Muthen (2001) failed to find support for residence as a mediator of the relationship between prior (high school) problem behaviors and college drinking, suggesting the housing effect is not merely indexing a selection effect. Thus, existing data suggest that not only do higher-risk students self-select into residence halls, but there is an additional influence of residence beyond this selection (a finding we also see with regard to membership in Greek organizations as discussed below).

Greek System

Involvement in Greek social organizations has been thought to be among the strongest risk factors in college drinking. More extensive alcohol use among fraternity and sorority members compared with other students has been well documented across various measures of alcohol involvement. A substantial body of research on multicampus samples has consistently reported a higher proportion of drinkers among fraternity and sorority members (Engs, Diebold, & Hanson, 1996; Wechsler, Kuh, & Davenport, 1996), as well as a higher quantity of alcohol consumption (Alva, 1998; Cashin, Presley, & Meilman, 1998; Engs et al., 1996), a higher frequency of drinking (Alva, 1998), a higher proportion of heavy drinkers (Cashin et al., 1998; Engs et al., 1996; Wechsler et al., 1996), and a higher proportion of frequent heavy drinkers (Wechsler et al., 1996; McCabe et al., 2005) than among students who were not involved in Greek organizations. Also, Greek members report more negative consequences from alcohol use (Cashin et al., 1998; Engs et al., 1996), and higher rates of alcohol use disorders (Knight et al., 2002) than non-Greek members.

Using longitudinal data from MTF, McCabe et al. (2005) found that fraternity and sorority members increased their frequency of binge drinking at a higher rate than students not involved in the Greek system. Moreover, rates of binge drinking tracked membership in the Greek system over time, such that Greek members who became inactive later during college experienced a decrease in alcohol use. Wechsler et al. (2002) found that Greek members and Greek house residents remained the groups most at risk for heavy drinking compared with other residence groups despite significant decreases in the proportion of heavy drinkers among these groups over time. Also, Weitzman et al. (2003) found that involvement in the Greek system predicted initiation of binge drinking among first-year students. Moreover, using IMPACTS data, Park, Sher, and Krull (2008) found that changes in Greek status were associated with changes in alcohol-related environmental factors (peer norms and alcohol availability), as well as changes in alcohol use behaviors. As shown in Figure 7.1, students who were involved in the Greek system across the 3 years (i.e., constant Greeks) tended to experience a steeper increase in heavy drinking, alcohol consequences, and peer drinking norms compared to individuals who never joined the Greek system (i.e., constant non-Greeks). Also, late joiners tended to increase more in measures of drinking when compared to constant non-Greeks, suggesting that alcohol involvement tracks Greek status over time (Park et al., 2008).

Not all Greek members, however, are involved in risky alcohol use, and there are considerable differences in drinking behaviors among Greek members. Specifically, gender differences in drinking that are consistently found in the general population (e.g., Wilsnack, Vogeltanz, Wilsnack, & Harris, 2000) are also found within the Greek population, such that sorority members are less likely to be involved in risky alcohol use than fraternity members (Alva, 1998; Harrington, Brigham, & Clayton, 1997). Also, differences in drinking behaviors as a function of aspects of Greek life have been documented, including residence in a Greek house (Wechsler et al., 1996) and the house's reputation for alcohol consumption (Larimer, Irvine, Kilmer, & Marlatt, 1997). Moreover, Greek house leaders have been found to report more alcohol use than other members (Cashin et al., 1998). However, it is noteworthy that in the AHB study, the ostensible effect of Greek involvement on heavy drinking during the college years did not persist 3 and 7 years after college (Bartholow, Sher, & Krull, 2003; Sher, Bartholow, & Nanda, 2001), suggesting that the Greek effect is limited to college years and tends to disappear as individuals mature out of heavy drinking (Littlefield, Sher, & Wood, 2009).

Interestingly, entering freshmen who reported their intention to join a fraternity or sorority showed higher levels of alcohol involvement (Can-

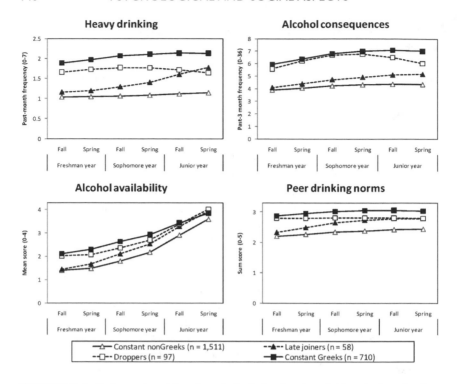

FIGURE 7.1. Estimated trajectories of alcohol-related variables during the first six semesters of college as a function of Greek status. Adapted from Park, Sher, and Krull (2008). Copyright 2008 by the American Psychological Association. Adapted by permission.

terbury et al., 1992; Werner & Greene, 1992) and higher negative consequences of drinking (Read, Wood, Davidoff, McLacken, & Campbell, 2002) when compared with other students who did not intend to join a fraternity or sorority. Similarly, O'Connor, Cooper, and Thiel (1996) found that freshmen who consumed alcohol in high quantities were more likely to pledge fraternities than students who drank lower quantities. These findings indicate a selection effect; that is, those students who are already involved in heavy drinking tend to seek out Greek affiliations. In addition, other researchers have found evidence of a socialization effect of Greek affiliation on alcohol involvement. For instance, Lo and Globetti (1993) found that involvement in a fraternity or sorority was one of the strongest predictors of initiating drinking during college among individuals who abstained during their senior year of high school. Several other studies have suggested that both selection and socialization causal effects of Greek affiliation are operating in drinking among Greek members (Baer et al., 1995; Park, Sher, & Krull, 2009a; Wechsler et al., 1996). For example, using multilevel data analysis to account for variability across residence units in the IMPACTS sample, Park, Sher, and Krull (2009a) investigated the self-selection and socialization effects of type of residence on drinking. Our findings showed a robust selection effect among women; that is, self-reported precollege binge drinking (i.e., frequency of five or more drinks per occasion) strongly predicted entering into the sorority system, even after controlling for selection into specific residence halls, college attendance motives, and cigarette use. A selection effect among men was also found that could be statistically accounted for by college attendance motives such as partying, dating/mating, edification, career, sports, and extracurricular activities. This implies that incoming students appear to seek out environments that facilitate the continuation or escalation of existing drinking behaviors and associated activities. Importantly, socialization effects were found among both men and women, with fraternity and sorority residents showing a higher increase in the frequency of binge drinking when compared to non-Greek individuals. However, this effect was stronger among individuals with lower levels of heavy drinking.

Given that there appear to be meaningful socialization effects, what specific factors within the Greek system predict future drinking? That is, how is the "Greek influence" on drinking transmitted? Clearly there are distinct aspects of the environment (Kodman & Sturmak, 1984) and culture (Kuh & Arnold, 1993) of Greek organizations (such as the role of alcohol in bonding processes and social pressure) that promote drinking. In addition, variables such as on-premise alcohol availability (especially in the freshman year; Park et al., 2008) and high rates of "fake ID" acquisition (Martinez, Rutledge, & Sher, 2007) facilitate the likelihood of obtaining alcohol. These environmental variables clearly affect drinking-relevant cognitions such as higher perceived peer norms for drinking (Baer, 1994; Baer, Stacy, & Larimer, 1991), higher positive alcohol expectancies (Alva, 1998; Cashin et al., 1998; Wechsler et al., 1996), and lower perceived risk of drinking (Tampke, 1990). Nevertheless, individual factors are also important, as discussed below.

INDIVIDUAL FACTORS PREDICTING DRINKING

Personality

The association between drinking and personality in college students is largely consistent with the broader literature (see Littlefield & Sher, 2010; Sher, Trull, Bartholow, & Vieth, 1999, for a review of this literature). Specifically, personality traits related to impulsivity/disinhibition appear to be robust correlates of both drinking and drinking problems, and traits related to neuroticism/negative emotionality are often, but inconsistently, associated with problematic alcohol involvement (Baer, 2002; Baer et al., 1995; Brennan, Walfish, & AuBuchon, 1986; Pullen, 1994; Schall, Weede, & Maltzman, 1991; Sher, Wood, Crews, & Vandiver, 1995). Although the relation between normal-range neuroticism/negative affectivity and problematic alcohol involvement is variable in existing studies, it appears that extremely high levels of negative affectivity are associated with drinking problems. For example, in the AHB study a diagnosis of alcohol abuse or dependence was nearly twice as likely among students with an anxiety disorder (Kushner & Sher, 1993). Also consistent with the broader literature, the association between consumption and extraversion/sociability has generally been weak (Baer, 2002). Those who are more sociable may be more likely to drink but are not more likely to experience alcohol-related problems (Baer, 2002).

With regard to alcohol dependence symptomatology, Grekin, Sher, and Wood (2006) analyzed data from IMPACTS using a well-validated five-factor model of personality (Costa & McCrae, 1992) and additional personality measures. Results indicated that novelty seeking and neuroticism predicted alcohol, drug, and tobacco dependence symptoms. These findings are consistent with previous research showing associations of substance use disorders with both disinhibition/impulsivity and neuroticism/negative affectivity (Sher et al., 1999). Moreover, alcohol symptomatology was also uniquely predicted by low openness to experience and by extraversion. These findings suggest that beyond a common vulnerability to diverse forms of substance use, additional factors may help us to understand specific forms of substance dependence.

Drinking Motives and Expectancies

The college student literature examining the association between alcohol involvement and alcohol expectancies and drinking motives also parallels the general literature (for a review, see Goldman, Darkes, & Del Boca, 1999). In general, research on college students has supported two motives for drinking: drinking for social purposes and drinking for escape or relief (Baer, 2002; Brennan et al., 1986). Cronin (1997) noted that social motives were more likely to predict consumption, whereas mood enhancement motives were more likely to predict alcohol problems and problem drinking. Similarly, Brown (1985) found that social drinkers expect social enhancement from alcohol, whereas problem drinkers expect tension reduction.

Regardless of the nature of the outcome expected from alcohol's effects, positive expectancies are more predictive of drinking than negative expectancies (Leigh & Stacy, 1993), and heavier drinkers report more positive expectancies (Leigh, 1987). Consistent with this finding, Wood, Sher, and Strathman (1996) found that when college students were asked to generate expectancies about the effects of alcohol, more positive expectancies were generated by those with more, compared to fewer, alcohol dependence symptoms. Moreover, in the AHB study, Sher, Wood, Wood, and Raskin (1996) found that positive expectancies predicted and were predicted by alcohol use in a 3-year period in which expectancies decreased while alcohol use remained stable. (For greater detail on expectancies, see Reich & Goldman, Chapter 5, this volume.)

PERSON–ENVIRONMENT CORRELATION AND INTERACTION

There are multiple mechanisms through which personality might be related to alcohol use. One of those mechanisms that may have relevant implications for college drinking is environment selection. Using data from IMPACTS, Park, Sher, Wood, and Krull (2009b) indicated that selection into the Greek system was strongly influenced by personality traits. As shown in Figure 7.2, some of these traits (i.e., novelty seeking) were directly related to precollege heavy alcohol use (measured by the frequency of having 12 or more drinks in a single sitting in the last 30 days), whereas other traits (i.e., extraversion and neuroticism) were not. However, the latter traits predicted Greek affiliation at college, which in turn predicted both heavy drinking at the first semester and a linear increase in heavy drinking over the following 3 years of college. This implies that extraversion and neuroticism promoted selection into the Greek system among individuals without heavy precollege alcohol use. However, those individuals entered an environment that increased their risk for developing heavy drinking during college (also measured by the frequency of having 12 or more drinks in a single sitting). Thus, when considering personality-based selection into heavy drinking environments, it is important to consider the multiple facets of that environment. While the Greek system is associated with heavy drinking and poses a significant environmental risk factor, it is also associated with prosocial activities, such as campus and community service, and it offers a range of opportunities for socialization. Thus, individuals can select into this environment for diverse (and multiple) reasons.

Overall, personality traits may interact with environmental factors in predicting heavy drinking. For example, Grekin and Sher (2006) analyzed data from IMPACTS, finding that an interaction between Greek status and behavioral undercontrol predicted dependence symptoms. The

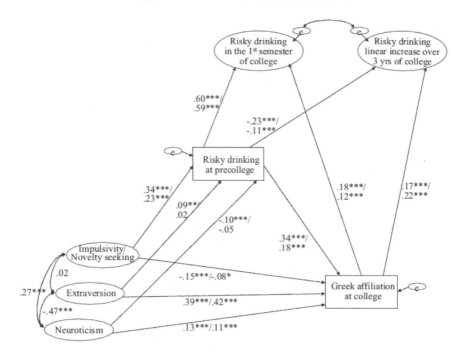

FIGURE 7.2. Latent growth model characterizing personality-based self-selection into Greek systems, mediated by precollege risky drinking. Numbers on the left side of the slash are estimates for a model of 5 or more drinks; numbers on the right are for 12 or more drinks. The effects of three personality traits on college drinking growth factors and the effects of sex on all variables in the models were controlled for (paths are not shown). The circled letter *e* indicates an error term (i.e., residual variance). $^*p < .05$; $^{**}p < .01$; $^{***}p < .001$. From Park, Sher, Wood, and Krull (2009b). Copyright 2009 by the American Psychological Association. Reprinted by permission.

pattern of the interaction was such that the association between behavioral undercontrol and number of symptoms of dependence was stronger among Greek members than among nonmembers. Moreover, Park, Sher, and Krull (2006) studied the interaction between public and private self-consciousness (i.e., the trait of attending to private aspects of the self) and Greek status in the AHB sample. Their results showed that sorority members were more likely to increase their drinking when private self-consciousness increased, whereas fraternity members increased their drinking when private and public self-consciousness decreased. These results demonstrate that there are identifiable differences among students in their susceptibility to Greek influence. These results resemble interactions between personality and environment found in other populations (e.g., Hill et al., 2010).

SUMMARY AND CONCLUSIONS

Epidemiological data indicate that the college years, a period in the life course referred to as "emerging adulthood" (Arnett, 2004), represents the time in the life cycle most associated with heavy alcohol consumption and alcohol-related problems. Within this period of life, those attending traditional 4-year residential campuses appear to be at particularly high risk for heavy alcohol involvement and alcohol problems. Among those attending college, students involved in the Greek system appear to be at the highest risk. While much of the risk associated with Greek involvement appears to be attributable to selection of heavier drinkers into the Greek system, there appear to be nontrivial socialization effects of being in the Greek system that occur early in the course of affiliation but persist over the course of college (Park, Sher, Wood, & Krull, 2009b). It is important to note that, in addition to precollege drinking, there are personality-based selection biases into the Greek system due to multiple appeals of Greek life. However, individuals affiliating with the Greek system for reasons independent of alcohol-related motivation are still at situational risk for excessive drinking and alcohol-related problems. While the effects of Greek affiliation do not tend to persist following disaffiliation (Park et al., 2008) or graduation (Bartholow et al., 2003; Sher et al., 2001), acute harms associated with excessive consumption mean that we still need to take this subpopulation seriously.

It is important to bear in mind that the primary mission of colleges and universities is to educate students via a specified curriculum. Surprisingly, the effects of structural aspects of the curriculum on drinking have not received much empirical attention. We have shown that the "thirsty Thursday" phenomenon is due, in part, to the permissive class scheduling that accommodates heavy drinking during the week. Based in part on these findings, a number of campuses have attempted to promote the offering of early Friday morning classes (e.g., University of Iowa; see Vu, 2007; National Institute on Alcohol Abuse and Alcoholism, 2007), although we are not aware of a formal evaluation of these policy interventions. Such evaluations would be extremely valuable and would provide an evidence base for this type of policy change.

Environmental manipulations can take other forms as well. Risky environments on campus such as Greek societies and residences promote heavy drinking because of the social needs they serve. Developing and extending attractive competing environments that are "pro health" and incompatible with drinking but that also promote socialization should be a high priority. For example, student recreational facilities (especially weight rooms and other large areas that host a good amount of fitness equipment, as well as swimming pools) provide a setting for student socialization and, in part, serve needs similar to those met by the "bar scene" (i.e., opportunities to see and be seen in an appealing context). Indeed, many universities have invested large sums of money in improving these facilities in order to compete for incoming students (June, 2006; Reisberg, 2001). However, the hours of operation of these types of facilities are usually limited, so they do not compete with drinking venues late in the evening and in the early morning hours. It would be useful to evaluate the effectiveness of extending the hours of operation for these types of facilities to cover prime drinking periods (e.g., late night/early morning, weekends).

While the typical personality predictors of alcohol consumption and alcohol-related problems among college students are similar to those of nonstudents and individuals at other life stages, there may be some factors that are differentially relevant in college students (Park, Sher, Wood, & Krull, 2009b; Park et al., 2006). Thus, when seeking to understand those environmental variables that appear to promote drinking on campus, we need to consider the role of personality with respect to both exposure to those environments and the effects of those environments on the drinker.

Using AHB data, recent studies have shown that the "maturing out" of alcohol problems that typically occurs soon after college is associated with personality change (Littlefield et al., 2009; Littlefield, Sher, & Wood, 2010). This finding has two clear implications for addressing college student drinking. First, experiences that promote personality maturation (i.e., assumption of adult roles and increased responsibilities; Caspi, Roberts, & Shiner, 2005; Roberts & Mroczek, 2008) could be given greater consideration in designing the college experience. Second, to the extent that high levels of impulsivity and negative affectivity indicate risk for drinking problems, clinicians might want to consider monitoring ongoing personality risk in the individuals they treat. Ostensible improvement in drinking outcomes in the presence of high levels of personality risk may require additional ongoing monitoring.

REFERENCES

Alva, S. A. (1998). Self-reported alcohol use of college fraternity and sorority members. *Journal of College Student Development, 39*, 3–10.

Arnett, J. J. (2004). *Emerging adulthood: The winding road from late teens through the twenties.* New York: Oxford University Press.

Baer, J. S. (1994). Effects of college residence on perceived norms for alcohol consumption: An examination of the first year in college. *Psychology of Addictive Behaviors, 8,* 43–50.

Baer, J. S. (2002). Student factors: Understanding individual variation in college drinking. *Journal of Studies on Alcohol*(Suppl. 14), 40–53.

Baer, J. S., Kivlahan, D. R., & Marlatt, G. A. (1995). High-risk drinking across the transition from high school to college. *Alcoholism: Clinical and Experimental Research, 19,* 54–61.

Baer, J. S., Stacy, A., & Larimer, M. (1991). Biases in the perception of drinking norms among college students. *Journal of Studies on Alcohol, 52,* 580–586.

Bartholow, B. D., Sher, K. J., & Krull, J. L. (2003). Changes in heavy drinking over the third decade of life as a function of collegiate fraternity and sorority involvement: A prospective, multilevel analysis. *Health Psychology, 22,* 616–626.

Brennan, A. F., Walfish, S., & AuBuchon, P. (1986). Alcohol use and abuse in college students: I. A review of individual and personality correlates. *International Journal of the Addictions, 21,* 449–474.

Brown, S. A. (1985). Expectancies versus background in the prediction of college drinking patterns. *Journal of Consulting and Clinical Psychology, 53,* 123–130.

Canterbury, R. G., Gressard, C. F., Vieweg, W. V. R., Grossman, S. J., McKelway, R. B., & Westerman, P. S. (1992). Risk-taking behavior of college students and social forces. *American Journal of Drug and Alcohol Abuse, 18,* 213–223.

Cashin, J., R., Presley, C. A., & Meilman, P. W. (1998). Alcohol use in the Greek system: Follow the leader? *Journal of Studies on Alcohol, 59,* 63–70.

Caspi, A., Roberts, B. W., & Shiner, R. L. (2005). Personality development: Stability and change. *Annual Review of Psychology, 56,* 453–484.

Costa, P. T., & McCrae, R. R. (1992). The five factor model of personality and its relevance to personality disorders. *Journal of Personality Disorders, 6,* 343–359.

Cronin, C. (1997). Reasons for drinking versus outcome expectancies in the prediction of college student drinking. *Substance Use and Misuse, 32,* 1287–1311.

Crowley, J. E. (1991). Educational status and drinking patterns: How representative are college students? *Journal of Studies on Alcohol, 52,* 10–16.

Dawson, D. A., Grant, B. F., Stinson, F. S., & Chou, P. S. (2004). Another look at heavy episodic drinking and alcohol use disorders among college and noncollege youth. *Journal of Studies on Alcohol, 65,* 477–488.

Debro, J. (1991). Drug use and abuse at historical black colleges. In L. Harris (Ed.), *Problems of Drug Dependence 1990: Proceedings of the 52nd annual scientific meeting of the Committee on Problems of Drug Dependence* (NIDA Research Monograph 105, pp. 460–467). Rockville, MD: National Institute on Drug Abuse.

Engs, R. C., Diebold, B. A., & Hanson, D. J. (1996). The drinking patterns and problems of a national sample of college students, 1994. *Journal of Alcohol and Drug Education, 41,* 13–33.

Gfroerer, J. C., Greenblatt, J. C., & Wright, D. A. (1997). Substance use in the US college-age population: Differences according to educational status and living arrangement. *American Journal of Public Health, 87,* 62–65.

Globetti, G., Stern, J. T., Marasco, F., & Haworth-Hoeppner, S. (1988). Student residence arrangements and alcohol use and abuse: A research note. *Journal of College and University Student Housing, 18,* 28–33.

Goldman, M. S., Darkes, J., & Del Boca, F. K. (1999). Expectancy mediation of biopsychosocial risk for alcohol use and alcoholism. In E. I. Kirsch (Ed.), *How expectancies shape experience* (pp. 233–262). Washington, DC: American Psychological Association.

Grant, B. F. (1997). Convergent validity of DSM-III-R and DSM-IV alcohol dependence: Results from the national longitudinal alcohol epidemiologic survey. *Journal of Substance Abuse, 9,* 89–102.

Grekin, E. R., & Sher, K. J. (2006). Alcohol dependence symptoms among college freshmen: Prevalence, stability and person/environment interactions. *Experimental and Clinical Psychopharmacology, 14,* 329–338.

Grekin, E. R., Sher, K. J., & Wood, P. K. (2006). Personality and substance dependence symptoms: Modeling substance-specific traits. *Psychology of Addictive Behavior, 20,* 415–424.

Harford, T. C., & Muthen, B. O. (2001). Alcohol use among college students: The effects of prior problem behaviors and change of residence. *Journal of Studies on Alcohol, 62,* 306–312.

Harford, T. C., Wechsler, H., & Muthen, B. O. (2002). The impact of current residence and high school drinking on alcohol problems among college students. *Journal of Studies on Alcohol, 63,* 271–279.

Harrington, N. G., Brigham, N. L., & Clayton, R. R. (1997). Differences in alcohol use and alcohol-related problems among fraternity and sorority members. *Drug and Alcohol Dependence, 47,* 237–246.

Hill, K. G., Hawkins, J. D., Bailey, J. A., Catalano, R. F., Abbott, R. D., & Shapiro, V. B. (2010). Person–environment interaction in the prediction of alcohol abuse and alcohol dependence in adulthood. *Drug and Alcohol Dependence, 110,* 62–69.

Johnston, L. D., O'Malley, P. M., & Bachman, J. G. (2002). *Monitorizing the Future National Survey results on drug use, 1975–2001: Vol. II. College students and adults ages 19–40* (NIH Publication No. 02-5107). Bethesda, MD: National Institute on Drug Abuse.

Johnston, L. D., O'Malley, P. M., Bachman, J. G., & Schulenberg, J. E. (2009). *Monitoring the Future national survey results on drug use, 1975–2008: Volume II, College students and adults ages 19–50* (NIH Publication No. 09–7403). Bethesda, MD: National Institute on Drug Abuse.

June, A. W. (2006, June 9). Facilities play a key role in students' enrollment decisions, study finds. *Chronicle of Higher Education,* p. A27.

Knight, J. R., Wechsler, H., Kuo, M., Seibring, M., Weitzman, E. R., & Schuckit, M. A. (2002). Alcohol abuse and dependence among U.S. college students. *Journal of Studies on Alcohol, 63,* 263–270.

Kodman, F., & Sturmak, M. (1984). Drinking patterns among college fraternities: A report. *Journal of Alcohol and Drug Education, 29,* 65–69.

Kuh, G. D., & Arnold, J. C. (1993). Liquid bonding: A cultural analysis of the role of alcohol in fraternity pledgeship. *Journal of College Student Development, 34*, 327–334.

Kushner, M. G., & Sher, K. J. (1993). Comorbidity of alcohol and anxiety disorders among college students: Effects of gender and family history of alcoholism. *Addictice Behaviors, 18*, 543–552.

Larimer, M. E., Irvine, D. L., Kilmer, J. R., & Marlatt, G. A. (1997). College drinking and the Greek system: Examining the role of perceived norms for high-risk behavior. *Journal of College Student Development, 38*, 589–596.

Leigh, B. C. (1987). Beliefs about the effects of alcohol on self and others. *Journal of Studies on Alcohol, 48*, 467–475.

Leigh, B. C., & Stacy, A. W. (1993). Alcohol outcome expectancies: Scale construction and predictive utility in higher order confirmatory models. *Psychological Assessment, 5*, 216–229.

Littlefield, A., & Sher, K. J. (2010). The multiple, distinct ways that personality contributes to alcohol use disorders. *Social and Personality Psychology Compass, 4*, 767–782.

Littlefield, A., Sher, K. J., & Wood, P. K. (2009). Is "maturing out" of problematic alcohol involvement related to personality change? *Journal of Abnormal Psychology, 118*, 360–374.

Littlefield, A., Sher, K. J., & Wood, P. K. (2010). Do changes in drinking motives mediate the relation between personality change and "maturing out" of problem drinking? *Journal of Abnormal Psychology, 119*, 93–105.

Lo, C. C., & Globetti, G. (1993). A partial analysis of the campus influence on drinking behavior: Students who enter college as nondrinkers. *Journal of Drug Issues, 23*, 715–725.

Maggs, J. L. (1997). Alcohol use and binge drinking as goal-directed action during the transition to postsecondary education. In J. E. M. Schulenberg, J. L. Maggs, & K. Hurrelmann (Eds.), *Health risks and developmental transitions during adolescence* (pp. 345–371). Cambridge, UK: Cambridge University.

Martinez, J. A., Rutledge, P. C., & Sher, K. J. (2007). Fake ID ownership and heavy drinking in underage college students: Prospective findings. *Psychology of Addictive Behaviors, 21*, 226–232.

McCabe, S. E., Schulenberg, J. E., Johnston, L. D., O'Malley, P. M., Bachman, J. G., & Kloska, D. D. (2005). Selection and socialization effects of fraternities and sororities on U.S. college student substance use: A multi-cohort national longitudinal study. *Addiction, 100*, 512–524.

Meilman, P. W., Presley, C. A., & Cashin, J. R. (1995). The sober social life at the historically black colleges. *Journal of Blacks in Higher Education, 9*, 98–100.

National Center for Education Statistics. (2003, July). Distance education at degree-granting postsecondary institutions: 2000–2001. Retrieved from *nces.ed.gov/surveys/peqis/publications/2003017*.

National Institute on Alcohol Abuse and Alcoholism. (2007). *College drinking: Changing the culture*. Retrieved from *www.collegedrinkingprevention.gov/ StatsSummaries/4tier.aspx*.

O'Connor, R. M. J., Cooper, S. E., & Thiel, W. S. (1996). Alcohol use as a predictor of potential fraternity membership. *Journal of College Student Development, 37*, 669–675.

O'Hare, T. M. (1990). Drinking in college: Consumption patterns, problems, sex differences and legal drinking age. *Journal of Studies on Alcohol, 51*, 536–541.

Park, A., Sher, K. J., & Krull, J. (2006). Individual differences in the Greek effect on risky drinking: The role of self-consciousness. *Psychology of Addictive Behaviors, 20*, 85–90.

Park, A., Sher, K. J., & Krull, J. (2008). Risky drinking in college changes as fraternity/sorority affiliation changes: A person–environment perspective. *Psychology of Addictive Behaviors, 22*, 219–229.

Park, A., Sher, K. J., & Krull, J. (2009a). Selection and socialization of risky drinking during the college transition: The importance of micro-environments associated with specific living units. *Psychology of Addictive Behaviors, 23*, 428–442.

Park, A., Sher, K. J., Wood, P. K., & Krull, J. (2009b). Dual mechanisms underlying accentuation of risky drinking via fraternity/sorority affiliation: The role of personality, peer norms, and alcohol availability. *Journal of Abnormal Psychology, 118*, 241–245.

Presley, C. A., Meilman, P. W., & Cashin, J. R. (1996). *Alcohol and drugs on America's college campuses: Use, consequences, and perceptions of the campus environment* (Vol. 4, 1992–1994). Carbondale: Southern Illinois University.

Presley, C. A., Meilman, P. W., & Leichliter, J. S. (2002). College factors that influence drinking. *Journal of Studies on Alcohol*(Suppl. 14), 82–90.

Pullen, L. M. (1994). The relationship among alcohol abuse in college students and selected psychological/demographic variables. *Journal of Alcohol and Drug Education, 40*, 36–50.

Read, J. P., Wood, M. D., Davidoff, O. J., McLacken, J., & Campbell, J. F. (2002). Making the transition from high school to college: The role of alcohol-related social influence factors in students' drinking. *Substance Abuse, 23*, 53–65.

Reisberg, L. (2001, February 9). Colleges replace drab gyms with sleek, playful facilities. *Chronicle of Higher Education*, p. A38.

Roberts, B. W., & Mroczek, D. (2008). Personality trait change in adulthood. *Current Directions in Psychological Science, 17*, 31–35.

Schall, M., Weede, T. J., & Maltzman, I. (1991). Predictors of alcohol consumption by university students. *Journal of Alcohol and Drug Education, 37*, 72–80.

Sher, K. J., Bartholow, B. D., & Nanda, S. (2001). Short- and long-term effects of fraternity and sorority membership on heavy drinking: A social norms perspective. *Psychology of Addictive Behaviors, 15*, 42–51.

Sher, K. J., & Rutledge, P. (2007). Heavy drinking across the transition to college: Predicting first-semester heavy drinking from college variables. *Addictive Behaviors, 32*, 819–835.

Sher, K. J., Trull, T. J., Bartholow, B. D., & Vieth, A. (1999). Personality and alcoholism: Issues, methods, and etiological processes. In K. E. B. Leonard & H. T. Blane (Eds.), *Psychological theories of drinking and alcoholism* (2nd ed., pp. 54–105). New York: Guilford Press.

Sher, K. J., Walitzer, K. S., Wood, P., & Brent, E. E. (1991). Characteristics of children of alcoholics: Putative risk factors, substance use and abuse, and psychopathology. *Journal of Abnormal Psychology, 100,* 427–448.

Sher, K. J., Wood, M., Crews, T., & Vandiver, T. A. (1995). The Tridimensional Personality Questionnaire: Reliability and validity studies and derivation of a short form. *Psychological Assessment, 7,* 195–208.

Sher, K. J., Wood, M. D., Wood, P. K., & Raskin, G. (1996). Alcohol outcome expectancies and alcohol use: A latent variable cross-lagged panel study. *Journal of Abnormal Psychology, 105,* 561–574.

Shore, E. R., Rivers, P. C., & Berman, J. J. (1983). Resistance by college students to peer pressure to drink. *Journal of Studies on Alcohol, 44,* 352–361.

Tampke, D. R. (1990). Alcohol behavior, risk perception, and fraternity and sorority membership. *NASPA Journal, 28,* 71–77.

Vu, P. (2007, October 3). Colleges go on offense against binge drinking. *Stateline.org.* Retrieved from *www.stateline.org/live/details/story?contentId=245335.*

Wechsler, H., Davenport, A., Dowdall, G., Moeykens, B., & Castillo, S. (1994). Health and behavioral consequences of binge drinking in college: A national survey of students at 140 campuses. *Journal of the American Medical Association, 272,* 1672–1677.

Wechsler, H., Kuh, G., & Davenport, A. E. (1996). Fraternities, sororities and binge drinking: Results from a national study of American colleges. *NASPA Journal, 33,* 260–279.

Wechsler, H., & Kuo, M. (2003). Watering down the drinks: The moderating effect of college demographics on alcohol use of high-risk groups. *American Journal of Public Health, 93,* 1929–1933.

Wechsler, H., Lee, J. E., Kuo, M., & Lee, H. (2000). College binge drinking in the 1990s: A continuing problem—Results of the Harvard School of Public Health 1999 College Alcohol Study. *Journal of American College Health, 48,* 199–210.

Wechsler, H., Lee, J. E., Kuo, M., Seibring, M., Nelson, T. F., & Lee, H. (2002). Trends in college binge drinking during a period of increased prevention efforts: Findings from 4 Harvard School of Public Health College Alcohol Study Surveys: 1993–2001. *Journal of American College Health, 50,* 203–217.

Wechsler, H., & Nelson, T. F. (2008). What we have learned from the Harvard School of Public Health College Alcohol Study: Focusing attention on college student alcohol consumption and the environmental conditions that promote it. *Journal of Studies on Alcohol and Drugs, 69,* 481–490.

Weitzman, E. R., & Chen, Y. Y. (2005). Risk modifying effect of social capital on measures of heavy alcohol consumption, alcohol abuse, harms, and second-hand effects: National survey findings. *Journal of Epidemiology and Community Health, 59,* 303–309.

Weitzman, E. R., Nelson, T. F., & Wechsler, H. (2003). Taking up binge drinking in college: The influences of person, social group, and environment. *Journal of Adolescent Health, 32,* 26–35.

Werner, M. J., & Greene, J. W. (1992). Problem drinking among college freshmen. *Journal of Adolescent Health, 13,* 487–492.

White, H. R., McMorris, B., Catalano, R. F., Fleming, C. B., Haggerty, K. P., & Abbott, R. W. (2006). Increases in alcohol and marijuana use during the transition out of high school into emerging adulthood: The effects of leaving home, going to college, and high school protective factors. *Journal of Studies on Alcohol, 67,* 810–822.

Wilsnack, R. W., Vogeltanz, N. D., Wilsnack, S. C., & Harris, T. R. (2000). Gender differences in alcohol consumption and adverse drinking consequences: Cross-cultural patterns. *Addiction, 95,* 251–265.

Wood, M. D., Sher, K. J., & Strathman, A. (1996). Alcohol outcome expectancies and alcohol use and problems. *Journal of Studies on Alcohol, 57,* 283–288.

Wood, P. K., Sher, K. J., & Rutledge, P. C. (2007). College student alcohol consumption, day of the week, and class schedule. *Alcoholism: Clinical and Experimental Research, 31,* 1195–1207.

PART IV

PREVENTION AND INTERVENTION STRATEGIES

CHAPTER 8

Brief Individual-Focused Alcohol Interventions for College Students

Jessica M. Cronce *and* Mary E. Larimer

Most young adults, particularly college students, consume alcohol at least occasionally (Johnston, O'Malley, Bachman, & Schulenberg, 2009). Many of those who consume alcohol misuse it, engaging in *heavy episodic consumption*, or *binge drinking*, which directly and indirectly contributes to a host of harmful consequences (Perkins, 2002). What constitutes a binge or heavy episode of drinking has been differentially defined across studies, with a shared focus on number of drinks consumed. The most commonly used definition, by Wechsler, Dowdall, Davenport, and Castillo (1995), denotes a binge episode as consumption of five or more drinks for men and four or more drinks for women on a single occasion.

Although most college students mature out of heavy drinking around age 21 or 22 (Johnston et al., 2009), negative consequences experienced as a result of heavy drinking, most of which are acute, such as impaired academic performance or physical injury, may significantly alter the natural course of students' development, leading to long-term harm. In an effort to reduce or prevent long-term harm associated with alcohol use and misuse, numerous prevention programs have been developed to target factors associated with college student drinking, including positive beliefs about alcohol's effects (i.e., alcohol expectancies), personal reasons or motives for drinking, perceived norms for the prevalence and acceptability of drinking in the college culture at large and more proximal peer groups, deficient knowledge or use of protective behavioral skills (e.g., drink refusal, monitoring and spacing consumption), and inherent ambivalence regarding drinking behavior (Baer, 2002; Presley, Meilman, & Leichliter, 2002).

Multiple reviews have been published summarizing the outcomes from individual-focused preventive interventions targeting college student drinking (Carey, Scott-Sheldon, Carey, & DeMartini, 2007; Larimer & Cronce, 2002, 2007; Walters & Neighbors, 2005; White, 2006). Since the most recent reviews (Carey et al., 2007; Larimer & Cronce, 2007), there has been a rapid expansion of research in this area. In order to draw specific conclusions and make recommendations for future research based on the current state of the science, this chapter presents a summary of prior reviews and a qualitative review of subsequently published individual prevention studies. Consistent with prior reviews, studies were included if they utilized a randomized controlled trial approach, randomly assigning individual participants (or intact groups) to one or more experimental conditions, including active interventions or ostensibly inert controls (e.g., assessment only).

INDIVIDUAL-FOCUSED PREVENTIVE INTERVENTIONS 1984–2007

Larimer and Cronce (2002, 2007) reviewed the outcome of individual-focused preventive interventions published between 1984 and early 2007. There was a consistent *lack* of support for education and awareness programs comprising solely didactic (instructive) and values clarification approaches. Programs that fall in the didactic category focus on provision of alcohol information/knowledge. For example, such programs may focus on teaching students about the consequences of alcohol use, including the personal and collateral impact of drunk driving, negative effects on academic performance, and acute and long-term effects on health. Information on the specific effects associated with a range of blood alcohol concentrations (BACs) is also often included, as well as information debunking myths regarding how alcohol is absorbed and oxidized (e.g., coffee may affect subjective intoxication, but will not decrease BAC). Values clarification programs may include alcohol information, but they focus on helping students to consider their own personal goals (e.g., to maintain good relationships) and evaluate how choices related to alcohol use influence attainment of these goals (see Goodstadt & Sheppard, 1983, for more details on alcohol education and values clarification programs).

In contrast to the absence of positive findings for didactic and values clarification approaches, there was consistent evidence supporting the efficacy of cognitive-behavioral skills-based interventions, including behavioral self-monitoring, *in vivo* alcohol expectancy challenge, and multicomponent skills training. Most cognitive-behavioral programs incorporate elements of information/knowledge, values clarification, and normative reeducation programs but focus on teaching skills to modify beliefs or behaviors related to high-risk drinking. Some programs focus on teaching specific skills. For example, behavioral self-monitoring involves consistently tracking alcohol use as a means of increasing awareness of behavior, whereas BAC feedback/discrimination teaches students how to determine their BAC using external information (e.g., BAC chart, breathalyzer) and internal cues associated with different levels of intoxication (see Caddy & Lovibond, 1976, for more details on BAC feedback/discrimination).

Alcohol expectancy challenge (AEC), another specific skill program, involves evaluation of the effects attributable to alcohol versus an individual's expectations for how alcohol will affect him or her. *In vivo* (experiential) AEC incorporates actual and perceived alcohol administration to intervention participants as a means of demonstrating the influence of expectancies (see Darkes & Goldman, 1993, 1998, for more details). As the name implies, multicomponent skills-training programs focus on teaching a broad range of alcohol-related skills including behavioral self-monitoring, expectancy challenge, harm reduction strategies, and drink refusal skills.

In addition to cognitive-behavioral skills programs, there was strong support for the efficacy of brief motivational interventions (BMIs) in reducing alcohol use and consequences. BMIs are usually delivered over one or two sessions, and are led by a facilitator whose goal is to increase the student's motivation and commitment to change risky drinking behavior. In service of this goal, facilitators utilize a motivational interviewing (MI) style (Miller & Rollnick, 2002). MI is a therapeutic approach built around a core *spirit*, or way of being, marked by (1) fostering collaboration with the client, (2) supporting/respecting the client's autonomy, and (3) evoking motivation/goals from the client versus imposing these on the client. Consistent with this spirit, MI has four guiding *principles*: (1) express genuine empathy, (2) develop discrepancy between clients' values/goals and their current behavior, (3) roll with resistance to change, and (4) support clients' self-efficacy. Adherence to these principles is evident in the facilitator's strategic use of four specific MI *skills*: (1) asking open-ended questions, (2) affirming clients' strengths/values, (3) listening reflectively, and (4) summarizing clients' responses. Adherence to MI style serves to elicit self-motivational statements (*change talk*).

BMIs most often utilize personalized feedback (often referred to as Personalized Feedback Interventions, or PFIs) regarding drinking and related consequences, alcohol expectancies, and drinking motives in order to facilitate discussion of personal behavior. PFIs provide a written summary and graphic representation of an individual's drinking behavior, including his or her typical and peak frequency, quantity, and calculated BACs. Information on an individual's typical and peak BACs is presented in relation to BAC-specific effects so that risk for consequences, including motor impairment and alcohol poisoning, is apparent. BMIs also typically include didactic presentation of general alcohol education (e.g., the cognitive effects of alcohol; impact of alcohol expectancies on behavior), as well as discussion of alcohol-specific coping and harm reduction skills (e.g., how to prevent high BACs; how to reduce tolerance).

The Brief Alcohol Screening and Intervention for College Students (BASICS) program is a prototypical example of a BMI (see Dimeff, Baer, Kivlahan, & Marlatt, 1999, for a description of BASICS and a sample of personalized feedback). PFIs delivered as part of a BMI or as a stand-alone intervention generally also include personalized normative feedback (PNF) contrasting self-reported drinking behavior with the typical drinking behavior of a relevant reference group (e.g., typical female student, typical fraternity member). Inclusion of PNF facilitates examination and development of discrepancies between an individual's perception of his or her drinking as "typical" and actual drinking behavior among the referent group, which is generally much more moderate (see Dimeff et al., 1999, and Neighbors, Larimer, & Lewis, 2004, for samples of PFI and PNF, respectively). PNF shares similarities with normative reeducation programs (classically considered a traditional alcohol-information-focused intervention) insofar as it presents accurate drinking norms for an appropriate reference group (e.g., college students at a given campus). However, PNF differs from normative reeducation programs in that it juxtaposes an individual's personal drinking behavior with his or her perception of the drinking norms for the reference group and the accurate drinking norms. Many normative reeducation programs also incorporate discussion of the acceptability of drinking behavior in addition to its prevalence, whereas this information is not typically included in PNF (see Mallett, Bachrach, & Turrisi, 2009, for more details). As with PFI, PNF can be used as a stand-alone intervention without a facilitator to lead review and discussion of the feedback, and has demonstrated reductions in drinking and/or consequences, which (for PNF) were mediated through changes in normative perceptions (Larimer & Cronce, 2007).

Carey and colleagues (2007) separately reviewed randomized clinical trials of college student alcohol interventions that were published during roughly the same time period covered by the reviews by Larimer and Cronce (i.e., 1985 to early 2007). The primary findings from this meta-analysis are generally consistent with those of Larimer and Cronce (2002, 2007), but differentially note that significant intervention effects on alcohol consumption appear to peak prior to 6-month follow-up and effects on alcohol-related negative consequences tend to emerge later (after 6 months), lasting through long-term follow-up (up to 3.75 years). In particular, individual interventions that (1) incorporated motivational enhancement, (2) included PFI/PNF, and (3) included exercises elaborating decisional balance (i.e., pros and cons of drinking behavior) were more efficacious in reducing alcohol-related consequences relative to different comparison groups. Carey et al. (2007) observed that this specific combination of intervention components is frequently present in approaches modeled after BASICS (Dimeff et al., 1999).

INDIVIDUAL-FOCUSED PREVENTIVE
INTERVENTIONS 2007–2010

As previously indicated, the remainder of this chapter comprises a qualitative review of individual-focused alcohol intervention studies published subsequent to the reviews by Carey et al. (2007) and Larimer and Cronce (2007). Many of these studies evaluated the efficacy of multicomponent BMIs adapted from BASICS, most of which incorporated personalized feedback containing normative feedback (PFI/PNF). Additional studies evaluated PFI/PNF delivered alone in the absence of a trained facilitator. Delivery of BMIs with PFI/PNF and PFI/PNF-only interventions was achieved via in-person group and individual sessions, mailed printed material, and Web-based content, and many were conducted in special settings (e.g., a primary care provider's office, in the student's home before he or she entered college) or targeted high-risk student subpopulations (mandated/sanctioned students, freshmen, athletes). A concise summary of the studies included in this chapter is available in Table 8.1.

Intervention effect sizes are reported for each study that included effect size estimates in the original report or included sufficient postintervention data to calculate between-group estimates (with the latter denoted as *estimated* in the text to differentiate it from the former). Effect sizes reported include Cohen's d (Cohen, 1988), which denotes the standardized difference between the mean of the intervention and comparison groups, Cohen's h (Cohen, 1988), which denotes the difference between two proportions, and eta squared (η^2), which denotes the proportion of total variability in the dependent variable attributable to the effect of the independent variable, or partial eta squared (η_p^2). According to Cohen's (1988, 1992) definitions of effect size, small, medium, and large effects

TABLE 8.1. Comparison of Larimer and Cronce (2002, 2007) and Studies Reviewed in This Chapter

Prevention and treatment categories	Number of studies providing support/total studies			
	Larimer & Cronce (2002)	Larimer & Cronce (2007)	Cronce & Larimer (2011)	Total
Education/awareness programs				
Information/knowledge programs	1/7	1/10	0/4	2/21
Values clarification programs	2/5	0/3	*	2/8
In-person normative reeducation programs	1/2	2/4	*	3/6
Personalized normative feedback (PNF) alone	*	4/4	3/4[a]	7/8
Cognitive-behavioral skills-based programs				
Alcohol-specific skills				
Expectancy challenge interventions	2/3	2/7	2/2	6/12
Self-monitoring/self-assessment	3/3	1/1	0/1	4/5
BAC feedback	*	*	1/3	1/3
Multicomponent alcohol skills training	7/10	4/8	2/4	13/22
General life skills training/lifestyle balance/coping skills	2/2	0/1	1/1	3/4
Motivational/feedback-based approaches				
Brief motivational intervention (BMI) with or without PFI/PNF	8/8	10/14	16/18	34/40
Personalized feedback intervention (PFI) with or without PNF	3/3	7/8	10/14	20/25
Multicomponent education-focused programs	*	*	3/7	3/7
Intensive treatment and medication				
	1/1	0/0	*	1/1

Note. Ratio indicates the number of studies showing support for the efficacy of a given intervention in reducing, or exhibiting a protective effect against, relevant behavioral outcomes (e.g., quantity or frequency of alcohol consumption; alcohol-related negative consequences) out of the total number of studies including this type of intervention as an experimental or comparison group. Limitations of each study should be considered when evaluating the strength of the evidence in support of a particular intervention. The number of studies listed in the table may exceed the number of studies listed in the text, as some authors tested more than one intervention in a given study.

[a]Includes event-specific interventions.

*No studies in this category were included.

for d and h are considered to be 0.20, 0.50, and 0.80, respectively, and for η^2 and η_p^2 are 0.01, 0.06, and 0.14, respectively.

PFI/PNF and PNF-Only Compared with a Control Group

A total of 12 studies evaluated the impact of 10 PFI/PNF and 4 PNF-only interventions on college student drinking, most of which utilized an assessment-only comparison group. For example, Geisner, Neighbors, Lee, and Larimer (2007) found that mailed PFI including PNF along with general tips for moderating alcohol use significantly reduced perception of drinking norms ($d = 0.60$) relative to assessment only in a sample of mildly depressed students. Furthermore, reductions in perceived drinking norms were significantly associated with reductions in alcohol use and consequences. However, an overall main effect of the intervention on alcohol use or alcohol-related consequences was not evident.

Weitzel, Bernhardt, Usdan, Mays, and Glanz (2007) evaluated PFI against assessment only using wireless handheld computer devices. Both groups used the devices for daily self-monitoring of alcohol use, and individuals in the PFI group were additionally sent personalized alcohol-risk-reduction text messages. PFI was associated with reduced drinks per drinking day *during the intervention period*, but not at 2-week follow-up. At follow-up, PFI participants reported expecting to experience fewer consequences as a result of their drinking. However, no differences in actual negative consequences were evident. In comparison, Bewick, Trusler, Mulhern, Barkham, and Hill (2008) tested the efficacy of a Web-based PFI including PNF, information on general alcohol-related health risks, and moderate drinking guidelines, relative to assessment only. At 12-week follow-up, PFI participants experienced significant reductions in drinks per drinking occasion ($d = 0.29$), though they did not report reductions in overall weekly drinking or CAGE questionnaire scores.

Lewis, Neighbors, Oster-Aaland, Kirkeby, and Larimer (2007) tested the efficacy of a computerized PNF intervention among freshmen, contrasting the effect of gender-specific versus gender-neutral drinking norms against the effect of assessment only. Gender-specific PNF led to significant reductions in drinks per week and drinking frequency at 5-month follow-up. Gender-neutral PNF led to reductions in drinking frequency, but was not different from control with respect to drinks per week. Gender-neutral but not gender-specific norms at 3-month follow-up mediated intervention effects on alcohol quantity but not frequency at 5-month follow-up.

Likewise, Neighbors, Lee, Lewis, Fossos, and Walter (2009) tested the efficacy of PNF relative to assessment only to reduce drinking related to celebration of participants' 21st birthdays. PNF including 21st birth-day drinking intentions and protective behavioral strategies was delivered in conjunction with an e-card with a moderation message 2 days prior to participants' birthdays. Results at 4-day post-birthday follow-up indicate that PNF was effective in reducing estimated BACs ($d = 0.33$), especially among those with baseline intentions to reach higher BACs ($d = 0.41$). Lewis, Neighbors, Lee, and Oster-Aaland (2008) also evaluated the effect of an event-specific intervention with written PNF regarding 21st birth-day drinking intentions. Although significant reductions in normative misperceptions were associated with the birthday card intervention ($\eta_p^2 = 0.11$), no reductions in drinking or consequences were evident relative to assessment only.

Hustad, Barnett, Borsari, and Jackson (2010) tested the efficacy of Electronic Checkup to Go (*e-Chug*), an online program that incorporates alcohol information with extensive, immediately available PFI with PNF, in comparison to AlcoholEdu for College (a multicomponent alcohol-education-focused intervention) and assessment only. Participants in the two interventions showed reductions or a protective effect (i.e., limited increases) from baseline to 1-month follow-up across a number of typi-cal and peak drinking indices relative to controls (e-Chug $d = 0.54$ to 0.85, AlcoholEdu for College $d = 0.59$ to 0.75). Individuals who received AlcoholEdu for College showed a significant reduction in alcohol-related consequences ($d = 0.56$), and there was a nonsignificant trend ($p = .09$) for reduced consequences among those who received e-Chug ($d = 0.34$) relative to controls. Using a freshman sample, Doumas and Andersen (2009) similarly evaluated e-Chug in comparison to assessment only. At 3-month follow-up, high-risk drinkers who received e-Chug reduced their frequency of drinking to the point of intoxication ($d = 0.85$) and alcohol-related negative consequences ($d = 0.80$). No group differences were found for low-risk drinkers.

Doumas and Haustveit (2008) compared Web-based PFI with PNF to alcohol education in a sample of athletes. Among high-risk student-athletes, participation in the PFI was associated with reduc-tions in weekly ($\eta^2 = 0.14$) and peak drinking quantity ($\eta^2 = 0.15$), and frequency of drinking to intoxication ($\eta^2 = 0.20$), at 6-week and 3-month follow-up relative to the education condition. Drinking reduc-tions were positively associated with changes in normative perceptions of typical student drinking. Doumas, McKinley, and Book (2009) com-pared the same Web-based PFI program to a different online alcohol education program (the Judicial Educator) in a sample of mandated students. Results indicated the PFI was more effective than education in reducing alcohol use (weekly, $\eta^2 = 0.07$, and peak drinking quantity, $\eta^2 = 0.08$, and frequency of drinking to intoxication, $\eta^2 = 0.07$), with a trend toward a reduction in alcohol consequences. Changes in drinking were mediated by reductions in perceived peer norms for alcohol consumption.

White, Mun, and Morgan (2008) similarly evaluated the effect of a PFI with PNF among mandated students. Participants who reported very high-risk drinking at baseline were excluded and referred for other services. Eligible participants were randomized to receive PFI/PNF immediately or after the 2-month follow-up assessment (delayed). Significant within-individual decreases in alcohol use and problems were evident. However, no significant differences emerged between the immediate and delayed intervention groups at 2- or 7-month follow-up ($d = 0.01$–0.12 and 0.06–0.15, respectively). As noted by the authors, the absence of an intervention effect may be due in part to the exclusion of the heaviest drinkers (high-risk students).

Finally, Saitz et al. (2007) evaluated the effect of two versions of Web-based PFI among high-risk drinking freshmen: a *minimal* version including PNF along with alcohol and health education, and an *enhanced* version including the minimal intervention elements plus BAC education, feedback on negative drinking-related consequences with normative comparison, and information quantifying alcohol use in terms of money, calories, and exercise needed to offset calories. High-risk drinking decreased from post-intervention to 1-month follow-up across both intervention groups, but the absence of an assessment-only control group limits conclusions regarding the effect of the PFI.

PFI/PNF-Only Compared with BMI

Four additional studies directly compared PFI/PNF alone to BMI with or without PFI/PNF components. For example, Butler and Correia (2009) compared in-person BMI with PFI to computerized PFI alone and assessment only. Both interventions were efficacious in reducing frequency ($\eta_p^2 = 0.13$) and quantity ($\eta_p^2 = 0.17$) of typical drinking and frequency of binge drinking ($\eta_p^2 = 0.15$) relative to control at 4-week follow-up, with no differences between the two interventions. There was also a trend toward reduction in alcohol-related consequences in both intervention conditions relative to control. Likewise, Doumas and Hannah (2008) compared BMI with PFI to PFI alone and assessment only interventions in a sample of working young adults ages 18 to 24 (75% college students). Among high-risk drinkers, participation in either intervention was associated with equivalent reductions in weekend drinking ($\eta_p^2 = 0.07$) and frequency of drinking to intoxication ($\eta_p^2 = 0.04$) at 30-day follow-up relative to control. No group differences were evident among low-risk drinkers.

Walters, Vader, Harris, Field, and Jouriles (2009) compared a BMI with PFI to a BMI without PFI, Web-based PFI only, and assessment only among heavy-drinking students. The PFI-only and BMI without PFI groups did not differ from control. However, BMI combined with PFI was associated with significant reductions in a drinking composite variable capturing typical drinking, peak BAC, and alcohol-related consequences as compared to control and the other two intervention groups at 6-month follow-up ($d = 0.54$). The effect of the BMI combined with PFI was mediated by changes in normative drinking perceptions. White, Mun, Pugh, and Morgan (2007) similarly compared a BMI with PFI to written PFI only among mandated students and found that both interventions resulted in comparable reductions in alcohol use and problems at 4-month follow-up. Reductions were not maintained, with increases in use and problems evident in both groups from 4- to 15-month follow-up. However, individuals who received the BMI reported experiencing fewer alcohol problems relative to those who received PFI only. The absence of an assessment-only group necessarily limits conclusions regarding intervention effects. A follow-up study (Mun, White, & Morgan, 2009) comparing those students who improved from baseline to follow-up to those who did not improve showed that individuals who experienced a serious alcohol-related incident or had higher baseline levels of alcohol problems were more likely to benefit from the BMI with PFI versus the written PFI only.

BMIs in Special Settings or with High-Risk Subpopulations

Ten additional studies have further evaluated the effects of 13 BMIs (most including PFI/PNF elements) in special settings and/or among high-risk subpopulations. For example, Schaus, Sole, McCoy, Mullett, and O'Brien (2009) tested a BMI with PFI facilitated by primary care providers among high-risk drinkers identified in a college health care setting against an alcohol education control. Significant overall trends were evident for BMI participants from baseline to 12-month follow-up for reduced typical and peak drinking, typical and peak BAC, and number of times drunk in a typical week. Group differences in favor of the BMI on these indices were evident at 3-month (estimated $d = 0.27, 0.25, 0.28, 0.37$, and 0.42, respectively) and 6-month (estimated $d = 0.41, 0.36, 0.35, 0.49$, and 0.50, respectively) follow-up. A significant overall trend for reduced alcohol-related negative consequences from baseline to 12-month follow-up was also found in the BMI group, with significant group differences in favor of the BMI evident at 6-month (estimated $d = 0.23$) and 9-month (estimated $d = 0.29$) follow-up.

Stahlbrandt, Johnsson, and Berglund (2007) evaluated the efficacy of a group BMI in comparison to a 12-step intervention (TSI) and assessment only among residence hall students. Students who were unable to attend the in-person BMI (37%) or in-person TSI (75%) sessions were mailed a 22-page manual or CD-ROM, respectively, containing the intervention material. BMI participants who reported high-risk drinking at baseline evidenced greater reductions in Alcohol Use Disorders Identification Test (AUDIT) scores relative to control (estimated $d = 0.27$). However, overall group differences were not evident at 2-year follow-up on indices of alcohol use, alcohol consequences, and alcohol psychopathology.

In a sample of sanctioned students, Carey, Henson, Carey, and Maisto (2009) compared BMI with PFI/PNF to a computer-based multicomponent alcohol-education-focused program (Alcohol 101 Plus) and found reductions in alcohol use at 1-month follow-up (estimated $d = 0.21$–0.38 across indices) but not consequences among women who received the BMI. Reductions in alcohol use evident among men in the BMI group were not different from control. Intervention effects were not maintained at 12-month follow-up. Cimini et al. (2009) evaluated a group BMI against an interactive peer theatrical presentation on alcohol use and an in-person multicomponent alcohol-education-focused program in a sanctioned-student sample, and similarly found no intervention effects on alcohol use or problems at 6-month follow-up. However, significant correlations were found between alcohol outcomes and changes in normative drinking perceptions ($r = .17$ to $.70$ across indices) and use of protective behavioral strategies ($r = -.11$ to $-.20$ across indices). Amaro et al. (2009) also evaluated a BMI for mandated students, in the context of a novel University Assistance Program (UAP). Participants randomized to UAP received BMI with PFI in addition to supplemental interventions (coping skills, stress management, solution-focused therapy) as indicated. Compared to services as usual in the counseling center, growth curve analyses indicated UAP participants reduced their weekday alcohol use ($d = 1.06$) and alcohol-related consequences ($d = 0.65$), and increased their alcohol protective behavioral strategies ($d = 1.98$) from baseline to 6-month follow-up.

LaBrie and colleagues (2008, 2009) found that a group BMI significantly reduced typical ($d = 0.34$) and heavy episodic drinking ($d = 0.42$), and evidenced a trend ($p = .05$) toward reduced alcohol consequences ($d = 0.28$) among freshmen women at 10-week follow-up relative to assessment only. The intervention was found to be especially effective in reducing typical and peak drinking among women higher in social motives ($d = 0.44$ and 0.35, respectively) and enhancement motives ($d = 0.34$ and 0.33, respectively) for drinking. However, data collected at 6-month follow-up (Labrie et al., 2009) suggest an absence of long-term intervention effects. Turrisi et al. (2009) compared the relative efficacy of a parenting handbook intervention focused on facilitating parent–child communication around alcohol, a BMI alone and in combination with the parenting handbook, and assessment only among college freshmen who were high school athletes. The combined parenting handbook/BMI group showed reduced typical and peak alcohol use and alcohol-related problems at 10-month follow-up relative to the parenting group ($d =$ 0.14–0.18, 0.17, and 0.13, respectively) and control ($d = 0.16$–0.20, 0.26 and 0.20, respectively), and reduced alcohol-related problems relative to BMI only ($d = 0.20$). These effects were mediated through correction of descriptive and injunctive normative misperceptions. The BMI-only group also showed significant reductions in peak BAC relative to assessment only ($d = 0.16$), and in number of drinks per weekend relative to assessment only ($d = 0.18$) and the parenting handbook condition ($d = 0.16$). Wood, Fairlie, and Fernandez (2010) randomized students to receive a BMI, a parent-based intervention (PBI), combined BMI and PBI, or assessment only prior to college matriculation. At 10- and 22-month follow-up, BMI participation was associated with lower likelihood of initiating heavy episodic consumption ($h = 0.02$ and 0.22, respectively) and experiencing the onset of alcohol-related consequences ($h = 0.07$ and 0.15, respectively). Participation in the combined BMI/ PBI evidenced a protective effect against the onset of alcohol-related consequences that was greater than the independent effect of the two component interventions. Changes in perceptions of descriptive norms mediated the observed effects of the BMI on likelihood of heavy episodic drinking and consequence onset.

Hansson, Rundberg, Zetterlind, Johnsson, and Berglund (2007) randomized student drinkers who reported having one or more parents with an alcohol use disorder to one of three conditions: a BMI, a cognitive-behavioral coping skills intervention, or a program combining both interventions. Comparison of data gathered at 12- and 24-month follow-up suggests an advantage for the combined program relative to coping skills or BMI alone in terms of decreased alcohol psychopathology ($d = 0.60$ and 0.52, respectively) and drinking consequence scores ($d = 0.42$ and 0.72, respectively), as well as an advantage for the combined program relative to coping skills alone with respect to estimated BACs ($d = 0.49$). A quantitative comparison of changes from baseline to 12-month follow-up was not presented. However, figures displaying group means suggest a potential short-term effect of the BMI in reducing estimated BACs.

Finally, Wood, Capone, Laforge, Erickson, and Brand (2007) compared a BMI, an experiential alcohol expectancy challenge (AEC) protocol, and a combined BMI and AEC to assessment only among heavy-drinking students. At 1-, 3-, and 6-month follow-up, results indicate that the BMI led to significant reductions in total alcohol use (d = 0.18, 0.25, and 0.16, respectively), heavy episodic consumption (d = 0.19, 0.26, and 0.18, respectively), and alcohol consequences (d = 0.33, 0.32, and 0.29, respectively), while the AEC was associated with significant reductions in alcohol use alone (total alcohol use d = 0.11, 0.20, and –0.01, respectively; heavy episodic consumption d = 0.15, 0.22, and 0.00, respectively). Changes in perceived drinking norms mediated the relation between BMI and alcohol problems, but not alcohol use. The combined condition was no more effective than the individual components in reducing use and problems, and all intervention effects were time limited, with significant differences evident at short-term (1- and 3-month) but not long-term (6-month) follow-up.

Cognitive-Behavioral Skills-Based Approaches

AEC interventions, which are considered to be more skills-based than motivational, have previously demonstrated efficacy in male populations, but have received more mixed findings among women. Accordingly, Lau-Barraco and Dunn (2008) tested the efficacy of a gender-specific experiential AEC protocol in same-sex groups of heavy-drinking students. Relative to a computer-based, multicomponent alcohol-education-focused program (Alcohol 101) and assessment only, AEC was associated with reductions in typical drinks per week (d = 0.30 and 0.35, respectively) and frequency of heavy episodic drinking (d = 0.36 and 0.34, respectively) from pre- to post-intervention, with no differences between the alcohol education and control groups. Reductions in alcohol expectancies mediated the effect of the AEC on drinking outcomes. As detailed above, Wood et al. (2007) similarly found an experiential AEC was associated with significant reductions in alcohol use.

BAC feedback is another cognitive-behavioral skills-based approach used to intervene with college students. Glindemann, Ehrhart, Drake, and Geller (2007) randomized six fraternities, each hosting two parties, to participate in an incentive-based BAC-reduction program or assessment only. Baseline BAC readings were collected at the first party. Flyers distributed at the second party to both control and intervention groups advertised entry into a raffle for $100 for participating in the research. However, the intervention flyer stipulated that entry was dependent upon having a BAC below 0.05 g%. Individuals at the three intervention parties also received a gender-specific nomogram (BAC calculation card) and a flyer listing protective behavioral strategies. The intervention was associated with lower BACs (estimated d = 0.31) relative to control and an increased percentage of individuals with a BAC below 0.08 g% from baseline to follow-up (estimated d = 0.20). However, the percentage of individuals with a BAC below 0.08 g% at the second party did not differ between intervention and control.

By comparison, Thombs et al. (2007) evaluated BAC feedback in conjunction with normative reeducation in comparison to BAC feedback alone in two freshmen residence halls. All participants provided BAC samples on self-selected evenings and were provided with feedback regarding their BAC the next morning. Individuals in the intervention hall also received feedback regarding the mean BAC of their fellow hall residents, information on BAC interpretation, motivational enhancement elements, and referral sources. The overall observed BAC was higher in the intervention than in the control hall; however, the authors note both means indicate low intoxication (≤ 0.02 g%) and the effect size was small ($d = 0.30$).

Alcohol-Education-Only and Multicomponent Education-Focused Programs

During the past 3 years, only one primary evaluation of an education-only intervention was identified in the literature. Thadani, Huchting, and LaBrie (2009) found that the education-only component of a multicomponent alcohol intervention resulted in increased alcohol knowledge among freshmen women ($d = 0.73$) but was not predictive of alcohol use outcomes at 6-month follow-up in comparison to assessment only. Three additional studies included education-focused comparison groups (Doumas & Haustveit, 2008; Doumas et al., 2009; Schaus et al., 2009), with equivocal or negative results given the absence of group differences and/or lack of an assessment-only control group. Finally, four previously detailed studies included multicomponent alcohol-education-focused programs as comparison conditions, one with positive (Hustad et al., 2010) and three with negative (Carey et al., 2009; Cimini et al., 2009; Lau-Barraco & Dunn, 2008) results.

Three additional studies directly tested the efficacy of multicomponent education-focused programs on alcohol outcomes. Although different programs were tested across studies, each included elements typically associated with efficacious BMI and PFI/PNF interventions, including personalized feedback, correction of normative misperceptions of drinking behavior, discussion of alcohol expectancies, and tips for harm reduction, in addition to general alcohol information. For example, Croom et al. (2008) compared AlcoholEdu for College against an assessment/wait-list control. At 4–6 weeks postmatriculation follow-up, AlcoholEdu was associated with increased alcohol knowledge (estimated $d = 0.52$), but no group differences were evident on alcohol use or problems. With respect to risk behaviors, AlcoholEdu participants reported lower participation in drinking games (estimated $d = 0.12$) but less likelihood of using safer sex strategies. Among students who drank prior to college, AlcoholEdu was associated with consumption of higher-alcohol drinks and greater likelihood of hangovers than the control group.

In contrast, Bersamin, Paschall, Fearnow-Kenney, and Wyrick (2007) evaluated the College Alc program against assessment only and found reductions in frequency of binge drinking at 3-month follow-up relative to control among freshmen reporting past 30-day alcohol consumption at baseline ($d = 0.15$).

Finally, Lovecchio, Wyatt, and DeJong (2010) evaluated the efficacy of AlcoholEdu (2007 version) against assessment only. As expected, AlcoholEdu was associated with greater alcohol knowledge relative to control ($d = 0.11$). Both groups increased their alcohol use from baseline to 1-month follow-up. However, the increase in the AlcoholEdu group was significantly less than in the control group. AlcoholEdu participants also reported fewer alcohol-related consequences ($d = 0.59$), decreased acceptance of others' drinking ($d = 0.65$), and lower positive alcohol expectancies at follow-up ($d = 0.07$). In contrast, AlcoholEdu participants also reported larger decreases in responsible drinking behaviors relative to controls ($d = 0.28$), an effect that cannot be explained by reduced need for such strategies given their overall increase in drinking.

As previously mentioned, although broadly focused on alcohol education, the College Alc and AlcoholEdu programs (most recent versions) include elements of PFI/PNF, including graphic presentation of drinking behavior, correction of normative misperceptions of others' drinking behavior, and personalized harm reduction tips. As such, it is not possible to disentangle the effect of the education-focused component of these interventions from the PFI/PNF elements.

CONCLUSIONS AND RECOMMENDATIONS

Several conclusions and recommendations can be drawn from this review. Of the 18 PFI/PNF and PNF-only interventions evaluated, 11 (Bewick et al., 2008; Butler & Correia, 2009; Doumas & Hannah, 2008; Doumas & Haustveit, 2008; Doumas et al., 2009; Hustad et al., 2010; Lewis et al., 2007 [2 PNF]; Neighbors et al., 2009; Saitz et al., 2007 [2 PFI/PNF]) were associated with reductions in drinking but not drinking-related consequences at follow-up, and 2 (Doumas & Andersen, 2009; White et al., 2007) were associated with both reductions in drinking and consequences. PNF-only interventions were also associated with reductions in perceived drinking norms and increased readiness for behavior change. However, some of these effects were short-term.

Comparatively, of the 19 BMI conditions evaluated, most of which incorporated PFI and/or PNF, 13 (Amaro et al., 2009; Butler & Correia, 2009; Carey et al., 2009; Doumas & Hannah, 2008; Hansson et al., 2007 [1 of 2 BMI]; LaBrie et al., 2008; Schaus et al., 2009; Stahlbrandt et al., 2007; Turrisi et al., 2009 [2 BMI]; Walters et al., 2009 [1 of 2 BMI]; White et al., 2007; Wood et al., 2007 [1 of 2 BMI]) were associated with reductions in alcohol consumption, alcohol-related negative consequences, and/or associated psychopathology. Consistent with findings by Carey et al. (2007), one study (Schaus et al., 2009) evidenced short-term reductions in alcohol consumption with subsequently emerging reductions in alcohol-related negative consequences. One additional study testing two BMI conditions (Wood et al., 2010) found significant protective effects of BMI participation against the likelihood of onset of heavy episodic drinking and related negative consequences.

Findings regarding the efficacy of BMIs in specialized settings and high-risk subpopulations indicate that primary care is a feasible venue, and group BMI or BMI with adjunctive parental communications coaching (via a self-administered manual) is effective in reducing alcohol consumption among freshmen. Although BMI is consistently effective for nonmandated students, findings of recent studies are more mixed for mandated students, with some documented benefit for female students (Carey et al., 2009) and students who receive additional services including coping skills, problem solving, and stress management training (Amaro et al., 2009), as well as short-term reductions in alcohol use and problems with a potential long-term protective effect against alcohol-related consequences (White et al., 2007).

Two studies included AEC protocols, both resulting in reductions in alcohol use but not alcohol-related negative consequences (Lau-Barraco & Dunn, 2008; Wood et al., 2007). Two studies utilized BAC feedback and education in conjunction with other elements, one of which demonstrated a positive intervention effect (Glindemann et al., 2007), and the other demonstrated a potentially iatrogenic effect (Thombs et al., 2007). Finally, 11 studies evaluated alcohol education interventions or multi-component alcohol-education-focused programs, or included education-only comparison groups, only two of which were associated with reductions in drinking and/or alcohol consequences (Bersamin et al., 2007; Hustad et al., 2010), and one evidenced a potential protective effect against increased drinking relative to control (Lovecchio et al., 2010). However, the effective multicomponent alcohol-education-focused programs (AlcoholEdu, 2007 version; AlcoholEdu for College; College Alc) included PF1/PNF elements, making it impossible to disentangle the effect of education alone.

Overall, consistent with prior reviews (Carey et al., 2007; Larimer

& Cronce, 2002, 2007; Walters & Neighbors, 2005; White, 2006), these studies provide support for the efficacy of brief, personalized, individual motivational feedback interventions (BMI with PFI/PNF), AEC interventions, and stand-alone PFI/PNF, with much more limited support for multicomponent alcohol-education-focused interventions that include elements of PFI/PNF, and an absence of support for programs focused exclusively on alcohol education.

Despite the preponderance of evidence supporting the efficacy of BMI and PFI/PNF-only interventions, further research is needed to (1) determine which intervention components and/or delivery modalities are associated with behavior change, (2) identify moderators of intervention efficacy (i.e., what individual variables predict increased/decreased efficacy of in-person BMI relative to PFI/PNF-only and/or PNF-only interventions), and (3) determine conclusively the efficacy of these brief preventive interventions in reducing long-term risk for alcohol misuse and associated problems. Findings (Carey et al., 2007; Schaus et al., 2009) demonstrating emergent effects on alcohol-related consequences, particularly for in-person BMI (Carey et al., 2007; White et al., 2007) suggest that the addition of longer-term follow-up assessments is necessary to adequately gauge efficacy. Modification of existing interventions and/or evaluation of supplemental interventions may also be needed to extend demonstrable short-term effects on alcohol consumption and consequences. Finally, additional research is needed to evaluate the efficacy of brief individual-focused preventive interventions in combination with other alcohol interventions, such as social marketing campaigns targeting campuswide normative misperceptions, environmental interventions targeting sale and distribution of alcohol on or near college campuses, and parenting practices regarding discussion of alcohol use. Ultimately, multiple intervention strategies may be necessary to produce long-term effects on college student drinking.

As support for the *efficacy* of BMIs and other interventions with PFI/PNF components is increasingly evident, additional efforts should be devoted to increasing the *reach* and *effectiveness* of these interventions on college campuses. Based on results of the current review as well as several prior reviews of this literature (Carey et al., 2007; Larimer & Cronce, 2002, 2007; Walters & Neighbors, 2005; White, 2006), implementation of screening and BMI/PFI interventions on college campuses as part of a comprehensive alcohol prevention and intervention strategy is recommended. Options include in-person BMI as well as Web-based or written/mailed PFI/PNF approaches, and it is likely that both in-person and feedback-only approaches have utility in the continuum of care. These services may be most useful when integrated into natural points of contact with students, including health and counseling venues as well as residence halls, fraternity/sorority organizations, athletic teams, and freshman orientation.

Unfortunately, college administrators and health personnel face a number of barriers to implementation of efficacious individual-focused alcohol interventions. Specifically, with the exception of commercially available products such as e-Chug, CollegeAlc, or AlcoholEdu for College, most intervention protocols are neither published nor easily accessible from program developers. Necessary measures and feedback programs are typically not available or not immediately usable in the absence of expensive software. Those seeking to implement BASICS (Dimeff et al., 1999) have access to a published manual and measures. However, they may not have sufficient resources (e.g., expertise to train and supervise therapists, access to programs that can generate tailored feedback) to implement the program with fidelity. Even gathering normative data for inclusion in PFI/PNF protocols may pose a significant challenge.

Despite these challenges, many campuses are instituting BASICS and related BMIs, as well as Web-based PFI/PNF approaches, into routine practice. For example, some studies reviewed above (Amaro et al., 2009; Schaus et al., 2009) integrated BASICS and related interventions into usual care settings with favorable results. Further, many barriers identified above can be overcome by pairing health and counseling personnel with faculty in academic departments who may have expertise in program evaluation and implementation. Simple feedback programs can be created using word processing and spreadsheet/database programs, and/or via the Web with the assistance of tech-savvy students. Distance learning methods (e.g., static Web content, real-time Web-based audio/video, and telephone consultation) have been successfully developed for dissemination of evidence-based interventions for other pressing public health problems such as depression treatment, and they could be adapted to support skill development of individuals seeking to implement in-person BMIs on their campus.

Barriers to intervention implementation also necessitate further research into effective, broad dissemination of evidence-based BMI/PFI approaches. This includes a need for more research evaluating the training and assessment necessary to ensure interventions are delivered with adequate fidelity, methods to improve impact and portability of interventions, and research testing the efficacy of these interventions for young adults from different cultural backgrounds and in contexts outside the traditional, mainstream college setting. The majority of efficacy trials have focused on ethnic majority populations in 4-year colleges, and there is a need to expand our research and prevention focus to young adults in community college settings, tribal colleges and universities, historically black colleges and universities, other minority-serving institutions, and the workplace. Meaningful community partnerships will need to be developed in order to support the adaptation of efficacious prevention approaches for these settings, as well as to develop new approaches that will be maximally relevant to more diverse populations.

ACKNOWLEDGMENTS

Production of this chapter was supported in part through funding from the National Institute on Alcohol Abuse and Alcoholism (Grant No. T32 AA007455, Psychology Training in Alcohol Research).

REFERENCES

Amaro, H., Ahl, M., Matsumoto, A., Prado, G., Mulé, C., Kemmemer, A., et al. (2009). Trial of the university assistance program for alcohol use among mandated students. *Journal of Studies on Alcohol and Drugs*(Suppl. 16), 45–56.

Baer, J. S. (2002). Student factors: Understanding individual variation in college drinking. *Journal of Studies on Alcohol* (Suppl. 14), 40–53.

Bersamin, M., Paschall, M. J., Fearnow-Kenney, M., & Wyrick, D. (2007). Effectiveness of a web-based alcohol-misuse and harm-prevention course among high- and low-risk students. *Journal of American College Health, 55*, 247–254.

Bewick, B. M., Trusler, K., Mulhern, B., Barkham, M., & Hill, A. J. (2008). The feasibility and effectiveness of a web-based personalised feedback and social norms alcohol intervention in UK university students: A randomised control trial. *Addictive Behaviors, 33*, 1192–1198.

Butler, L. H., & Correia, C. J. (2009). Brief alcohol intervention with college student drinkers: Face-to-face versus computerized feedback. *Psychology of Addictive Behaviors, 23*, 163–167.

Caddy, G. R., & Lovibond, S. H. (1976). Self-regulation and discriminated aversive conditioning in the modification of alcoholics' drinking behavior. *Behavior Therapy, 7*, 223–230.

Carey, K. B., Henson, J. M., Carey, M. P., & Maisto, S. A. (2009). Computer versus in-person intervention for students violating campus alcohol policy. *Journal of Consulting and Clinical Psychology, 77*, 74–87.

Carey, K. B., Scott-Sheldon, L. A. J., Carey, M. P., & DeMartini, K. S. (2007). Individual-level interventions to reduce college student drinking: A meta-analytic review. *Addictive Behaviors, 32*, 2469–2494.

Cimini, M. D., Martens, M. P., Larimer, M. E., Kilmer, J. R., Neighbors, C., & Monserrat, J. M. (2009). Assessing the effectiveness of peer-facilitated interventions addressing high-risk drinking among judicially mandated college students. *Journal of Studies on Alcohol and Drugs*(Suppl. 16), 57–66.

Cohen, J. (1988). *Statistical power analysis for the behavioral sciences*. Hillsdale, NJ: Erlbaum.

Cohen, J. (1992). A power primer. *Psychological Bulletin, 112*, 155–159.

Croom, K., Lewis, D., Marchell, T., Lesser, M. L., Reyna, V. F., Kubicki-Bedford, L., et al. (2008). Impact of an online alcohol education course on behavior and harm for incoming first-year college students: Short-term evaluation of a randomized trial. *Journal of American College Health, 57*, 445–454.

Darkes, J., & Goldman, M. S. (1993). Expectancy challenge and drinking reduction: Experimental evidence for a mediational process. *Journal of Consulting and Clinical Psychology, 61*, 344–353.

Darkes, J., & Goldman, M. S. (1998). Expectancy challenge and drinking reduction: Process and structure in the alcohol expectancy network. *Experimental and Clinical Psychopharmacology, 6*, 64–76.

Dimeff, L. A., Baer, J. S., Kivlahan, D. R., & Marlatt, G. A. (1999). *Brief Alcohol Screening and Intervention for College Students (BASICS): A harm reduction approach*. New York: Guilford Press.

Doumas, D. M., & Andersen, L. L. (2009). Reducing alcohol use in first-year university students: Evaluation of a Web-based personalized feedback program. *Journal of College Counseling, 12*, 18–32.

Doumas, D. M., & Hannah, E. (2008). Preventing high-risk drinking in youth in the workplace: A Web-based personalized feedback program. *Journal of Substance Abuse Treatment, 34*, 263–271.

Doumas, D. M., & Haustveit, T. (2008). Reducing heavy drinking in intercollegiate athletes: Evaluation of a Web-based personalized feedback program. *The Sport Psychologist, 22*, 212–228.

Doumas, D. M., McKinley, L. L., & Book, P. (2009). Evaluation of two web-based alcohol interventions for mandated college students. *Journal of Substance Abuse Treatment, 36*, 65–74.

Geisner, I. M., Neighbors, C., Lee, C. M., & Larimer, M. E. (2007). Evaluating personal alcohol feedback as a selective prevention for college students with depressed mood. *Addictive Behaviors, 32*, 2776–2787.

Glindemann, K. E., Ehrhart, I. J., Drake, E. A., & Geller, E. S. (2007). Reducing excessive alcohol consumption at university fraternity parties: A cost-effective incentive/reward intervention. *Addictive Behaviors, 32*, 39–48.

Goodstadt, M. S., & Sheppard, M. A. (1983). Three approaches to alcohol education. *Journal of Studies on Alcohol, 44*, 362–380.

Hansson, H., Rundberg, J., Zetterlind, U., Johnsson, K. O., & Berglund, M. (2007). Two-year outcome of an intervention program for university students who have parents with alcohol problems: A randomized controlled trial. *Alcoholism: Clinical and Experimental Research, 31*, 1927–1933.

Hustad, J. T. P., Barnett, N. P., Borsari, B., & Jackson, K. M. (2010). Web-based alcohol prevention for incoming college students: A randomized controlled trial. *Addictive Behaviors, 35*, 183–189.

Johnston, L. D., O'Malley, P. M., Bachman, J. G., & Schulenberg, J. E. (2009). *Monitoring the Future national survey results on drug use, 1975–2008: Vol. II. College students and adults ages 19–50* (NIH Publication No. 09-7403). Bethesda, MD: National Institute on Drug Abuse.

LaBrie, J. W., Huchting, K. K., Lac, A., Tawalbeh, S., Thompson, A. D., & Larimer, M. E. (2009). Preventing risky drinking in first-year college women: Further validation of a female-specific motivational enhancement group intervention. *Journal of Studies on Alcohol and Drugs*(Suppl. 16), 77–85.

LaBrie, J. W., Huchting, K., Tawalbeh, S., Pedersen, E. R., Thompson, A. D., Shelesky, K., et al. (2008). A randomized motivational enhancement prevention group reduces drinking and alcohol consequences in first-year college women. *Psychology of Addictive Behaviors, 22*, 149–155.

Larimer, M. E., & Cronce, J. M. (2002). Identification, prevention, and treatment: A review of individual-focused strategies to reduce problematic alcohol consumption by college students. *Journal of Studies on Alcohol* (Suppl. 14), 148–163.

Larimer, M. E., & Cronce, J. M. (2007). Identification, prevention, and treatment revisited: Individual-focused college drinking prevention strategies 1999–2006. *Addictive Behaviors, 32*, 2439–2468.

Lau-Barraco, C., & Dunn, M. E. (2008). Evaluation of a single-session expectancy challenge intervention to reduce alcohol use among college students. *Psychology of Addictive Behaviors, 22*, 168–175.

Lewis, M. A., Neighbors, C., Lee, C. M., & Oster-Aaland, L. (2008). 21st birthday celebratory drinking: Evaluation of a personalized normative feedback card intervention. *Psychology of Addictive Behaviors, 22*, 176–185.

Lewis, M. A., Neighbors, C., Oster-Aaland, L., Kirkeby, B. S., & Larimer, M. E. (2007). Indicated prevention for incoming freshmen: Personalized normative feedback and high-risk drinking. *Addictive Behaviors, 32*, 2495–2508.

Lovecchio, C. P., Wyatt, T. M., & DeJong, W. (2010). Reductions in drinking and alcohol-related harms reported by first-year college students taking an online alcohol education course: A randomized trial. *Journal of Health Communication, 15*, 805–819.

Mallett, K. A., Bachrach, R. L., & Turrisi, R. (2009). Examining the unique influence of interpersonal and intrapersonal drinking perceptions on alcohol consumption among college students. *Journal of Studies on Alcohol and Drugs, 70*, 178–185.

Miller, W. R., & Rollnick, S. (2002). *Motivational interviewing: Preparing people for change* (2nd ed.). New York: Guilford Press.

Mun, E. Y., White, H. R., & Morgan, T. J. (2009). Individual and situational factors that influence the efficacy of personalized feedback substance use interventions for mandated college students. *Journal of Consulting and Clinical Psychology, 77*, 88–102.

Neighbors, C., Larimer, M. E., & Lewis, M. A. (2004). Targeting misperceptions of descriptive drinking norms: Efficacy of a computer-delivered personalized normative feedback intervention. *Journal of Consulting and Clinical Psychology, 72*, 434–447.

Neighbors, C., Lee, C. M., Lewis, M. A., Fossos, N., & Walter, T. (2009). Internet-based personalized feedback to reduce 21st birthday drinking: A randomized controlled trial of an event-specific prevention intervention. *Journal of Consulting and Clinical Psychology, 77*, 51–63.

Perkins, H. W. (2002). Surveying the damage: A review of research on consequences of alcohol misuse in college populations. *Journal of Studies on Alcohol* (Suppl. 14), 91–100.

Presley, C. A., Meilman, P. W., & Leichliter, J. S. (2002). College factors that influence drinking. *Journal of Studies on Alcohol (Suppl. 14)*, 82–90.

Saitz, R., Palfai, T. P., Freedner, N., Winter, M. R., MacDonald, A., Lu, J., et al. (2007). Screening and brief intervention online for college students: The iHealth study. *Alcohol and Alcoholism, 42*(1), 28–36.

Schaus, J. F., Sole, M. L., McCoy, T. P., Mullett, N., & O'Brien, M. C. (2009). Alcohol screening and brief intervention in a college student health center: A randomized controlled trial. *Journal of Studies on Alcohol and Drugs* (Suppl. 16), 131–141.

Stahlbrandt, H., Johnsson, K. O., & Berglund, M. (2007). Two-year outcome of alcohol interventions in Swedish university halls of residence: A cluster randomized trial of a brief skills training program, twelve-step-influenced intervention, and controls. *Alcoholism: Clinical and Experimental Research, 31*, 458–466.

Thadani, V., Huchting, K., & LaBrie, J. (2009). Alcohol-related information in multi-component interventions and college students' drinking behavior. *Journal of Alcohol and Drug Education, 53*, 31–51.

Thombs, D. L., Olds, R. S., Osborn, C. J., Casseday, S., Glavin, K., & Berkowitz, A. D. (2007). Outcomes of a technology-based social norms intervention to deter alcohol use in freshman residence halls. *Journal of American College Health, 55*, 325–332.

Turrisi, R., Larimer, M. E., Mallett, K. A., Kilmer, J. R., Ray, A. E., Mastroleo, N. R., et al. (2009). A randomized clinical trial evaluating a combined alcohol intervention for high-risk college students. *Journal of Studies on Alcohol and Drugs, 70*, 555–567.

Walters, S. T., & Neighbors, C. (2005). Feedback interventions for college alcohol misuse: What, why and for whom? *Addictive Behaviors, 30*, 1168–1182.

Walters, S. T., Vader, A. M., Harris, T. R., Field, C. A., & Jouriles, E. N. (2009). Dismantling Motivational Interviewing and feedback for college drinkers: A randomized clinical trial. *Journal of Consulting and Clinical Psychology, 77*, 64–73.

Wechsler, H., Dowdall, G. W., Davenport, A., & Castillo, S. (1995). Correlates of college student binge drinking. *American Journal of Public Health, 85*, 921–926.

Weitzel, J. A., Bernhardt, J. M., Usdan, S., Mays, D., & Glanz, K. (2007). Using wireless handheld computers and tailored text messaging to reduce negative consequences of drinking alcohol. *Journal of Studies on Alcohol and Drugs, 68*, 534–537.

White, H. R. (2006). Reduction of alcohol-related harm on United States college campuses: The use of personal feedback interventions. *International Journal of Drug Policy, 17*, 310–319.

White, H. R., Mun, E. Y., & Morgan, T. J. (2008). Do brief personalized feedback interventions work for mandated students or is it just getting caught that works? *Psychology of Addictive Behaviors, 22*, 107–116.

White, H. R., Mun, E. Y., Pugh, L., & Morgan, T. J. (2007). Long-term effects of brief substance use interventions for mandated college students: Sleeper effects of an in-person personal feedback intervention. *Alcoholism: Clinical and Experimental Research, 31*, 1380–1391.

Wood, M. D., Capone, C., Laforge, R., Erickson, D. J., & Brand, N. H. (2007). Brief motivational intervention and alcohol expectancy challenge with heavy drinking college students: A randomized factorial study. *Addictive Behaviors, 32*, 2509–2528.

Wood, M. D., Fairlie, A. M., & Fernandez, A. C. (2010). Brief motivational and parent interventions for college students: A randomized factorial study. *Journal of Consulting and Clinical Psychology, 78*, 349–361.

CHAPTER 9

Brief Interventions
for Marijuana Use

Scott T. Walters, Christine M. Lee,
and Denise D. Walker

WHAT'S HAPPENING ON CAMPUS?

Marijuana is the most common illicit substance used by college students, with 46.8% of U.S. students reporting lifetime use, 32.3% reporting past-year use, and 17.0% reporting past-month use (Johnston, O'Malley, Bachman, & Schulenberg, 2009). There are several factors that make young adults, and in particular young college students, more prone to marijuana use. In general, young adults tend to use more marijuana than other age groups (Chen & Kandel, 1995; Substance Abuse and Mental Health Services Administration [SAMHSA], 2008). Among college students, initiation of marijuana use peaks around age 18 (Chen & Kandel, 1995; Wagner & Anthony, 2002), and highest monthly use occurs between the ages of 19 and 22 (Chen & Kandel, 1995). Young adults also have the highest risk of dependence, with approximately 7.4% of young adults meeting DSM-IV criteria for past-year cannabis dependence (Chen, Kandel, & Davies, 1997). In a study of first-year college students at one university, Caldeira, Arria, O'Grady, Vincent, and Wish (2008) found that nearly 10% of past-year marijuana users met criteria for a cannabis use disorder, with 10.1% of at-risk users (defined as using marijuana five or more times in the past year) meeting a clinical definition of dependence and 14.5% meeting criteria for abuse.

While young adults commonly view marijuana as a low-risk drug, there are in fact a number of short- and long-term consequences that tend to follow use. Short-term or acute effects of marijuana include decreased cognitive functioning (e.g., trouble thinking, problem solving), respiratory problems, and increased heart rate (National Institute on Drug Abuse [NIDA], 2002; Taylor, Poulton, Moffitt, Ramankutty, & Sears, 2000). Marijuana use is also associated with poorer school performance and attendance (Bell, Wechsler, & Johnston, 1997; Buckner, Ecker, & Cohen, 2010; Lynskey & Hall, 2000), violence against others (Moore & Stuart, 2005), and risky sexual behavior (Simons, Maisto, & Wray, 2010). Among first-year college students using marijuana five or more times in the past year, over 40% reported concentration problems, 18.6% reported driving after using, and 14% reported oversleeping and missing class as a result of marijuana use (Caldeira et al., 2008). Buckner et al. (2010) found that college students who used marijuana reported on average nearly three problems related to marijuana use in the last 3 months, including procrastination, memory loss, and lower energy. Further, marijuana use has been associated with mental health problems such as depression and anxiety (Buckner et al., 2010).

Marijuana use most often occurs alongside other substance use. Mohler-Kuo, Lee, and Wechsler (2003) reported that college students who used marijuana in the last 30 days were also more likely to have smoked cigarettes and engaged in heavy drinking (cf. Bell et al., 1997; Gledhill-Hoyt, Lee, Strote, & Wechsler, 2000). Other research shows that college student drinkers are much more likely to use marijuana than nondrinkers (O'Malley & Johnston, 2002), and students who use both alcohol and marijuana are more likely to experience negative consequences compared to students who only drink (Shillington & Clapp, 2006; Simons & Carey, 2006). For example, after controlling for age, gender, ethnicity, and number of drinks, students who use alcohol and marijuana are nearly six times as likely to report trouble with police compared to those who use only alcohol (Shillington & Clapp, 2006).

FACTORS THAT INFLUENCE USE

Numerous studies have found that being male, younger in age, and white are associated with greater marijuana use (Buckner et al., 2010; Mohler-Kuo et al., 2003). The activities in which college students participate also predict increased risk of marijuana use, particularly participating in fraternities or sororities (Bell et al., 1997; Mohler-Kuo et al., 2003). With regard to residential status, college students who live off campus, not with parents, in fraternity or sorority houses or in coeducational residences tend to report higher rates of marijuana use (Bell et al., 1997; Mohler-Kuo et al., 2003). For example, students living in fraternity or sorority houses were more than twice as likely to have used marijuana compared to other students (Bell et al., 1997). Finally, students who rated religion as less important and students who rated parties as more important are more likely to use marijuana (Bell et al., 1997).

Institutional characteristics also predict marijuana use. In a survey of 119 colleges and universities, Mohler-Kuo et al. (2003) found that 17% of students reported using marijuana in the past month. However, rates varied significantly between colleges, from 0% to 45%. In particular, schools that were primarily non-commuter, non-religiously affiliated, and located in the northeast United States had higher rates of marijuana use. Not surprisingly, the authors also noted a strong relationship between institutional rates of marijuana use, tobacco use, and alcohol use. In fact, the correlation between schools' rates of 30-day marijuana use and tobacco use was $r = .56$, while the relationship between marijuana and binge drinking was $r = .58$. In examining rates of use over time, the authors noted an overall increase in daily, weekly, and annual rates from 1993 to 2001. In particular, they found disproportionate increases in African American and Asian/Pacific Islander students. Interestingly, these increases occurred at a time when binge drinking and tobacco use rates were stable or declining on the same survey. This might indicate that marijuana is being perceived by students as a less risky drug, or that colleges may be devoting fewer resources to marijuana and other illicit substance use prevention.

Beyond demographic and institutional factors, motivational factors also influence marijuana use. For example, Lee, Neighbors, Hendershot, and Grossbard (2009) found that students who used marijuana because they believed it was relatively low risk, or who used for enjoyment, help with sleep, boredom relief, or for altered perceptions, tended to use more frequently than those who used for other reasons. In terms of marijuana-related problems, those who used marijuana to help with sleep or to cope with stress were more likely to experience problems. Conversely, students who used primarily for experimentation reasons tended to use less marijuana and experienced fewer problems as a result of their use (Lee et al., 2009). Interestingly, it is not uncommon for young people to report that they use marijuana because they believe that it is less risky than alcohol or cigarettes (Lee, Neighbors, & Woods, 2007; Lee et al., 2009), even when they report some degree of adverse consequences as a result of their use (Kilmer, Hunt, Lee, & Neighbors, 2007).

Finally, norm perceptions also strongly influence marijuana use. Most college students overestimate the percentage of students who use marijuana on their campus (Kilmer et al., 2006; Page & Scanlan, 1999;

Perkins, Meilman, Leichliter, Cashin, & Presley, 1999; Wolfson, 2000). This overestimation is related to use; those who use marijuana are more likely to overestimate the number of others who also use (Page & Scanlan, 1999; Wolfson, 2000). Perceived injunctive norms, or the perceived *acceptability* of marijuana use among peers, also predict greater use (e.g., Conner & McMillan, 1999; Cook, Lounsbury, & Fontenelle, 1980; Morrison, Golder, Keller, & Gillmore, 2002). As discussed below, approaches that correct misperceptions about alcohol have shown promise in reducing college student alcohol use (Larimer et al., 2009; Neighbors, Larimer, & Lewis, 2004; Walters, Vader, & Harris, 2007), and there is some rationale for their use with marijuana as well.

TREATMENT FOR MARIJUANA ABUSE AND DEPENDENCE

Though it is the most widely used illicit substance, there have only been a handful of treatment trials for marijuana abuse or dependence. McRae, Budney, and Brady (2003) hypothesize that the lack of treatment research stems from a historical assumption that marijuana use typically did not present as a primary disorder, but rather occurred in the presence of alcohol or other drug use. Hence, it was believed that treatment providers mainly saw marijuana use as secondary to other kinds of alcohol or drug use. Further, many researchers believed that marijuana use did not produce a true dependence syndrome, and so treatment for marijuana was seen as less of a priority. (Anecdotally, it seems to us that it has sometimes been more difficult to secure NIH funding for marijuana-related treatment research, which may also explain the scant number of research trials.) Despite these historical beliefs, there is good evidence that many people have selected marijuana as their single or primary drug of abuse, and that many users do exhibit significant dependence symptoms.

Starting with two recent reviews (Budney, Roffman, Stephens, & Walker, 2007; Denis, Lavie, Fatseas, & Auriacombe, 2006), we identified nine independent research studies for adult marijuana use and dependence. (We excluded studies that primarily focused on children or adolescents under the age of 18.) All studies used random assignment to condition and reported on behavioral outcomes, such as treatment completion or abstinence from marijuana. Eight of these studies used a general community sample, while only one (Lee, Neighbors, Kilmer, & Larimer, 2010) was conducted specifically with college students. Table 9.1 summarizes the nine studies.

Most studies included individual meetings, ranging from 1 to 14 contacts. Almost all studies used two behavioral treatments adapted from alcohol treatment: motivational enhancement therapy (MET) and cognitive-behavioral therapy (CBT). Briefly, MET is an intervention format that involves the presentation of a personalized feedback profile, delivered in the clinical style of motivational interviewing (discussed in more detail below). A typical MET sequence involves between one and four individual meetings in which a counselor uses the results of a feedback profile, as well as other motivational techniques, to guide the participant toward increased motivation to change. The one study with college students used a Web-based personalized feedback profile (discussed below) similar to the feedback used in an MET session.

CBT, usually delivered in 6–14 sessions of individual or group counseling, focuses on changing thought patterns to reduce the likelihood of drug-use initiation and relapse. CBT may also involve teaching skills relevant to avoiding marijuana use, such as identifying triggers for cravings, problem-solving skills, and stress management. Some recent studies have also examined whether contingency management (CM) might increase the effectiveness of MET or CBT. CM, a technique adapted from studies of cocaine dependence, uses prizes or vouchers paid to participants based on abstinence from drug use. In a typical scenario, a participant might submit twice-weekly urine samples over the course of the study. For each clean urine sample, the participant might receive a small amount of money (e.g., $5) or a voucher that can be exchanged for prizes. Typically, the value of the prize escalates with each week of sustained abstinence, but is reset to the minimum value if a person relapses.

Taken together, these nine studies suggest that cannabis-using adults respond well to at least three types of behavioral interventions—CBT, MET, and CM. Across studies, 1-year abstinence rates ranged from 9 to 28% for MET and from 19 to 29% for MET/CBT, with a somewhat larger number of participants reporting a reduction in use and associated problems (but not necessarily complete abstinence). Where included, corresponding abstinence rates for delayed treatment groups ranged from 0 to 9%. In the single study published with college students, Lee et al. (2010) did not find an overall intervention effect. However, there was a significant effect of the intervention for students with a family history of drug problems and, to a smaller extent, students who were in the contemplation stage with regard to their marijuana use.

From this review, we can draw three additional conclusions. First, generally speaking, participants in all groups (including the control group) tended to use less marijuana over time. This may relate to the typical participant profile in these studies, which most often included cannabis users who were seeking treatment. Second, *reduced use* was a more common outcome than complete abstinence. This might suggest that, although desired by the treatment provider, total abstinence may

TABLE 9.1. Published Trials of Cannabis Use/Dependence

Study	Participants	Intervention approach	Outcome
Stephens, Roffman, & Simpson, 1994	212 adult users	1. 10-session group CBT/relapse prevention, or 2. 10-session social support group	Both groups reduced use, with no significant differences between them.
Budney et al. (2000)	60 cannabis-dependent adults	1. 4-session MET, 2. 14-session MET + CBT, or 3. 14-session MET + CBT + CM	MET + CBT + CM reduced use over other two conditions.
Stephens, Roffman, & Curtin (2000)	291 adult users	1. 14-session CBT group, 2. 2-session MET, or 3. Delayed treatment	CBT and MET showed reductions over delayed treatment.
Copeland, Swift, Roffman, & Stephens (2001)	229 adult users	1. 1-session CBT, 2. 6-session CBT, or 3. Delayed treatment	CBT conditions showed reductions over delayed treatment.
Marijuana Treatment Project Research Group (2004)	450 cannabis-dependent adults	1. 2-session MET, 2. 9-session MET + CBT, or 3. Delayed treatment	Both active conditions showed reductions over delayed treatment. CBT + MET produced greater long-term abstinence than MET alone.
Sinha, Easton, Renee-Aubin, & Carroll (2003)	65 probation-referred young adults	1. 3-session MET, or 2. 3-session MET + CM	Both groups reported reductions in use. MET + CM showed better treatment completion rates.
Budney, Moore, Rocha, & Higgins (2006)	90 cannabis-dependent adults	1. 14-session MET + CBT, 2. 14-session MET + CBT + CM vouchers, or 3. 14-session CM alone	CM conditions had better short-term abstinence rates. MET + CBT + CM had better long-term abstinence rates.

(continued)

TABLE 9.1. (continued)

Study	Participants	Intervention approach	Outcome
Kadden, Litt, Kabela-Cormier, & Petry (2007)	240 cannabis-dependent adults	1. 9-session MET + CBT, 2. 9-session MET + CBT + CM, 3. 9-session CM alone, or 4. Case management	CM conditions had better short-term abstinence rates. MET + CBT + CM had better long-term abstinence rates.
Lee et al. (2010)	341 marijuana-using freshman college students	1. Web-based personalized feedback, or 2. Assessment only	No differences between groups. Family-history-positive users in the feedback group showed reduced use.

not be a realistic goal for all participants. Ironically, in contrast to the voluminous literature on moderation and harm reduction for alcohol (Marlatt & Witkiewitz, 2002), there is virtually no research on harm reduction approaches for marijuana use. Despite this, the literature suggests that many users do, in fact, choose this route. Third, treatment sequences that were longer or multicomponent tended to produce better outcomes. Although MET and CBT tended to produce similar outcomes when tested alone, the results tended to be superior when the two approaches were combined. Although no one study has directly compared the two approaches alone and combined, this observation seems to hold generally. This also fits philosophically with the intent of the two approaches; while MET is designed to raise interest in change, CBT helps to teach skills for making changes. Similarly, when CM was combined with the other two approaches, it tended to improve outcomes, especially in rates of continuous abstinence. For example, Budney, Higgins, Radonovich, and Novy (2000) reported abstinence rates of 5% for MET, 10% for MET + CBT, and 35% for MET + CBT + CM. When considering only brief interventions (the focus of this chapter), there was some support for the effectiveness of MET delivered in one to three contacts.

In relating these results to college student marijuana use, it is important to note that the intervention research is currently limited to only one study that found only partial support for the intervention. Thus, at this point, most college interventions must still rely on evidence from general-population marijuana studies or intervention studies of alcohol (and other drug) use among college students.

MARIJUANA TREATMENT ON THE COLLEGE CAMPUS

As previously discussed, a significant number of college students are using marijuana and combining marijuana with other substances (especially alcohol and cigarettes), and may be experiencing significant harm as a result of their use. Unfortunately, risk perception remains low; most students who would benefit from a change do not seek help. Buckner et al. (2010) found that among college students who used marijuana, a clear majority (86%) said they were uninterested in receiving formal treatment. Even among students who reported experiencing more than one problem related to their use, only 23% said they were interested in receiving treatment (Buckner et al., 2010). Caldeira et al. (2009) found that over 96% of students who met the criteria for a substance use disorder (SUD) did not perceive the need for help regarding their substance use. What this means on the college campus is that marijuana-using students will most often come to the attention of campus personnel through referral sources such as residence life or judicial affairs, or by presenting at student health or counseling centers for related problems, and as a result, problem recognition may be low compared to college alcohol users.

Although most brief interventions for college student marijuana use have been adapted from an alcohol model, there are a few special considerations when addressing marijuana use in a prevention or intervention context. One difference is the legal status of marijuana. For example, while drinking alcohol under the age of 21 is technically illegal in the United States, marijuana possession and use tends to result in greater legal consequences for individuals. In addition, while many campuses are developing policies to address marijuana violations on campus, it is unclear whether a harm reduction approach to intervention and treatment would be consistent and feasible within current policies and laws. For example, a harm reduction approach might include determining what level of use would be feasible and appropriate for an individual. It also is unclear to what extent the political climate on college campuses would be compatible with endorsing programs where abstinence may not be the primary goal.

TWO BRIEF INTERVENTION FORMATS

Personalized Feedback

In the research literature, computer and Web-based interventions have ranged from relatively simple formats such as assessment with tailored feedback (Neighbors et al., 2004; Walters et al., 2007), to more complex formats that involve interactive assessments, goal setting, skills practice, and self-monitoring (Lustria, Cortese, Noar, & Glueckauf, 2009). Several automated interventions have shown efficacy at reducing alcohol consumption and marijuana use among young people (Kypri et al., 2004; Neighbors, Larimer, & Lewis, 2004; Walters et al., 2007), with effects in some instances that are comparable to in-person interventions (Butler & Correia, 2009; Kay-Lambkin, Baker, Lewin, & Carr, 2009). As highlighted above, the literature on Web-based interventions for marijuana use in college students is currently limited to a single study, and thus the current thinking is clearly adapted from alcohol intervention studies.

Web-based feedback interventions are attractive because of their relatively low cost, high transportability, and appeal to young people (Elliott, Carey, & Bolles, 2008). As discussed by Hester and Miller (2006), automated interventions have several potential advantages over face-to-face interventions: (1) they require little or no staff contact, which may increase cost-effectiveness; (2) they allow for automatic data collection and follow-up; and (3) they can be disseminated with little loss of fidelity. According to the literature, personalized feedback programs are one promising Web-based intervention format for marijuana use. As mentioned above, personalized feedback approaches are similar to MET interventions in their emphasis on increasing motivation via the presentation of discrepant information. After students completed a self-assessment on marijuana (and possibly other behaviors), the program would provide feedback such as: (1) a summary of use; (2) information on marijuana-related problems, such as effects on academic performance or economic cost; (3) a comparison of one's use to national or campus norms; (4) details about related behaviors such as alcohol use; and (5) information and suggestions for quitting marijuana use.

In a review of feedback interventions for college alcohol use, Walters and Neighbors (2005) concluded that personalized feedback can have a modest impact on drinking whether delivered over the Internet or via a face-to-face interview. Eleven of the 13 reviewed studies (77%) reported significant reductions in drinking when compared to baseline or, when available, compared to a control or comparison condition. At the time of that review, Web-based feedback approaches showed clear effects at 6 months, with little short-term difference between Web-based and in-person feedback (e.g., MET) approaches. More recently, studies have suggested that feedback can effectively reduce drinking at follow-ups of up to 12 months (Butler & Correia, 2009; Doumas & Haustveit, 2008; Larimer et al., 2007). For instance, Larimer et al. (2007) reported that after 12 months, those who did not receive feedback were 1.4 times as likely to engage in heavy drinking as were those who received feedback. One of the difficulties noted by Walters and Neighbors (2005) was the widely varying content employed by the different studies. Feedback varied from relatively simple reports on how one's drinking compared to that of others, to accounts that included much more information about drinking, consequences, and related behaviors. Since studies have used a variety of forms, it is impossible to say which elements were responsible for the change. However, since the time of the review, several studies have suggested that normative feedback is the most likely mediator of drinking changes. In general, changes in normative perceptions tend to mediate changes in drinking (Larimer et al., 2009; Neighbors et al., 2004; Walters et al., 2007), and experimental studies have suggested that gender-specific normative comparisons may be especially effective for women (Lewis & Neighbors, 2007). However, it is important to note again that, with only one exception (Lee et al., 2010), information about feedback has come from alcohol studies; as previously mentioned, marijuana users may differ from alcohol users in their profile of use, perceptions of risk, and motivations for use, and thus it is difficult to determine the extent to which positive effects would generalize to marijuana users.

At the time of this writing, neither the feedback reports used in studies of MET nor the one study that employed Web-based marijuana feedback were commercially available. However, we were able to identify two sources of Web-based feedback for marijuana use. One program, eCheckup to Go, is distributed by San Diego State University Research Foundation (*www.echeckuptogo.com*). The program, which can be used either as stand-alone feedback or as an adjunct to an individual MET session, contains elements such as a summary of use, time spent under the influence, a comparison of use to other activities, money spent on marijuana, and normative comparisons. Another program marketed by BluSKY is designed to generate a feedback profile to supplement a BASICS-style feedback intervention (*www.basicsfeedback.com*). The survey and feedback portions of the program can be customized to the individual campus. Both programs generate feedback similar to the reports used in the aforementioned studies.

Motivational Enhancement Therapy

Another promising format for brief interventions is MET, and its related approach—the "Marijuana Check-Up." As previously mentioned, MET is a treatment format that combines motivational interviewing (MI) and a personalized feedback profile. MI is a "client-centered, directive style of interacting with a person to help explore and resolve ambivalence about change" (Miller & Rollnick, 2002). Because MI is an interaction style rather than a set of techniques, it is usually introduced in terms of its stylistic approach: (1) Express Empathy; (2) Develop Discrepancy; (3) Roll with Resistance; and (4) Support Self-Efficacy. MI borrows from client-centered counseling in its emphasis on empathy, optimism, and respect for client choice (Rogers, 1961). MI also draws from self-perception theory, which says that a person becomes more or less committed to an action based on the verbal stance he or she takes (Bem, 1972). Thus, a client who talks about the benefits of change is more likely to make that change, whereas a client who argues and defends the status quo is more likely to continue with present behavior. Finally, MI is also logically connected to the Stages of Change model, which suggests that people go through a sequence of stages when thinking about change (Prochaska, DiClemente, & Norcross, 1992). Although a full technical explanation is outside the scope of this chapter, briefly, MI involves the strategic use of reflective listening strategies such as open questions and reflections to guide a client's choice of language. In fact, there is good evidence that through elements such as the counselor's MI—choice of questions, his or her reflections, and the session tone—can influence the kind of language clients use during a counseling session, and that client language is related to later outcome (Moyers et al., 2007; Moyers, Martin, Houck, Christopher, & Tonigan, 2009).

When used as part of an MI session, personalized feedback helps demonstrate to clients, using their own responses, the ways that marijuana might be interfering with important goals or values. For instance, one section of the feedback might show the amount of time that the student has been under the influence of marijuana in the last month compared to the time spent studying for school. Another section might show the student's marijuana use in relation to other students. In an MET session, the counselor uses questions and reflections to elicit the student's reaction to this feedback. In essence, feedback becomes a motivational tool for eliciting pro-change talk (or reducing anti-change talk). However, in the case of marijuana, more work is needed to identify which feedback variables are most relevant to college student marijuana users.

An adaptation of MET for nontreatment seekers is the "Check-up" approach (Walker, Roffman, Picciano, & Stephens, 2007). This format was originally designed to attract adults who were experiencing negative consequences from their drinking but were not necessarily looking for treatment. MET and the Check-up share the same format but functionally they serve different groups. Whereas MET can be appropriate for those who are not actively considering change (e.g., disciplinary referrals), the Check-up can be advertised to those who might be interested in exploring their marijuana use (though not necessarily convinced that they need to change). For instance, in the original Drinker's Check-up (DCU) study (Miller, Sovereign, & Krege, 1988), a group of participants were recruited to participate in a free assessment and feedback service for drinkers who wanted to find out whether alcohol was harming them. In order to attract participants, the Check-up was promoted not as treatment, but rather as an opportunity to "take stock" of their behavior. Participants completed a structured interview battery and then received feedback on their alcohol consumption, delivered in an MI style. The personalized feedback report used in Check-up studies typically includes a summary of information from the baseline assessment, a comparison to population norms, identification of risk factors, and negative consequences of the behavior (Walker et al., 2007). Although most of these variables are essentially borrowed from an alcohol feedback model, based on our literature review there is some reason to think that at least some of the variables, such as injunctive and descriptive norms, would be effective in a marijuana profile as well. Likewise, a summary of negative consequences resulting from use, such as respiratory effects, difficulty concentrating, and money spent, might also be motivating to users. Finally, it might also be possible to incorporate motives for marijuana use, such as comparative risk, sleep facilitation, or stress reduction, in the overall profile.

Two books give detailed protocols for conducting MET sessions with college drinkers. The BASICS manual (Dimeff, Baer, Kivlahan, & Marlatt, 1999) presents a two- to three-session individual format that integrates personalized feedback with skills training, relapse prevention, and other activities. Another book, *Talking with College Students about Alcohol* (Walters & Baer, 2006), describes a one-session format organized closely along the lines of MET. While neither of the books focuses specifically on marijuana use, either method can be adapted for use with marijuana users. Finally, there are manuals available online for the adult Marijuana Treatment Project and the adolescent Cannabis Youth Treatment Series (*kap.samhsa.gov/products/manuals*). Both manuals describe a multiweek individual treatment sequence.

CLINICAL CONSIDERATIONS IN WORKING WITH MARIJUANA USERS

Brief interventions, and specifically adaptations of MI and feedback, are a particularly good fit for marijuana-using college students, as these approaches are useful with people who are ambivalent about making a behavior change because of the time, energy, or commitment involved. As previously mentioned, because very few college students self-refer to treatment but instead come to the attention of counseling services via residence life, judicial affairs, or other systems, such ambivalence is likely to be quite common. Developmentally, college students are enjoying a time when they are becoming more independent and self-sustaining. Therefore, using an approach that values their desire for autonomy (e.g., where the counselor avoids advice giving or taking on an expert role) can reduce defensiveness when talking about marijuana.

As previously mentioned, young people receive a host of mixed messages around marijuana use. On one side, many national organizations devoted to the study and treatment of alcohol and drugs (e.g., NIDA, SAMHSA) have detailed marijuana's addictive potential and its harmful effects on the brain, lungs, and heart. On the other side, organizations such as the National Organization for the Reform of Marijuana Laws (NORML) tend to emphasize the benefits of use and the ways in which laws surrounding marijuana use create injustices for those who use. Consequently, many youth have come to believe that marijuana is not as harmful as other drugs (Johnston et al., 2009). In our experience, young people often defend their use by saying that marijuana is a plant, a "natural" substance, and is not addictive. These views have been hotly debated despite an empirical literature that has demonstrated a range of problems and a reliable withdrawal syndrome associated with heavy marijuana use (Budney & Hughes, 2006). Thus, young adults can be confused about the information they receive about marijuana, which may in turn reduce motivation to change.

Clinically, these topics invariably make their way into counseling conversations. Many students will acknowledge and want to debate the more benign or even positive aspects of marijuana, such as the medicinal value for some chronic health problems or the relaxed laws surrounding personal use in some states—none of which may relate to the student's actual use. While it can be tempting to debate with the student, strong arguments tend to increase a student's resistance. When confronted with such information, it is important to try and appreciate the student's viewpoint, while at the same time keeping the discussion focused on the student's *personal experiences* with marijuana. Similarly, it may be helpful to consider rules of thumb around personal disclosure. The counselor's perspective on the topic should only be included if the student asks for it *and* there is therapeutic merit in disclosing such information. Sessions can easily turn into policy debates if the purpose of the conversation is not tightly focused on how marijuana has impacted the student.

In terms of clinical strategy, there are more similarities than differences between marijuana and other drugs of abuse. Like other substances of abuse, we assume that people who use marijuana can experience unwanted consequences, as well as abuse and dependence symptoms. In fact, despite marijuana's reputation as a "soft" drug, students can and often do find that marijuana use is creating unwanted consequences (e.g., memory problems, respiratory difficulties) or it is in conflict with present or future goals (e.g., class or job performance). The use of a feedback profile is one way to help a student identify these items of concern. Additionally, MI-consistent techniques like open-ended questions and reflections are designed to elicit talk about ways that marijuana use is inconsistent with personal values or goals. In this process, it is essential to be tuned in to what students may say spontaneously about the downside of their personal experience.

CONCLUSION

With nearly a third of students reporting past year use, marijuana is the most commonly encountered substance of abuse on the college campus. Heavy marijuana use has been linked to both acute and long-term consequences, such as respiratory and memory difficulties, poorer school performance, legal problems, and risk for cannabis dependence. In fact, a significant number of marijuana users report at least some problems related to their use. Despite this, most people's perceptions of their own risk remain low when compared to perceptions of risk from alcohol or cigarettes, and thus very few marijuana users self-refer for treatment. This means that most often, marijuana users come to the attention of counseling services through the residence life, judicial, or health systems. In addition, the host of mixed messages around marijuana use means that students are far more likely to resist messages to reduce or quit use.

However, despite these tendencies, college students can and do change their use. In fact, the most common pattern for young people is to mature out of marijuana use as they age into their 20s. The most promising intervention formats for young adult users involve cognitive-behavioral, motivational, and feedback approaches. In particular, when having conversations with students around marijuana, we have suggested that providers: (1) use evidence-based strategies such as motivational interviewing and feedback; (2) steer clear of debates about the general benefits/risks of marijuana; (3) keep the focus on the student's own experiences with the drug; and (4) look for ways that a student's use is resulting in problems, or is in conflict with personal values or norms. In some instances, the resulting problems (or risk for problems) may be very minor (at least in the student's mind), but the concept of increased motivation for change remains the principle target.

With regard to legality and tolerance for moderate use outcomes, it must be up to the discretion of the individual university and counselor to determine what approach is tolerable. We have specifically avoided this issue because of the rapidly changing state laws with regard to marijuana possession and use. Finally, it is striking that only a single treatment study of marijuana use with college students has been conducted, even though marijuana is the most common illicit substance among college students. Future research on marijuana interventions would likely mirror the research agenda 10 years ago with respect to alcohol interventions. For interventions to become more efficacious, researchers will need to identify the specific mechanisms that underlie successful interventions, and then work to tailor these to different kinds of students.

ACKNOWLEDGMENTS

We wish to acknowledge Jason Kilmer and Betsy Foy for their contributions to earlier drafts of this chapter.

REFERENCES

Bell, R., Wechsler, H., & Johnston, L. (1997). Correlates of college student marijuana use: Results of a US national survey. *Addiction, 92*(5), 571–581.

Bem, D. J. (1972). Self-perception theory. In L. Berkowitz (Ed.), *Advances in experimental social psychology* (Vol. 6, pp. 1–62). New York: Academic Press.

Buckner, J. D., Ecker, A. H. & Cohen, A. S. (2010). Mental health problems and interest in marijuana treatment among marijuana-using college students. *Addictive Behaviors, 35*, 826–833.

Budney, A. J., Higgins, S. T., Radonovich, K. J., & Novy, P. L. (2000). Adding voucher-based incentives to coping skills and motivational enhancement improves outcomes during treatment for marijuana dependence. *Journal of Consulting and Clinical Psychology, 68*(6), 1051–1061.

Budney, A. J., & Hughes, J. R. (2006). The cannabis withdrawal syndrome. *Current Opinion in Psychiatry, 19*(3), 233–238.

Budney, A. J., Moore, B. A., Rocha, H. L., & Higgins, S. T. (2006). Clinical trial of abstinence-based vouchers and cognitive-behavioral therapy for cannabis dependence. *Journal of Consulting and Clinical Psychology, 74*(2), 307–316.

Budney, A. J., Roffman, R., Stephens, R. S., & Walker, D. (2007). Marijuana dependence and its treatment. *Addiction Science & Clinical Practice, 4*(1), 4–16.

Butler, L. H., & Correia, C. J. (2009). Brief alcohol intervention with college student drinkers: Face-to-face versus computerized feedback. *Psychology of Addictive Behaviors, 23*(1), 163–167.

Caldeira, K. M., Arria, A. M., O'Grady, K. E., Vincent, K. B., & Wish, E. D. (2008). The occurrence of cannabis use disorders and other cannabis-related problems among first-year college students. *Addictive Behaviors, 33*, 397–411.

Caldeira, K., Kasperski, S., Sharma, E., Vincent, K., O'Grady, K., Wish, E., et al. (2009). College students rarely seek help despite serious substance use problems. *Journal of Substance Abuse Treatment, 37*(4), 368–378.

Chen, K., & Kandel, D. B. (1995). The natural history of drug use from adolescence to the mid-thirties in a general population sample. *American Journal of Public Health, 85*, 41–47.

Chen, K., Kandel, D. B., & Davies, M. (1997). Relationships between frequency and quantity of marijuana use and last year proxy dependence among adolescents and adults in the United States. *Drug and Alcohol Dependence, 46*, 53–67.

Conner, M., & McMillan, B. (1999). Interaction effects in the theory of planned behavior: Studying cannabis use. *British Journal of Social Psychology, 38*(2), 195–222.

Cook, P. M., Lounsbury, W. J., & Fontenelle, A. G. (1980). An application of Fishbein and Ajzen's attitude-subjective norms model to the study of drug use. *The Journal of Social Psychology, 110*, 193–201.

Copeland, J., Swift, W., Roffman, R., & Stephens, R. (2001). A randomized controlled trial of brief cognitive-behavioral interventions for cannabis use disorder. *Journal of Substance Abuse Treatment, 21*(2), 55–64.

Denis, C., Lavie, E., Fatseas, M., & Auriacombe, M. (2006). Psychotherapeutic interventions for cannabis abuse and/or dependence in outpatient settings. *Cochrane Database of Systematic Reviews, 3*, CD005336.

Dimeff, L. A., Baer, J. S., Kivlahan, D. R., & Marlatt, G. A. (1999). *Brief Alcohol Screening and Intervention for College Students (BASICS): A harm reduction approach*. New York: Guilford Press.

Doumas, D. M., & Haustveit, T. (2008). Reducing heavy drinking in intercollegiate athletes: Evaluation of a Web-based personalized feedback program. *Sport Psychologist, 22*(2), 212–228.

Elliott, J. C., Carey, K. B., & Bolles, J. R. (2008). Computer-based interventions for college drinking: A qualitative review. *Addictive Behaviors, 33*(8), 994–1005.

Gledhill-Hoyt, J., Lee, H., Strote, J., & Wechsler, H. (2000). Increased use of marijuana and other illicit drugs at US colleges in the 1990s: Results of three national surveys. *Addiction, 95*, 1655–1667.

Hester, R. K., & Miller, J. H. (2006). Computer-based tools for diagnosis and treatment of alcohol problems. *Alcohol Research and Health, 29*(1), 36–40.

Johnston, L. D., O'Malley, P. M., Bachman, J. G., & Schulenberg, J. E. (2009). *Monitoring the Future national results on adolescent drug use: Overview of key findings* (NIH Publication No. 09-7401). Bethesda, MD: National Institute on Drug Abuse.

Kadden, R. M., Litt, M. D., Kabela-Cormier, E., & Petry, N. M. (2007). Abstinence rates following behavioral treatments for marijuana dependence. *Addictive Behaviors, 32*(6), 1220–1236.

Kay-Lambkin, F. J., Baker, A. L., Lewin, T. J., & Carr, V. J. (2009). Computer-based psychological treatment for comorbid depression and problematic alcohol and/or cannabis use: A randomized controlled trial of clinical efficacy. *Addiction, 104*(3), 378–388.

Kilmer, J. R., Hunt, S. B., Lee, C. M., & Neighbors, C. (2007). Marijuana use, risk perception, and consequences: Is perceived risk congruent with reality? *Addictive Behaviors, 32*, 3026–3033.

Kilmer, J. R., Walker, D. D., Lee, C. M., Palmer, R. S., Mallett, K. A., Fabiano, P., et al. (2006). Misperceptions of college student marijuana use: Implications for prevention. *Journal of Studies on Alcohol, 67*, 277–281.

Kypri, K., Saunders, J. B., Williams, S. M., McGee, R. O., Langley, J. D., Cashell-Smith, M. L., et al. (2004). Web-based screening and brief intervention for hazardous drinking: A double-blind randomized controlled trial. *Addiction, 99*(11), 1410–1417.

Larimer, M. E., Kaysen, D. L., Lee, C. M., Kilmer, J. R., Lewis, M. A., Dillworth, T., et al. (2009). Evaluating level of specificity of normative referents in relation to personal drinking behavior. *Journal of Studies on Alcohol and Drugs* (Suppl. 16), 115–121.

Larimer, M. E., Lee, C. M., Kilmer, J. R., Fabiano, P. M., Stark, C. B., Geisner, I. M., et al. (2007). Personalized mailed feedback for college drinking prevention: A randomized clinical trial. *Journal of Consulting and Clinical Psychology, 75*(2), 285–293.

Lee, C. M., Neighbors, C., Hendershot, C. S., & Grossbard, J. (2009). Development and preliminary validation of a comprehensive marijuana motives questionnaire. *Journal of Studies on Alcohol and Drugs, 70*, 279–287.

Lee, C., Neighbors, C., Kilmer, J., & Larimer, M. (2010). A brief, Web-based personalized feedback selective intervention for college student marijuana use: A randomized clinical trial. *Psychology of Addictive Behaviors, 24*(2), 265–273.

Lee, C. M., Neighbors, C., & Woods, B. A. (2007). Marijuana motives: Young adults' reasons for using marijuana. *Addictive Behaviors, 32*, 1384–1394.

Lewis, M. A., & Neighbors, C. (2007). Optimizing personalized normative feedback: The use of gender-specific referents. *Journal of Studies on Alcohol and Drugs, 68*(2), 228–237.

Lustria, M. L., Cortese, J., Noar, S. M., & Glueckauf, R. L. (2009). Computer-tailored health interventions delivered over the web: Review and analysis of key components. *Patient Education and Counseling, 74*(2), 156–173.

Lynskey, M., & Hall, W. (2000). The effects of adolescent cannabis use on educational attainment: A review. *Addiction, 95*, 1621–1630.

Marijuana Treatment Project Research Group. (2004). Brief treatments for cannabis dependence: Findings from a randomized multisite trial. *Journal of Consulting and Clinical Psychology, 72*(3), 455–466.

Marlatt, G. A., & Witkiewitz, K. (2002). Harm reduction approaches to alcohol use: Health promotion, prevention, and treatment. *Addictive Behaviors, 27*(6), 867–886.

McRae, A. L., Budney, A. J., & Brady, K. T. (2003). Treatment of marijuana dependence: A review of the literature. *Journal of Substance Abuse Treatment, 24*(4), 369–376.

Miller, W. R., & Rollnick, S. (2002). *Motivational interviewing: Preparing people for change* (2nd ed.). New York: Guilford Press.

Miller, W. R., Sovereign, R. G., & Krege, B. (1988). Motivational Interviewing with problem drinkers: II. The Drinker's Check-Up as a preventive intervention. *Behavioural Psychotherapy, 16*(4), 251–268.

Mohler-Kuo, M., Lee, J. E., & Wechsler, H. (2003). Trends in marijuana and other illicit drug use among college students: Results from 4 Harvard School of Public Health College Alcohol Study surveys: 1993–2001. *Journal of American College Health, 52*(1), 17–24.

Moore, T. M., & Stuart, G. L. (2005). A review of the literature on marijuana and interpersonal violence. *Addictive Behaviors, 10,* 171–192.

Morrison, D. M., Golder, S., Keller, T. E., & Gillmore, M. R. (2002). The theory of reasoned action as a model of marijuana use: Tests of implicit assumptions and applicability to high-risk young women. *Psychology of Addictive Behaviors, 16,* 212–224.

Moyers, T. B., Martin, T., Christopher, P. J., Houck, J. M., Tonigan, J. S., & Amrhein, P. C. (2007). Client language as a mediator of motivational interviewing efficacy: Where is the evidence? *Alcoholism: Clinical and Experimental Research, 31*(Suppl. 3), 40s–47s.

Moyers, T. B., Martin, T., Houck, J. M., Christopher, P. J., & Tonigan, J. S. (2009). From in-session behaviors to drinking outcomes: a causal chain for motivational interviewing. *Journal of Consulting and Clinical Psychology, 77*(6), 1113–1124.

National Institute on Drug Abuse. (2002). *Marijuana abuse* (NIH Publication No. 02-3859). Bethesda, MD: Author.

Neighbors, C., Larimer, M. E., & Lewis, M. A, (2004). Targeting misperceptions of descriptive drinking norms: Efficacy of a computer-delivered personalized normative feedback intervention. *Journal of Consulting and Clinical Psychology 72*(3), 434–447.

Neighbors, C., Larimer, M. E., & Lewis, M. A. (2004). Targeting misperceptions of descriptive drinking norms: Efficacy of a computer-delivered personalized normative feedback intervention. *Journal of Consulting and Clinical Psychology, 72*(3), 434–447.

O'Malley, P. M., & Johnston, L. D. (2002). Epidemiology of alcohol and other drug use among American college students. *Journal of Studies on Alcohol* (Suppl. 14), 23–39.

Page, M. R., & Scanlan A. (1999). Perceptions of the prevalence of marijuana use among college students: A comparison between current users and nonusers. *Journal of Child and Adolescent Substance Abuse, 9,* 1–13.

Perkins, H. W., Meilman, W. P., Leichliter, S. J., Cashin, R. J., & Presley, A. C. (1999). Misperceptions of the norms for the frequency of alcohol and other drug use on college campuses. *Journal of American College Health, 47,* 253–261.

Prochaska, J. O., DiClemente, C. C., & Norcross, J. C. (1992). In search of how people change: Applications to addictive behaviors. *American Psychologist, 47*(9), 1102–1114.

Rogers, C. R. (1961). *On becoming a person: A therapist's view of psychotherapy.* Boston: Houghton Mifflin.

Shillington, A., & Clapp, J. (2006). Heavy alcohol use compared to alcohol and marijuana use: Do college students experience a difference in substance use problems? *Journal of Drug Education, 36*(1), 91–103.

Simons, J. S., & Carey, K. B. (2006). An affective and cognitive model of marijuana and alcohol problems. *Addictive Behaviors, 31,* 1578–1592.

Simons, J. S., Maisto, S. A., & Wray, T. B. (2010). Sexual risk among young adult dual alcohol and marijuana users. *Addictive Behaviors, 35,* 533–536

Sinha, R., Easton, C., Renee-Aubin, L., & Carroll, K. M. (2003). Engaging young probation-referred marijuana-abusing individuals in treatment: A pilot trial. *American Journal on Addictions, 12*(4), 314–323.

Stephens, R. S., Roffman, R. A., & Curtin, L. (2000). Comparison of extended versus brief treatments for marijuana use. *Journal of Consulting and Clinical Psychology, 68*(5), 898–908.

Stephens, R. S., Roffman, R. A., & Simpson, E. E. (1994). Treating adult marijuana dependence: A test of the relapse prevention model. *Journal of Consulting and Clinical Psychology, 62*(1), 92–99.

Substance Abuse and Mental Health Services Administration (SAMHSA). (2008). *2004 National Survey on Drug Use and Health: Detailed tables.* Retrieved from *www.oas.samhsa.gov/nsduh/2k4nsduh/2k4tabs/sect1petabs1to66.htm# tab1.20b.*

Taylor, R. D., Poulton, R., Moffitt, E. T., Ramankutty, P., & Sears, R. M. (2000). The respiratory effects of cannabis dependence in young adults. *Addiction, 95,* 1669–1677.

Wagner, F. A., & Anthony, J. C. (2002). From first drug use to drug dependence: Developmental periods of risk for dependence upon marijuana, cocaine, and alcohol. *Neuropsychopharmacology, 26,* 479–488.

Walker, D. D., Roffman, R. A., Picciano, J. F., & Stephens, R. S. (2007). The check-up: In-person, computerized, and telephone adaptations of motivational enhancement treatment to elicit voluntary participation by the contemplator. *Substance Abuse Treatment Prevention, and Policy, 2,* 2–10.

Walters, S. T., & Baer, J. S. (2006). *Talking with college students about alcohol: Motivational strategies for reducing abuse.* New York: Guilford Press.

Walters, S. T., & Neighbors, C. (2005). Feedback interventions for college alcohol misuse: What, why and for whom? *Addictive Behaviors, 30*(6), 1168–1182.

Walters, S. T., Vader, A. M., & Harris, T. R. (2007). A controlled trial of Web-based feedback for heavy drinking college students. *Prevention Science, 8*(1), 83–88.

Wolfson, S. (2000). Students' estimates of the prevalence of drug use: Evidence for a false consensus effect. *Psychology of Addictive Behaviors, 14,* 295–298.

CHAPTER 10

Alcohol Interventions for College Student-Athletes

Matthew P. Martens

The public health problems associated with college student drinking are well known. For example, in 2005 there were 1,825 deaths and 599,000 injuries among college students that were directly or indirectly associated with alcohol use (Hingson, Zha, & Weitzman, 2009). Heavy-drinking college students also negatively impact other students and the surrounding campus community (Perkins, 2002; Wechsler et al., 2003). It is therefore important that researchers and clinicians develop effective strategies to confront this issue. One aspect of addressing the overall problem of college student drinking is to identify and develop targeted interventions for high-risk subgroups of students. One such subgroup is student-athletes, who have been shown to be particularly at risk for excessive alcohol use and its related consequences (Leichliter, Meilman, Presley, & Cashin, 1998; Nelson & Wechsler, 2001; Wechsler, Davenport, Dowdall, Grossman, & Zanakos, 1997). The purpose of this chapter is to (1) review the research on drinking rates among college athletes, (2) examine potential explanations for high-risk drinking among college athletes, (3) discuss intervention strategies for college athletes, and (4) address clinical/policy implications and future directions regarding efforts in this area. This chapter is limited to a focus on alcohol, as studies have generally shown that college athletes report either similar or lower rates of use of other drugs than nonathletes (for a review, see Martens, Dams-O'Connor, & Kilmer, 2007; for an exception involving performance enhancing drugs see Yusko, Buckman, White, & Pandina, 2008a). Thus, in comparison to their nonathlete peers, college athletes seem to be most at risk for the negative consequences associated with excessive alcohol consumption.

ALCOHOL USE AMONG COLLEGE ATHLETES

Three national studies have compared the alcohol use rates of college athletes and nonathletes, but in one study the way that *athlete* was defined may have allowed for students not participating in formal intercollegiate sports to be categorized as athletes (Wechsler et al., 1997). In that study two types of athletic involvement were outlined: those who reported participating in intercollegiate sports for 1 or more hours per day *and* who stated that participating in sports was important were classified as being "involved" in athletics; those who reported participating in intercollegiate sports for 1 or more hours per day but who did not report that participating in sports was important were classified as being "partially involved," as were those who stated that participating in sports was important but who did not participant in intercollegiate sports. Thus, depending upon their response to the importance question, college athletes could be classified as either involved or partially involved in athletics, while those not participating in athletics could be classified as either partially involved or not involved. Therefore, this review focuses on the two studies that more clearly differentiated between those who were and were not participating in college sports (Leichliter et al., 1998; Nelson & Wechsler, 2001).

Nelson and Wechsler compared 2,172 college athletes (defined as participating in intercollegiate athletics for at least 1 hour per day) and 10,605 nonathletes (including regular exercisers and intramural athletes) who completed the Harvard School of Public Health College Alcohol Study, while Leichliter et al. compared 8,749 college athletes (defined as "actively involved" or in a position of leadership in intercollegiate athletics) and 42,734 nonathletes who completed the Core Alcohol and Drug Survey. Nelson and Wechsler found that although overall past-year prevalence rates were similar for the two groups (83.1% of athletes versus 80.6% of nonathletes), the rate of heavy episodic drinking (five or more drinks for men/four or more drinks for women in one sitting) in the prior 2 weeks was considerably higher for athletes than nonathletes (52.9% of athletes versus 43.4% of nonathletes). They also found that athletes were more likely than nonathletes to report frequent heavy episodic drinking (defined as three or more instances) in the preceding 2 weeks (28.0% versus 21.4%). Leichliter et al. reported similar findings, although they divided their college athlete sample into team "leaders" (e.g., team captains) versus other athletes. They found that 58.0% of team leaders and 54.4% of team members reported heavy episodic drinking in the past 2 weeks (five or more drinks in one sitting for both men and women), versus only 36.3% of nonathletes. They also found that team leaders averaged 8.25 drinks per week, team members 7.34 drinks, and nonathletes only 4.12 drinks. In both studies athlete–nonathlete differences in drinking were consistent across gender. Finally, both studies showed that college athletes were more likely than nonathletes to experience numerous alcohol-related negative consequences, such as impaired academic work, getting into trouble with authorities, and doing something they later regretted. For example, Nelson and Wechsler found that, as a result of alcohol consumption, 46% of college athletes did something they later regretted, 31% had unprotected sexual activity, 16% got hurt/injured, and 11% got into trouble with the authorities, while corresponding percentages for nonathletes were 37%, 23%, 12%, and 6%, respectively. Leichliter et al. reported similar findings on their measure of alcohol-related problems. Other studies using smaller, local samples have generally reported a similar pattern of results (see Lisha & Sussman, 2010). The epidemiological findings are thus fairly clear: college athletes are more likely to engage in heavy drinking and experience negative alcohol-related consequences than their nonathlete counterparts.

REASONS FOR HEAVY DRINKING
IN COLLEGE ATHLETES

A number of theoretical explanations have been proposed in an effort to understand why a disproportionate number of college athletes engage in excessive drinking. Such explanations include (1) personality factors, (2) excessive stress, (3) characteristics of athletic teams, and (4) social opportunities associated with being an athlete. Unfortunately, research on these potential risk factors is relatively scarce. Each factor and the manner in which it might inform intervention efforts are reviewed below.

Personality Factors

One possible explanation for college athlete–nonathlete differences in alcohol use is that college athletes possess, on average, higher levels of personality characteristics that have been shown to be associated with alcohol use. One characteristic, which has been shown to be related to heavy alcohol consumption and has also been examined in research comparing athletes to nonathletes, is the impulsivity-related trait of sensation seeking (see Cyders, Flory, Rainer, & Smith, 2009; Cyders & Smith, 2008). Studies have shown that college athletes were more likely than other students to either report behaviors indicative of high sensation seeking or score higher than other students on measures of the construct (Gundersheim, 1987; Nattiv & Puffer, 1991; Nattiv, Puffer, & Green, 1997; Schroth, 1995). A more recent study with a relatively large sample of athletes and nonathletes found that athletes actually reported lower levels of sensation seeking than nonathletes, but that the relationship between sensation seeking and heavy drinking episodes was stronger among athletes than nonathletes (Yusko, Buckman, White, & Pandina, 2008b). Although these studies were limited by factors such as small sample size, non-random sampling, and/or lack of matching the athlete and nonathlete samples on relevant characteristics, they do suggest that high levels of sensation seeking may be a particular risk factor for heavy drinking among college athletes. Although more research is necessary before any definitive recommendations can be made, it may be that those developing interventions designed specifically for college athletes will need to consider the role of sensation seeking (and perhaps other impulsivity-related traits) in college athletes' drinking behaviors.

Excessive Stress

Sport psychology theorists have discussed excessive stress as a possible explanation for heavy alcohol use among college athletes (e.g., Damm & Murray, 1996; Tricker, Cook, & McGuire, 1989). The major premise of this argument is that athletes experience considerable stress and pressure due to their dual roles as both a student and an athlete. In addition to the typical academic demands placed on all college students, college athletes have a host of pressures associated with their competitive sport (e.g., concerns about playing time, balancing training, practice, and games with academic duties, relationship issues with coaches). If excessive stress were in fact an important cause of heavy drinking among college athletes, then intervention efforts could be targeted toward addressing that stress. Existing research, though, does not suggest that excessive stress is related to heavy drinking among college athletes. A national survey of 19,676 college athletes found that only 3.4% reported using alcohol primarily to deal with the stress of college athletics and college life, whereas 82.5% reported using alcohol primarily for recreational and social purposes (National Collegiate Athletic Association, 2006). One study showed that there were no differences between athletes and nonathletes on a measure of drinking to relax (Wilson, Pritchard, & Schaffer, 2004), while another showed no athlete–nonathlete differences on a measure of general stress and found that college athletes actually reported lower scores than nonathletes on a measure of coping-related drinking motives (Yusko et al., 2008b). Those college athletes who do endorse drinking for coping-related reasons or to otherwise deal with stress, pressure, or anxiety should be provided appropriate services, given the well-established relationship between drinking to cope and alcohol-related problems (Kuntsche, Knibbe, Gmel, & Engels, 2005). It does not appear, though, that excessive stress is a salient reason for heavy drinking among a large percentage of college athletes or meaningfully explains differences in drinking rates between athletes and nonathletes.

Characteristics of Athletic Teams

There are at least two characteristics associated with being on an athletic team that may be related to heavy drinking among college athletes. One possibility is that participating on an athletic team results in considerable explicit or implicit pressure to engage in heavy alcohol use. College athletes may perceive that it is "normal" for other athletes to drink heavily (i.e., descriptive norms) and/or perceive that other athletes have a favorable or permissive attitude toward heavy alcohol consumption (i.e., injunctive norms). The relationship between perceived descriptive and injunctive norms and college students' own drinking behavior has been well established (e.g., Larimer, Turner, Mallett, & Geisner, 2004; Neighbors, Lee, Lewis, Fossos, & Larimer, 2007), and research among college athletes has shown that perceived drinking among other athletes is a strong predictor of personal drinking behavior (Dams-O'Connor, Martin, Martens, & Martin, 2007). One study also found differences between college athletes and nonathletes in perceptions of the percentage of college students who engaged in heavy episodic drinking, with athletes reporting a higher percentage than nonathletes (Yusko et al., 2008b). Perhaps athletes drink more than other college students, at least in part, in order to conform to perceived expectations regarding elevated drinking.

Another possible team-related factor is competition among teammates when it comes to alcohol use. Athletes are used to engaging in competitive activities with both opponents and their teammates, so perhaps athletes are also drawn to competitive drinking activities. Research has shown that college athletes are more likely than other students to report engaging in drinking games (Grossbard, Geisner, Neighbors, Kilmer, & Larimer, 2007), and competition-related motives have been identified as a predictor of drinking game participation among college students in general (Johnson & Sheets, 2004). Further, one study from our lab found that general trait competitiveness was associated with alcohol use among a sample of elite and recreational college athletes (Serrao, Martens, Martin, & Rocha, 2008). These studies suggest that intervention efforts targeted specifically toward college athletes should consider dynamics unique to athletic teams that may be related to drinking behaviors among college athletes.

Social Opportunities

A final possible explanation of excessive drinking among intercollegiate athletes involves the existence of more social opportunities than other college students. Social events in college frequently involve alcohol, and it is possible that because of their status on campus athletes have more opportunities to engage in such events. For example, athletes may be more likely than other students to be invited to or be welcomed at parties and have others buy or otherwise supply them with drinks. An incident from graduate school comes to mind when, after the football team had won a game, I witnessed football players at a local establishment freely helping themselves to drinks from behind the bar. (It is unlikely that most college students will have such drinking-related opportunities!) Further, it is important to note that participating on an athletic team provides many college students with an established, extensive social network that could also facilitate opportunities for alcohol use. If college athletes are, in fact, presented with more opportunities to consume alcohol, particularly instances where others may be purchasing drinks for them or otherwise encouraging them to drink, then interventions addressing drinking refusal self-efficacy (e.g., Young, Hasking, Oei, & Loveday, 2007) or other related factors may be warranted.

INTERVENTION EFFORTS AMONG COLLEGE ATHLETES

The National Collegiate Athletic Association (NCAA) mandates that athletic departments conduct drug and alcohol prevention programming at least once a semester (National Collegiate Athletic Association, 2010). These programs are largely designed to increase an athlete's amount of information about alcohol and other drugs, focusing on components such as team, department, institution, and conference drug and alcohol policies and drug testing programs, reviewing lists of banned substances, and viewing an NCAA drug education/testing video. The NCAA also notes that individual athletic departments should have guidelines on alcohol and drug counseling or treatment options.

There are two somewhat contrary perspectives on this NCAA policy. On the one hand, it is encouraging that the NCAA has recognized the importance of addressing alcohol- and drug-related issues among intercollegiate athletes. On the other hand, the type of programming mandated by the NCAA is unlikely to have a significant impact on the alcohol use of intercollegiate athletes. Research has shown that information-only alcohol interventions are generally ineffective among college students (Larimer & Cronce, 2007). Therefore, unless individual athletic departments are implementing intervention strategies that go beyond the NCAA recommendations, the organization's mandate regarding information-based programming probably does not impact college athletes' behaviors regarding alcohol use. It is possible that NCAA and/or individual university drug testing policies may limit illicit drug use among college athletes. However, given the logistical difficulties associated with testing for alcohol use, it is unlikely that any benefits associated with drug testing programs would extend to alcohol-related outcomes.

If efforts mandated by college sports governing bodies like the NCAA are unlikely to be effective at reducing heavy drinking among college athletes, it is important that researchers and clinicians evaluate alternative intervention strategies. To date, though, there have only been a handful of studies examining the effectiveness of alcohol-related interventions among the college athlete population. Such interventions can be categorized into three groups: (1) skills-building interventions, (2) campuswide social norms interventions, and (3) personalized drinking feedback (PDF) interventions. (For more information on these interventions for college students, see Chapter 8 by Cronce & Latimer, this volume.)

Multicomponent Skills-Building Interventions

Studies in the general college student population have provided some support for the efficacy of multicomponent alcohol skills training programs (e.g., Fromme & Corbin, 2004; Kivlahan, Marlatt, Fromme, Coppel, & Williams, 1990), although many of the studies evaluating such interventions have been limited by a lack of appropriate control conditions (see Larimer & Cronce, 2007). There has been one published study examining the efficacy of this type of program specifically among college athletes (Marcello, Danish, & Stolberg, 1989). This trial examined the efficacy of a group-based intervention focusing on education, prevention skills training, and peer pressure skills training. Each component was presented in a single 2-hour session. The educational aspect of the intervention involved general and sport-related information about alcohol and other drugs. The prevention skills training component included stress management training, decision-making training regarding alcohol and drug use, and exercises designed to generalize the skills. Finally, peer pressure skills training included strategies for engaging in appropriate, assertive behavior, ideas for refusing alcohol or drug offers from peers, and general educational material on assertiveness training. Results from this study showed no differences between the intervention group and the delayed-treatment control condition on alcohol or drug use at an 8-week follow-up. These findings should be interpreted with caution, as the study was limited by low sample size and high dropout rate.

Another multicomponent program, MyPlaybook, has been developed specifically for college athletes (see *www.preventionstrategies.com/MP_researcbh.html*). MyPlaybook is a Web-based targeted intervention that covers topics such as alcohol's effects on athletic performance and NCAA policies regarding banned substances. Preliminary findings on the intervention support its effectiveness at limiting alcohol consumption among college athletes, but findings from the intervention have not yet been subjected to peer review (Wyrick, Fearnow-Kenney, & Milroy, 2009). Other skills-based programs for college athletes that include alcohol-related components have been described in the literature (e.g., Curry & Maniar, 2004; Meilman & Fleming, 1990), but they have also not been subjected to empirical evaluation. Thus, the efficacy of alcohol-related multicomponent skills-building interventions among college athletes has yet to be firmly established.

Social Norms Marketing Interventions

Campuswide social norms marketing interventions are designed to reduce alcohol use among college students by correcting misperceptions regarding the actual drinking behavior of other students (Perkins, 2002). Students generally overestimate the drinking rates of other college students, and some are presumably motivated to match their drinking habits to this perceived norm. Correcting the norm should thus result in reduced drinking behavior. The effectiveness of these types of interventions has been somewhat of a contentious topic (e.g., Perkins, Haines, & Rice, 2005; Wechsler et al., 2003), with the only randomized controlled trial examining a social norms marketing intervention showing a small but statistically significant effect of the intervention in comparison to a no-intervention control condition (DeJong et al., 2006).

There have been two studies examining social norms marketing campaigns directed toward college athletes. In one study, a social norms campaign that included, in part, messages targeted toward student-athletes was implemented on a single campus (Thombs & Hamilton, 2002). Approximately two-thirds of the athletes sampled on that campus reported being exposed to the campaign, and their drinking habits were compared to those of athletes on their own campus who reported not being exposed to the campaign and athletes from two other universities where no social norms campaign was implemented. Results indicated that those athletes exposed to the campaign reported a lower perceived drinking norm among other students, but actual drinking rates did not differ between the two groups. In the second study, college athletes at a single university were sampled on three occasions: baseline, 1 year posttest, and 2 years posttest (Perkins & Craig, 2006). A comprehensive social norms campaign targeted specifically toward athletes was implemented after the baseline assessment. The authors reported significant decreases in perceived student-athlete drinking norms and personal alcohol consumption from baseline to the posttest periods. They also reported a positive association between reported exposure to the social norms campaign and reductions in perceived student-athlete drinking norms and personal alcohol consumption. The authors therefore concluded that the social norms marketing campaign was effective at reducing alcohol consumption among college athletes.

What is to be made of these conflicting findings? First, it is important to note that both studies suffered from important methodological limitations. The Thombs and Hamilton (2002) study utilized non-random assignment, a heterogenous comparison group, and a posttest-only design. The degree to which the intervention was targeted specifically toward athletes was also relatively minimal. In contrast, Perkins and Craig (2006) implemented an intervention that was extensively targeted toward college athletes and collected longitudinal data. Important limitations of their study, though, included no control group, analysis of cohort-level rather than individual-level data, and combining multiple follow-up points into a single unit of analysis. Given the lack of pre–post analyses by Thombs and Hamilton and important concerns about the equivalence of their "control" group, it is difficult to make meaningful conclusions regarding their findings. The findings of Perkins and Craig may be considered encouraging regarding the effects of social norms marketing campaigns targeted specifically toward college athletes, but should, at best, be considered preliminary until more well-designed studies can be conducted among the population.

Personalized Drinking Feedback Interventions

PDF consists of providing an individual with detailed, personalized feedback about his or her drinking habits. Typical components of PDF include social norms comparisons, blood alcohol concentration (BAC) levels and associated risks based on reported alcohol use (e.g., BAC on one's heaviest drinking day in the past month), a summary of reported alcohol-related negative consequences, and other personalized alcohol-related information (e.g., Dimeff, Baer, Kivlahan, & Marlatt, 1999; Larimer et al., 2007; Marlatt et al., 1998). Because this information is personalized via data provided by the individual, it will theoretically be more likely to promote behavior change than just general information about alcohol and its related risks. PDF has most often been utilized in the context of a brief, in-person motivational-interviewing-based meeting, and research has generally supported the efficacy of this type of intervention (Carey,

Scott-Sheldon, Carey, & DeMartini, 2007; Larimer & Cronce, 2007). Other studies have examined the efficacy of PDF interventions where the individual receives PDF without meeting with a clinician. Several studies among college students in general have supported the efficacy of these "PDF-only" interventions in relation to a no-treatment control condition (e.g., Butler & Correia, 2009; Kypri et al., 2004; Larimer et al., 2007), although these findings are not uniform (Walters, Vader, Harris, Field, & Jouriles, 2009).

There have been two studies examining PDF-only interventions among intercollegiate athletes. Doumas and Haustveit (2008) examined the efficacy of a Web-based PDF intervention among a small sample (N = 52) of NCAA Division I athletes. Subjects were randomized to either the PDF condition or a general education control condition. Those in the PDF condition received personalized information on factors such as how their drinking compared to general college student norms, estimates of the amount of money they spent on alcohol, the number of calories from alcohol they consumed, and their risk status for alcohol-related negative consequences and problem drinking. Results indicated that among "high-risk" drinkers (defined as at least one heavy drinking episode in the preceding 2 weeks), those in the PDF condition reported greater reductions at 6-week and 3-month follow-ups on weekly drinking, peak alcohol consumption, and drinking to intoxication than those in the control condition. Although promising, the findings from this study are limited by the small sample size (N = 33) and relatively poor follow-up rate (64%).

My colleagues and I recently completed a study that expanded upon these promising findings (Martens, Kilmer, Beck, & Zamboanga, 2010). College athletes from three universities (N = 263) were randomized to one of three conditions that were delivered via the Web: a PDF condition targeted specifically for college athletes (PDF-targeted), a PDF condition that did not include information targeted specifically for athletes (PDF-standard), and an education-only condition that included educational information targeted specifically toward athletes. Both PDF conditions contained information consistent with other studies in the area (e.g., a summary of alcohol-related negative consequences, social norms comparisons, use of protective behavioral strategies). The PDF-targeted condition also included information designed to be particularly salient for college athletes, such as sport-related negative alcohol-related consequences (e.g., going to a game or practice with a hangover), the potential impact of one's drinking on athletic performance, and the link between alcohol use and injury risk. Athletes in the education-only condition also received alcohol-related information designed specifically for college athletes, but the information was not personalized. Results provided some support for the efficacy of the PDF-targeted intervention, particularly in terms of peak BAC over the past 30 days. Among the entire sample, those in the PDF-targeted condition reported a lower peak BAC at the 6-month follow-up than those in the PDF-standard or education-only condition (.072 versus .101 and .105, respectively). Among the at-risk drinkers in the sample (those who reported 10 or more drinks per week at baseline), those in the PDF-targeted condition reported a lower peak BAC at 1-month follow-up than those in the other conditions (.089 versus .159 and .164, respectively) and a lower peak BAC at 6-month follow-up than those in the education-only condition (.120 versus .196). We concluded that a PDF-targeted intervention could be particularly effective at impacting peak alcohol use among college athletes, since it is those types of drinking occasions that athletes might most associate with poor athletic performance. In sum, the results of these two studies provide preliminary support for the efficacy of PDF-only interventions among college athletes.

CLINICAL/POLICY IMPLICATIONS AND FUTURE DIRECTIONS

Research has established that college students participating in intercollegiate athletics are at risk for excessive alcohol use and resulting negative consequences, even within the high-risk population of college students in general. Although a number of theoretical explanations for this phenomenon have been put forth, well-designed research examining such explanations is lacking. Similarly, only a handful of studies have examined the efficacy of intervention strategies among intercollegiate athletes, although empirically supported models from both the general college student and athlete-specific literature do exist. The clinical and policy implications of this state of affairs are described below, as well as future directions for clinicians and researchers interested in curbing excessive alcohol use among intercollegiate athletes.

Implications for Governing Bodies

If governing bodies of college athletics like the NCAA are interested in reducing alcohol use among college athletes, then they may wish to consider modifying their guidelines regarding alcohol-related programming. These governing bodies hold considerable power in terms of mandating the behavior of member institutions, and could presumably specify the nature of alcohol-related interventions that should be delivered to college athletes. For example, instead of specifying that athletic departments simply provide largely educative programming regarding alcohol and other drugs, they could require that member institutions implement programs with demonstrated or promising empirical support. For example, given that some support exists for fairly low-cost interventions like Web-based PDF and targeted social norms marketing among both college athletes and students in general, the NCAA could mandate that member institutions, at minimum, develop and implement these types of interventions in their athletic departments. Although it would likely be difficult for a governing body to monitor these types of efforts at all its member institutions, such a policy would send a clear message to athletic departments regarding the importance of providing evidence-based alcohol-related programming for their athletes.

Implications for Athletic Departments

Any athletic department serious about providing effective alcohol-related programming for its athletes should consider a strategy that goes beyond providing general educational information. Given the host of demands placed on athletic departments, particularly the importance of athletic and academic success, it is easy to see how anything not directly tied to these areas is given only cursory attention. It is important that athletic departments recognize, though, that meaningfully impacting the drinking behavior of its athletes will require planning, time, and resources. Simply informing athletes of relevant alcohol- and drug-related policies is unlikely to make much of a difference on individual athlete behavior. One model for athletic departments would be to adopt a multifaceted approach that provides alcohol-related interventions at different levels and via different mechanisms. For example, a department could develop clear rules, standards, and enforcement policies regarding alcohol use among its athletes, perhaps in conjunction with team leaders or other well-respected athletes. A department could also provide preventative interventions like a targeted social norms marketing campaign and PDF-only interventions to all its athletes. Athletes who are identified as in some way engaging in problematic alcohol use but not in need of formal substance abuse treatment could be provided with more intensive interventions like a one-on-one motivational-interviewing-based intervention and/or short-term outpatient counseling. Finally, athletic departments could establish relationships with professionals and/or treatment centers for athletes in need of intensive alcohol or other drug treatment. Implementing this type of model would require time and effort by athletic department staff but should not be unduly expensive. PDF-only and social norms marketing interventions require no clinician support and could be implemented at relatively little cost. It is worth considering the costs, both financial and otherwise, to an athletic department that experiences a well-publicized incident involving alcohol among it athletes. Although by no means a guarantee, a comprehensive alcohol intervention strategy would reduce the likelihood of such negative events.

Implications for Clinicians

The most important implication of the information presented in this chapter for those engaging in clinical work with athletes is the preliminary support for the impact of PDF-based interventions on alcohol use among college athletes (Doumas & Haustveit, 2008; Martens et al., 2010). These findings, along with the efficacy data on PDF-based interventions among college students in general, suggest that clinicians who are in a position to address risky alcohol use with a college athlete should be versed in the delivery of an appropriate intervention strategy. One recommendation would be to become proficient in the delivery of motivational-interviewing-based strategies that include PDF (e.g., the BASICS intervention; Dimeff et al., 1999; Marlatt et al., 1998). There are free Web-based programs where PDF is available (e.g., *www.checkyourdrinking.net*), and clinicians could easily develop their own feedback sheets for any desired content not covered by other sources (e.g., athlete-specific personalized feedback). A second recommendation would be to work closely with other athletic department personnel when trying to develop and/or promote alcohol intervention programming within athletic departments. It may be particularly helpful to work with medical personnel like team physicians, athletic trainers, and strength coaches, who generally have a well-established role and high levels of credibility within an athletic department (Martens, Kilmer, & Beck, 2009). Buy-in from these professionals would likely increase political support if a clinician were trying to convince an athletic department to implement an alcohol-related intervention strategy. Further, athletic trainers and strength coaches have more day-to-day contact with athletes than mental health clinicians, and thus could be important sources in identifying those in need of a targeted intervention.

Future Directions for Researchers

Efforts focusing on several interrelated research areas could inform the development of alcohol intervention targeting college athletes. One important research direction would be to determine more precisely the relationship between alcohol use among college athletes and subsequent athletic performance. Alcohol use in general is known to inhibit athletic performance (for a review, see Martens, Dams-O'Connor, & Beck, 2006), but precise dose-response research is lacking. It would be useful to understand, for example, the ways in which varying types of drinking patterns among college athletes impact performance in both the long and short term. If researchers could provide athletic department personnel with more precise estimates regarding the deleterious impact of heavy drinking in areas like off-season training and in-season performance, then obtaining the necessary support for a comprehensive alcohol-related intervention may be an easier sell. A second important area would be to conduct studies that provide clearer information regarding why it is that college athletes tend to drink more than other students. Interventions targeted specifically toward college athletes have received promising initial support (Martens et al., 2010; Perkins & Craig, 2006), and a better understanding of factors unique to college athlete drinking would help inform additional targeted efforts. Finally, a third important area would be to examine the effects of additional intervention strategies on college athlete drinking. Such studies could include established interventions that have not yet been tested among college athletes (e.g., individual or group-based motivational interviewing) or novel interventions designed specifically for the athlete population.

One intriguing strategy could be to develop and examine the effects of an intervention that targeted college coaches. Coaches often play a parent-like role in the lives of their athletes, and studies have shown that parental behaviors can impact the drinking behaviors of college students (e.g., Turrisi, Jacard, Taki, Dunnam, & Grimes, 2001; Turrisi & Ray, 2010). Thus, it is possible that a coach-focused intervention incorporating components like general educational information about high-risk drinking among college athletes, strategies for talking to athletes about alcohol use, and ideas for establishing team-specific rules regarding alcohol use would impact the alcohol use of athletes playing for that coach.

CONCLUSION

There are a number of avenues that clinicians, researchers, policymakers, coaches, athletic department personnel, university administrators, and others who work with college athletes can explore to help address excessive drinking among this population. Research has established the nature of the problem and has provided initial ideas for intervention strategies designed to combat it, but more work in the area is needed. Like many complicated health-related problems, making a meaningful impact on the alcohol use habits of college athletes will likely require concerted and collaborative efforts among a diverse array of university stakeholders. These include additional research efforts to better understand and combat the problem, continued efforts to design and evaluate various intervention strategies, and willingness on the part of athletic department personnel and university administrators to promote comprehensive alcohol programming for its student athletes.

REFERENCES

Butler, L. H., & Correia, C. J. (2009). Brief alcohol intervention with college student drinkers: Face-to-face versus computerized feedback. *Psychology of Addictive Behaviors, 23*, 163–167.

Carey, K. B., Scott-Sheldon, L. A. J., Carey, M. P., & DeMartini, K. S. (2007). Individual level interventions to reduce college student drinking: A meta-analytic review. *Addictive Behaviors, 32*, 2469–2494.

Curry, L. A., & Maniar, S. D. (2004). Academic course for enhancing student-athlete performance in sport. *Sport Psychologist, 18*, 297–316.

Cyders, M. A., Flory, K., Rainer, S., & Smith, G. T. (2009). The role of personality dispositions to risky behavior in predicting first-year college drinking. *Addiction, 104*, 193–202.

Cyders, M.A., & Smith, G.T. (2008). Emotion-based dispositions to rash action: Positive and negative urgency. *Psychological Bulletin, 134*, 807–828.

Damm, J., & Murray, P. (1996). Alcohol and other drug use among college student-athletes. In E. F. Etzel, A. P. Ferrante, & J. W. Pinkney (Eds.), *Counseling college student-athletes: Issues and interventions* (2nd ed., pp. 185–220). Morgantown, WV: Fitness Information Technology.

Dams-O'Connor, K., Martin, J. L., & Martens, M. P. (2007). Social norms and alcohol consumption among intercollegiate athletes: The role of athlete and nonathlete reference groups. *Addictive Behaviors, 32*, 2657–2666.

DeJong, W., Schneider, S. K., Towvim, L. G., Murphy, M. J., Doerr, E. E., Simonsen, N. R., et al. (2006). A multisite randomized trial of social norms marketing campaigns to reduce college student drinking. *Journal of Studies on Alcohol, 67*, 868–879.

Dimeff, L. A., Baer, J. S., Kivlahan, D. R., & Marlatt, G. A. (1999). *Brief Alcohol Screening and Intervention for College Students (BASICS): A harm reduction approach*. New York: Guilford Press.

Doumas D. M., & Haustveit T. (2008) Reducing heavy drinking in intercollegiate athletes: Evaluation of a Web-based personalized feedback program. *Sport Psychology, 22*, 213–29.

Fromme, K., & Corbin, W. (2004). Prevention of heavy drinking and associated negative consequences among mandated and voluntary college students. *Journal of Consulting and Clinical Psychology, 72*, 1038–1049.

Grossbard, J., Geisner, I. M., Neighbors, C., Kilmer, J. R., & Larimer, M. E. (2007). Are drinking games sports? College athletes' participation in drinking games and alcohol-related problems. *Journal of Studies in Alcohol and Drugs, 68*, 97–105.

Gundersheim, J. (1987). Sensation seeking in male and female athletes and nonathletes. *International Journal of Sport Psychology, 18*, 87–99.

Hingson, R. W., Zha, W., & Weitzman, E. R. (2009). Magnitude of and trends in alcohol-related mortality and morbidity among U.S. college students ages 18–24, 1998–2005. *Journal of Studies on Alcohol and Drugs, 16,* 12–20.

Johnson, T. J., & Sheets, V. L. (2004). Measuring college students' motives for playing drinking games. *Psychology of Addictive Behaviors, 18,* 91–99.

Kivlahan, D. R., Marlatt, G. A., Fromme, K., Coppel, D. B., & Williams, E. (1990). Secondary prevention with college drinkers: Evaluation of an alcohol skills training program. *Journal of Consulting and Clinical Psychology, 58,* 805–810.

Kuntsche, E., Knibbe, R., Gmel, G., & Engels, R. (2005). Why do young people drink? A review of drinking motives. *Clinical Psychology Review, 25,* 841–861.

Kypri, K., Saunders, J. B., Williams, S. M., McGee, R. O., Langley, J. D., Cashall-Smith, M. L., et al. (2004). Web-based screening and brief intervention for hazardous drinking: A double-blind randomized controlled trial. *Addiction, 99,* 1410–1417.

Larimer, M. E., & Cronce, J. M. (2007). Identification, prevention, and treatment revisited: Individual-focused college drinking prevention strategies 1999–2006. *Addictive Behaviors, 32,* 2439–2468.

Larimer, M. E., Lee, C. M., Kilmer, J. R., Fabiano, P. M., Stark, C. B., Geisner, I. M., Mallett, K. A., Lostutter, T. W., Cronce, J. M., Feeney, M., & Neighbors, C. (2007). Personalized mailed feedback for college drinking prevention: A randomized clinical trial. *Journal of Consulting and Clinical Psychology, 75,* 285–293.

Larimer, M. E., Turner, A. P., Mallett, K. A., & Geisner, I. M. (2004). Predicting drinking behavior and alcohol-related problems among fraternity and sorority members: Examining the role of descriptive and injunctive norms. *Psychology of Addictive Behaviors, 18,* 203–212.

Leichliter, J. S., Meilman, P. W., Presley, C. A., & Cashin, J. R. (1998). Alcohol use and related consequences among students with varying levels of involvement with college athletics. *Journal of American College Health, 46,* 257–262.

Lisha, N. E., & Sussman, S. (2010). Relationship of high school and college sports participation with alcohol, tobacco, and illicit drug use: A review. *Addictive Behaviors, 35,* 399–407.

Marcello, R. J., Danish, S. J., & Stolberg, A. (1989). An evaluation of strategies developed to prevent substance abuse among student-athletes. *Sport Psychologist, 3,* 196–211.

Marlatt, G. A., Baer, J. S., Kivlahan, D. R., Dimeff, L. A., Larimer, M. E., Quigley, L. A., et al. (1998). Screening and brief intervention for high-risk college student drinkers: Results from a 2–year follow-up assessment. *Journal of Consulting and Clinical Psychology, 66,* 604–615.

Martens, M. P., Dams-O'Connor, K., & Beck, N. C. (2006). A systematic review of college student-athlete drinking: Prevalence rates, sport-related explanations, and interventions. *Journal of Substance Abuse Treatment, 31,* 305–316.

Martens, M. P., Dams-O'Connor, K., & Kilmer, J. (2007). Alcohol and drug abuse among athletes: Prevalence, etiology, and interventions. In G. Tenenbaum & R. C. Eklund (Eds.), *Handbook of sport psychology* (3rd ed., pp. 859–878). Hoboken, NJ: Wiley.

Martens, M. P., Kilmer, J. R., & Beck, N. C. (2009). Alcohol and drug use among college athletes. In E. Etzel (Ed.), *Counseling and psychological services for college student athletes* (pp. 451–475). Morgantown, WV: Fitness Information Technology.

Martens, M. P., Kilmer, J. R., Beck, N. C., & Zamboanga, B. L. (2010). The efficacy of a targeted personalized drinking feedback intervention among intercollegiate athletes: A randomized controlled trial. *Psychology of Addictive Behaviors, 24,* 660–669.

Meilman, P. W., & Fleming, R. L. (1990). A substance abuse prevention program for student-athletes. *Journal of College Student Development, 31,* 477–479.

National Collegiate Athletic Association. (2006). *NCAA study of substance use of college student-athletes.* Indianapolis, IN: Author.

National Collegiate Athletic Association. (2010). *NCAA minimum guidelines for institutional alcohol, tobacco, and other drug education programs.* Retrieved from the NCAA website *www.ncaa.org/wps/portal/ncaahome?WCM_ GLOBAL_CONTEXT=/ncaa/ncaa/academics+and+athletes/ personal+welfare/health+and+safety/drug+education+programs/inst_guidelines.*

Nattiv, A., & Puffer, J. C. (1991). Lifestyles and health risks of collegiate athletes. *Journal of Family Practice, 33,* 585–590.

Nattiv, A., Puffer, J. C., & Green, G. A. (1997). Lifestyles and health risks of collegiate athletes: A multi-center study. *Clinical Journal of Sport Medicine, 7,* 262–272.

Nelson, T. F., & Wechsler, H. (2001). Alcohol and college athletes. *Medicine and Science in Sports and Exercise, 33,* 43–47.

Neighbors, C., Lee, C. M., Lewis, M. A., Fossos, N., & Larimer, M. E. (2007). Are social norms the best predictor of outcomes among heavy-drinking college students? *Journal of Studies on Alcohol and Drugs, 68,* 556–565.

Perkins, H. W. (2002). Surveying the damage: A review of research on consequences of alcohol misuse in college populations. *Journal of Studies on Alcohol* (Suppl. 14), 91–100.

Perkins, H. W., & Craig, D. W. (2006). A successful social norms campaign to reduce alcohol misuse among college student-athletes. *Journal of Studies on Alcohol, 67,* 880–889.

Perkins, H. W., Haines, M. P., & Rice, R. (2005). Misperceiving the college drinking norm and related problems: A nationwide study of exposure to prevention information, perceived norms and student alcohol misuse. *Journal of Studies on Alcohol, 66,* 470–478.

Schroth, M. L. (1995). A comparison of sensation seeking among different groups of athletes and nonathletes. *Personality and Individual Differences, 18,* 219–222.

Serrao, H. F., Martens, M. P., Martin, J. L., & Rocha, T. L. (2008). Competitiveness and alcohol use among recreational and elite collegiate athletes. *Journal of Clinical Sport Psychology, 2,* 205–215.

Thombs, D. L., & Hamilton, M. J. (2002). Effects of a social norm feedback campaign on the drinking norms and behavior of Division I student-athletes. *Journal of Drug Education, 32,* 227–244.

Tricker, R., Cook, D. L., & McGuire, R. (1989). Issues related to drug abuse in college athletes: Athletes at risk. *Sport Psychologist, 3,* 155–165.

Turrisi, R., Jaccard, J., Taki, R., Dunnam, H., & Grimes, J. (2001). Examination of the short-term efficacy of a parent intervention to reduce college student drinking tendencies. *Psychology of Addictive Behaviors, 15,* 366–372.

Turrisi, R., & Ray, A. E. (2010). Sustained parenting and college drinking in first-year students. *Developmental Psychobiology, 52,* 286–294.

Walters, S. T., Vader, A. M., Harris, T. R., Field, C. A., & Jouriles, E. N. (2009). Dismantling motivational interviewing and feedback for college drinkers: A randomized clinical trial. *Journal of Consulting and Clinical Psychology, 77,* 64–73.

Wechsler, H., Davenport, A. E., Dowdall, G. W., Grossman, S. J., & Zanakos, S. I. (1997). Binge drinking, tobacco, and illicit drug use and involvement in college athletics. *Journal of American College Health, 45,* 195–200.

Wechsler, H., Nelson, T. F., Lee, J. E., Seibring, M., Lewis, C., & Keeling, R. P. (2003). Perception and reality: A national evaluation of social norms marketing interventions to reduce college students' heavy alcohol use. *Journal of Studies on Alcohol, 64,* 484–494.

Wilson, G. S., Pritchard, M. E., & Schaffer, J. (2004). Athletic status and drinking behavior in college students: The influence of gender and coping styles. *Journal of American College Health, 52,* 269–273.

Wyrick, D. L., Fearnow-Kenney, M., & Milroy, J. (2009). *Drug and alcohol prevention for NCAA student-athletes: Division II pilot study final report.* Greensboro, NC: Prevention Strategies.

Young, R. M., Hasking, P. A., Oei, T. P. S., & Loveday, W. (2007). Validation of the Drinking Refusal Self-Efficacy Questionnaire–Revised in an adolescent sample (DRSEQ-RA). *Addictive Behaviors, 32,* 862–868.

Yusko, D. A., Buckman, J. F., White, H. R., & Pandina, R. J. (2008a). Alcohol, tobacco, illicit drugs, and performance enhancers: A comparison of use by college student athletes and nonathletes. *Journal of American College Health, 57,* 281–289.

Yusko, D. A., Buckman, J. F., White, H. R., & Pandina, R. J. (2008b). Risk for excessive alcohol use and drinking-related problems in college student athletes. *Addictive Behaviors, 33,* 1546–1556.

CHAPTER 11

Community and Environmental Prevention Interventions

Robert F. Saltz

Other chapters in Part IV of this volume attest to the advances researchers and practitioners have made with respect to both prevention and treatment of alcohol and other drug problems among college students. On the prevention side, college administrators and staff have developed a number of strategies that have demonstrated efficacy in reducing alcohol consumption, especially among heavier-drinking students or those whose drinking behavior has resulted in one or more problems. For colleges and universities with ambition to significantly impact alcohol-related problems on and near their campus, however, prevention interventions designed to change individual drinking behavior should be part of a broader, comprehensive, and synergistic system of strategies that also aims to reduce drinking through changes at the community level, in addition to focusing more exclusively on students with problematic drinking. The public health approach sees the prevalence of a problem as a result of the combination of influences tied to an agent, a host, and the environment—in our case, alcoholic beverage (agent), the individual student's characteristics (host), and the characteristics of the local campus and community environment that may reduce or exacerbate risky drinking. This chapter focuses on issues related to adopting a public health perspective on college students' alcohol use, as well as interventions that derive from this perspective.

ENVIRONMENTAL-LEVEL
PREVENTION APPROACHES

The "environment" can encompass quite a lot, of course, but for alcohol prevention, it is helpful to think of it as comprising economic, physical, and social domains. The economic environment would include the price of alcoholic beverages (and the taxes paid), as well as the marketing and promotional activities associated with alcohol sales. The physical environment includes the density of alcohol outlets, the types of outlets (whether for consumption on-premise or off-premise), and the hours and days during which alcohol is available. The social environment would include the influence of peers and family, the living arrangement (e.g., fraternities or residence halls), and the broader normative and cultural environment related to alcohol use. Figure 11.1 provides one way to conceive of community-level forces that bear on alcohol consumption and its negative consequences.

The critical point here is that, apart from the variation in individual risk factors (e.g., family history of alcoholism, impulsivity, past history of alcohol use), there is another set of powerful forces largely extrinsic to the individual that are "overlaid" on those individual-level factors and help or hinder our efforts to reduce alcohol-related harm. In practical terms, we create safer and healthier environments via laws and policies that control the availability of alcohol (e.g., minimum drinking age, license restrictions), its cost, how it is marketed, and efforts to deter drinkers from becoming intoxicated or driving while impaired. Research over the past 30 years has been able to identify a host of universal population-level interventions that are effective in reducing problems (see Babor et al., 2010).

The National Institute on Alcohol Abuse and Alcoholism's (National Institute on Alcohol Abuse and Alcoholism [NIAAA]) task force on college student drinking was well aware of this evidence when it formed its recommendations (NIAAA, 2002). At the time, however, it could find no rigorous studies in which environmental strategies were evaluated in college communities. In creating a "tiered" set of recommendations, the task force was able to clearly identify the strategies that had been shown to reduce problematic drinking in college populations (Tier 1) while at the same time drawing attention to evidence-based environmental strategies known to work with general populations but unevaluated in college settings. Tier 1's three recommended strategies included combining cognitive-behavioral skills with norms clarification and motivational enhancement, brief motivational enhancement interventions, and alcohol expectancy challenges (see Cronce & Larimer, Chapter 8, this volume). Among the specific strategies recommended in Tier 2 (not yet evaluated

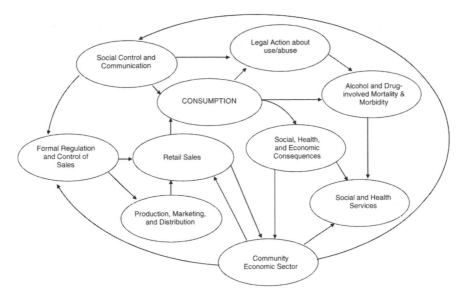

FIGURE 11.1. Community system of alcohol and drug use. Data from Holder (1992).

in college settings) were such alcohol control measures as enforcing laws related to the minimum drinking age, enforcing laws aimed at reducing alcohol-impaired driving, raising the price of alcoholic beverages, reducing the density of alcohol outlets, and promoting responsible beverage service among retailers (see DeJong & Langford, 2002). As these latter interventions typically require action at the community level, the task force went on to say that "formation of a campus and community coalition involving all major stakeholders may be critical to implement these strategies effectively" (NIAAA, 2002, p. 20).

Despite the importance of this recommendation, community prevention interventions seem difficult to design and implement, and even more difficult to evaluate. When the campus or community is the unit of intervention, a rigorous research design would require multiple intervention and comparison campuses, preferably with random assignment to intervention condition. It is little wonder that such studies are rare. Why not, then, be satisfied with just further developing and improving the Tier 1 interventions? There are at least a couple of points that compel our attention to community-level interventions. First, in their current form, most of the Tier 1 interventions are labor intensive and require skilled people to conduct them (although there are promising efforts being made to overcome these potential barriers). Having demonstrated their efficacy, developers of those programs are moving forward to address strategies related to the reach and implementation of the interventions (see other chapters in Part IV of this volume).

More importantly, those interventions are most appropriate for students whose drinking is already problematic or who are at least members of subgroups that drink more heavily than the general population (see Larimer & Cronce, 2002, 2007). However, alcohol-related harm is not limited to those whose drinking can be characterized as consistently heavy or risky (Gruenewald, Johnson, Light, Lipton, & Saltz, 2003; Weitzman & Nelson, 2004). At the population level, light and moderate drinkers so outnumber the heaviest drinkers that, even at their lower level of individual risk, they can be responsible for the majority of alcohol-related problems (see Kreitman, 1986). Figure 11.2, for example, shows a range of alcohol-related problems reported by a sample of college students. Those who drank five or more drinks more than once in the 2 weeks prior to the survey are highlighted in the lower portion of the bars. One can see that even if those students were to become abstainers, the total number of problems would be reduced by less than half. Thus, interventions aimed at risky drinkers should be complemented by universal prevention strategies as well.

Second, there is the possibility that ignoring the broader campus/community environment may actually sabotage the effectiveness of other prevention efforts. In looking for an explanation as to why a social norms marketing campaign failed to replicate original positive effects, DeJong et al. (2009) concluded that the intervention was thwarted at campuses that were surrounded by a high density of alcohol outlets. The intervention (which corrects students' overestimation of peer drinking) seemed unable to overcome the environmental risk produced by the number of places to buy alcohol. Finally, the prevalence and stability of college student drinking strongly suggests that reducing consumption and consequences will require a comprehensive set of effective strategies that will ultimately achieve a synergistic impact.

COMMUNITY-LEVEL INTERVENTION EXAMPLES

The task force commissioned a summary review of comprehensive community interventions by Hingson and Howland (2002). Among the variety of interventions described by the authors (which included health outcomes beyond alcohol) were three examples of community interventions that could serve as models for college community interventions. These examples are described below.

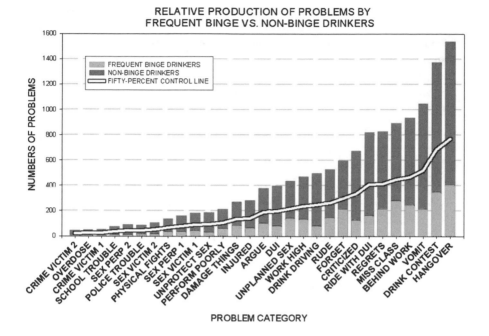

FIGURE 11.2. Alcohol-related problems are not limited to heavy drinkers. Unpublished data from Saltz.

The Massachusetts Saving Lives program targeted drunk driving and speeding through activities that included drunk-driving checkpoints, establishing speed-watch telephone hotlines, police training, alcohol-free prom nights, beer keg registration, business information campaigns, media campaigns, and increased surveillance of attempts by minors to buy alcohol. A great deal of attention was given to media advocacy to create and shape news stories in ways that supported the prevention efforts (Hingson et al., 1996). Self-reported driving after drinking among those under 20 dropped from 19 to 9%, the prevalence of speeding was cut by half, and alcohol-related traffic deaths were reduced by 45% in the treatment cities in comparison to the rest of the state over the project's 5-year period.

Communities Mobilizing for Change on Alcohol (CMCA) focused on alcohol availability to youth in seven small to midsized communities in Minnesota and Wisconsin (with another eight communities as comparison). A coordinator working with each community mobilized support for a variety of activities, including increased enforcement of laws prohibiting alcohol sales to minors and raising awareness of the problem and of the importance of enforcement to the community at large. As a result, alcohol sales to minors were reduced by 10–15% in the target communities; in addition, surveys of youth showed declines in attempts to purchase alcohol (25%), in providing alcohol to peers (about 17%), and in alcohol consumption (about 7%) (Wagenaar et al., 2000a; Wagenaar, Murray, & Toomey, 2000b). Drunk driving violations were also reduced among 18- to 20-year-olds in those communities. Interestingly, the program seemed to have the greatest effect on the oldest minors, that is, those of traditional college age (though this study was not targeted at college students per se).

Finally, the Community Trials Project targeted alcohol-related injury and deaths in three communities (each with a matched community for comparison). Specific components included responsible beverage service training and enforcement; increased enforcement of drunk driving laws (and public perception of that increase); enforcement of underage sales laws; reduced alcohol availability via curtailing outlet density; and mobilizing the community and its leaders in support of these interventions. The intervention reduced alcohol-involved crashes by more than 10% over the comparison communities, and reduced alcohol-related assaults by over 40% (Holder et al., 2000).

Although these community-level strategies differed in targets, components, and mobilizing strategies, they all worked to enhance existing alcohol control measures (whether for underage drinking or drinking and driving), which were coupled with publicity to magnify the effects of the enforcement. They also recruited or developed community coalitions or task forces to achieve the desired objectives. Successful community-level interventions such as these compelled the NIAAA task force to recommend similar efforts among college administrators. NIAAA also called for the research community to design evaluations of such strategies to confirm their utility to colleges and their neighboring communities. The report was followed by a commitment from NIAAA to fund more research on college student drinking problems. This funding, in turn, has helped produce research that has only recently become available to those interested in environmental prevention at colleges and universities.

DEVELOPMENTS SINCE THE NIAAA TASK FORCE REPORT

In the years since the NIAAA report, there have been a number of research studies that explored the influence of environmental factors on college student drinking and the efficacy of environmental prevention strategies. Many of these are observational (correlational) analyses of community or campus-level characteristics, and a few are opportunistic studies attempting to capture the possible impact of "natural experiments" when changes in policies or practices occurred independently of a research design. These studies are beyond the scope of this chapter but they and others are summarized in an excellent review by Toomey, Lenk, and Wagenaar (2007). Instead, this chapter focuses on purposeful, comprehensive campus/community prevention interventions. The remainder of the chapter describes the multicomponent, comprehensive prevention interventions that were designed, implemented and evaluated by a team of researchers.

In evaluating the American Medical Association's "A Matter of Degree" program, Weitzman, Nelson, Lee, and Wechsler (2004) compared 10 campuses selected as intervention sites with another set of 32 campuses that had similarly high rates of heavy episodic drinking. The intervention involved creating campus/community coalitions that would focus on environmental strategies to reduce alcohol availability (e.g., keg registration, mandatory server training at commercial or social settings), enhanced enforcement of local policies and laws (e.g., party patrols), limiting alcohol advertising and promotions, and promoting health via alcohol-free programming and campaigns. Individual campuses were given flexibility to adopt specific policies and practices that fell within these broader domains. Intervention sites were selected based in part on the willingness and interest of the campus personnel in collaborating on the intervention.

There were no significant differences in drinking between the 10 intervention and 32 comparison colleges. However, when the researchers examined a subset of five campuses that implemented the program with greater intensity, they found significantly lower rates of heavy drinking and alcohol-related negative consequences on these campuses (Weitzman et al., 2004).

Clapp and his colleagues (2005) evaluated a driving under the influence (DUI) prevention program on one campus that included enhanced enforcement via roadside checkpoints and patrols, accompanied by a media advocacy campaign and a social marketing effort. The primary emphasis of the intervention was on enhancing the perception of the risk of arrest for DUI. Self-reported DUI at that campus subsequently decreased (odds ratio of 0.55), while no change was reported among students at a comparison college. As the authors themselves note, the study was limited because it was not able to use random assignment and multiple campuses in a more rigorous design, but the results are suggestive of what might be possible in an enhanced replication.

The Western Washington University's "Neighborhoods Engaging with Students" (NEST) project employed a comprehensive strategy to decrease disruptive off-campus parties by increasing students' integration in and accountability to the neighborhoods in which they lived (Saltz, Welker, Paschall, Feeney, & Fabiano, 2009). The intervention increased publicity regarding "party emphasis patrols" and collaborated with the city to develop a regulatory mechanism to reduce repeat problematic party calls to the same address. Enforcement of laws prohibiting alcohol sales to minors was also increased for all outlets (for consumption on- and off-premise). The enforcement components were complemented by a neighborhood-based conflict mediation program, service-learning projects in the campus-contiguous neighborhoods, campus-based late-night activities for students, and an educational website designed to increase students' knowledge and skills around living safely and legally in the community. A second Washington State public university was simultaneously funded to initiate a campus community intervention largely based on the Western Washington University program described above. The evaluation included data from those two campuses with a third public school as a comparison site. Annual Web-based student surveys in 2005 and 2006 included measures of alcohol consumption, alcohol-related problems, and student perception of alcohol control and prevention activities. Hierarchical linear modeling (HLM) showed that the prevalence of heavy episodic drinking was significantly lower at the intervention schools (odds ratio of 0.73), with other measures approaching significance. The results strongly support conducting a replication with greater power and a more rigorous design.

The Study to Prevent Alcohol-Related Consequences (SPARC) was a comprehensive intervention using a community-organizing approach to implement environmental strategies in and around college campuses (Wolfson et al., 2007). The ultimate goal was to reduce high-risk drinking and alcohol-related consequences among college students. Eight public and two private universities in North Carolina were randomized to the intervention or comparison condition. A repeated cross-sectional design was used to assess impact of the intervention. Each intervention school was assigned a campus/community organizer. The organizer worked to form a campus community coalition, which then developed and implemented a unique strategic plan over a period of 3 years. Each campus was to address four general strategies: reduce alcohol availability, address price and marketing of alcoholic beverages, improve social norms (e.g., by correcting students' overestimates of heavy drinking among their peers), and minimize harm related to alcohol. Strategies were to be comprehensive in that they included policy, enforcement, and awareness. Within those general categories, campuses developed their own specific strategies, including restricting alcohol at campus events, promoting responsible beverage service, conducting compliance checks, creating a safe ride program, conducting a social norms marketing campaign, and/or creating alcohol-free programs.

The researchers found significant decreases in the intervention group but not the control group in two areas: the percent experiencing severe consequences due to students' own drinking (from 18 to 16%), and the number of alcohol-related injuries caused to others that required medical care (from 3.5 to 2%). With campus populations in the thousands, these reductions translate to significant numbers of students affected. In secondary analyses, higher levels of implementation of the intervention were associated with a reduction in interpersonal consequences due to others' drinking, and a decrease in alcohol-related injuries caused to others.

The Safer California Universities study was designed to test the efficacy of a community-based environmental alcohol risk management prevention strategy applied to college campuses (Saltz, Paschall, McGaffigan, & Nygaard, 2010). The study used a randomized control design involving 14 public universities, half of which were randomly assigned to the intervention condition. The comprehensive intervention included nuisance party enforcement operations (party patrols), minor decoy operations (where police send underage buyers into licensed businesses and cite when alcohol is sold), DUI checkpoints, nuisance party ordinances (i.e., heavier fines when police have to respond to nuisance parties at the same address), and the use of campus and local media to increase the visibility of environmental strategies. Annual surveys of randomly selected undergraduates measured: (1) the proportion of drinking occasions in which students drank to intoxication at six different settings (residence hall party, campus event, fraternity or sorority party, party at off-campus apartment or house, bar/restaurant, and outdoor setting) during the fall semester; (2) whether or not any intoxication occurred at each setting during the semester; and (3) whether students drank to intoxication the last time they went to each setting.

Significant reductions in the incidence and likelihood of intoxication at off-campus parties and bars/restaurants were observed for the intervention universities compared to controls. At Safer intervention universities, a lower likelihood of intoxication was also observed the last time students drank at an off-campus party (odds ratio 0.81), a bar or restaurant (0.76), or across all settings (0.80). No increase in drinking or intoxication (i.e., displacement) appeared in other settings. Furthermore, stronger intervention effects were achieved at intervention universities with the highest intensity of implementation. Given the average undergraduate student population of around 25,000 at these campuses, these reductions translate to approximately 6,000 fewer cases of intoxication at off-campus parties per semester at each campus, and 4,000 fewer cases of intoxication at off-campus bars and restaurants.

Recent Advances in Universal Educational Strategies

The NIAAA task force also drew attention (in their Tier 4 designation) to strategies that are not effective. These include purely educational interventions (i.e., providing information about alcohol and alcohol-related harms). Although all comprehensive interventions include an educational component, educational programs in isolation have been repeatedly shown to be ineffective. Nevertheless, there has been a great deal of interest in and development of online, electronic educational interventions that bear a resemblance to information strategies, but which incorporate features found in the effective cognitive-behavioral or brief motivational individual interventions. Those that have been evaluated in recent years include MyStudentBody, College Alc, Alcohol eCheckup to Go (e-Chug), and AlcoholEdu. Notably, they all incorporate personalized feedback based on students having entered data on their drinking behavior. The students are then shown how their own drinking compares to those of their peers. These programs typically incorporate interactive components along with information about alcohol and its effects. Some also provide students with tips or skills for monitoring and limiting their drinking (see Cronce & Larimer, Chapter 8, and Walters et al., Chapter 9, this volume, for more detail on these types of interventions).

In a recent evaluation of e-Chug alongside AlcoholEdu, Hustad, Barnett, Borsari, and Jackson (2010) provide a concise summary of the work done in this area. However, it is premature to draw definite conclusions, given the few evaluations and the methodological weaknesses (some minor and some major) that they contain (e.g., not controlling for campus-level differences, incompatible comparison groups, use of simple pre–post designs). Programs are under constant development as well, so the current version may not be the same as the one evaluated just 2 or 3 years before. Application of the programs also varies: some are being used as universal strategies required of all students, while in other studies the intervention is used for students who have been mandated to take the course because of their problematic drinking. Nevertheless, the evidence suggests that such strategies can reduce alcohol consumption and possibly also alcohol-related harms. In the evaluation cited above (Hustad et al., 2010), incoming freshman students from a small private university were randomly assigned to one of the intervention programs or to an assessment-only condition. The evaluation found that both programs reduced student alcohol consumption (several measures) at a 1-month follow-up (Hustad et al., 2010). These types of interventions show promise and are likely to improve with further development. Among the issues to be considered are whether the program works equally well for all types of students and at what time the students should be exposed to it. Given the low marginal cost of delivering these programs, demand for them is likely to be high.

WHAT LIES AHEAD?

It is clear that universal, community-level environmental interventions can reduce college student drinking and at least some negative outcomes. While we should be mindful that there are only a handful of such studies, the fact that positive results were produced by interventions quite different in their implementations provides some measure of confidence that the effects are due more to the substance than the style of intervention. There is, in other words, some measure of robustness in the principles underlying this collection of intervention studies.

This means that college administrators may have some confidence that a good-faith effort at controlling the availability of alcohol in both commercial and private settings, coupled with support for enforcing existing alcohol controls and accompanied by publicity, can be part of a successful, comprehensive program. While this strategy can be recommended now, there is, of course, a great deal of work ahead to develop efficient and optimal prevention programs that combine the best strategies currently available.

College administrators can take a lead in developing such holistic prevention programs. They can provide unambiguous support for the full range of interventions (from individual to community-level) and give sufficient authority and support to the professionals working in relevant departments to carry out the necessary steps to implement those interventions. While funding and staff are always sought after, when those direct resources are not available, administrators can give staff the flexibility to reshape their objectives at both the individual and department level. They can also facilitate coordination not only among college departments, but with the surrounding city agencies as well. Finally, most college administrators are fully aware that their influence is often limited to the "bully pulpit" and to opportunities where they can be visible leaders for change. This is not a trivial role, especially in a complex organization where staff want clarity of purpose.

In the case of community interventions, there is often a need to find the least expensive implementation (both in dollars and staff time), the optimal blend of alcohol control measures (DUI enforcement, enforcing sales to minors laws, etc.), and generally, the most effective way to achieve the greatest impact on student drinking.

As the other chapters in this volume suggest, there is a bright future ahead for those concerned with this issue. Many of the individual-level interventions are being developed to work less expensively (e.g., via the Web) and on a larger scale (e.g., LaBrie et al., 2009). At the same time, universal screening with brief intervention (e.g., Schaus, Sole, McCoy, Mullett, & O'Brien, 2009) will be improved upon and made more efficient as well. As attention shifts to focus on the best blend of prevention strategies, there will be the opportunity to integrate messages and reinforce skills at all levels of intervention.

In the meantime, college administrators and community leaders will need encouragement to make the necessary investment in prevention. Citing research evidence can help, but serious impact will only be possible when colleges and universities find ways to marshal resources and support from city councils, campus health and safety professionals, deans of students, parents, and, not incidentally, the students themselves. Though the NIAAA task force was referring to community interventions specifically, it is likely the case that no matter what the mix of interventions may be, the "formation of a campus and community coalition involving all major stakeholders may be critical to implement these strategies effectively" (NIAAA, 2002, p. 20). Universities, and even small colleges, will have people who can recruit and organize such coalitions. If those groups can maintain focus on well-defined and evidence-based strategies, coordinate the people and departments responsible for the range of prevention interventions, and emphasize follow-through on objectives and outcomes, we now have reason to expect they can achieve meaningful improvements in student health and safety.

REFERENCES

Babor, T., Caetano, R., Casswell, S., Edwards, G., Geisbrecht, N., Graham, K., et al. (2010). *Alcohol: No ordinary commodity: Research and public policy.* Oxford: Oxford University Press.

Clapp J., Johnson M., Voas, R. B., Lange J. E., Shillington A., & Russell, C. (2005). Reducing DUI among US college students: Results of an environmental prevention trial. *Addiction, 100,* 327–334.

DeJong, W., & Langford, L. M. (2002). A typology for campus-based alcohol prevention: Moving toward environmental management strategies. *Journal of Studies on Alcohol* (Suppl. 1), 140–147.

DeJong, W., Schneider, S. K., Towvim, L. G., Murphy, M. J., Doerr, E. E., Simonsen, N. R., et al. (2009). A multisite randomized trial of social norms marketing campaigns to reduce college student drinking: A replication study. *Substance Abuse, 30*(2), 127–140.

Gruenewald, P., Johnson, F., Light, J., Lipton, R., & Saltz, R. (2003). Understanding college drinking: Assessing dose response from survey self-reports. *Journal of Studies on Alcohol, 64*(4), 500–514.

Hingson, R. W., & Howland, J. (2002). Comprehensive community interventions to promote health: Implications for college-age drinking problems. *Journal of Studies on Alcohol* (Suppl. 14), 226–240.

Hingson, R. W., McGovern, T., Howland, J., Hereen, T., Winter, M., & Zakocs, R. (1996). Reducing alcohol-impaired driving in Massachusetts: The saving lives program. *American Journal of Public Health, 86*, 791–797.

Holder, H. D. (1992). What is a community and what are implications for prevention trials for reducing alcohol problems? In H. D. Holder & J. M. Howard (Eds.), *Community prevention trials for alcohol problems: Methodological issues* (pp. 15–33). Westport, CT: Praeger.

Holder, H. D., Gruenewald, P. J., Ponicki, W. R., Treno, A. J., Grube, J. W., Saltz, R. F., et al. (2000). Effect of community-based interventions on high-risk drinking and alcohol-related injuries. *Journal of the American Medical Association, 284*(18), 2341–2347.

Hustad, J. T. P., Barnett, N. P., Borsari, B., & Jackson, K. M. (2010). Web-based alcohol prevention for incoming college students: A randomized controlled trial. *Addictive Behaviors, 35*, 183–189.

Kreitman, N. (1986). Alcohol consumption and the preventive paradox. *British Journal of Addiction, 81*, 353–363.

LaBrie, J. W., Huchting, K. K., Lac, M. A., Tawalbeh, B. A., Thompson, B. A., & Larimer, M. E. (2009). Preventing risky drinking in first-year college women: Further validation of a female-specific motivational enhancement group intervention. *Journal of Studies on Alcohol and Drugs* (Suppl. 16), 77–85.

Larimer, M. E., & Cronce, J. M. (2002). Identification, prevention, and treatment: A review of individual-focused strategies to reduce problematic alcohol consumption by college students. *Journal of Studies on Alcohol* (Suppl. 14), 148–163.

Larimer, M. E., & Cronce, J. M. (2007). Identification, prevention, and treatment revisited: Individual-focused college drinking prevention strategies 1999–2006. *Addictive Behaviors, 32*(11), 2439–2468.

National Institute on Alcohol Abuse and Alcoholism (NIAAA). (2002). *A call to action: Changing the culture of drinking at U.S. colleges* (NIH Publication No. 02-5010). Bethesda, MD: Author.

Saltz, R. F., Paschall, M. J., McGaffigan, R. P., & Nygaard, P. M. O. (2010). Alcohol risk management in college settings: The Safer California Universities Randomized Trial. *American Journal of Preventive Medicine, 39*(6), 491–499.

Saltz, R. F., Welker, L. R., Paschall, M. J., Feeney, M. A., & Fabiano, P. M. (2009). Evaluating a comprehensive campus-community prevention intervention to reduce alcohol-related problems in a college population. *Journal of Studies on Alcohol and Drugs* (Suppl. 16), 21–27.

Schaus, J. F., Sole, M. L., McCoy, T. P., Mullett, N., & O'Brien, M. C. (2009). Alcohol screening and brief intervention in a college student health center: A randomized controlled trial. *Journal of Studies on Alcohol and Drugs* (Suppl. 16), 131–141.

Toomey, T. L., Lenk, K. M., & Wagenaar, A. C. (2007). Environmental policies to reduce college drinking: An update of research findings. *Journal of Studies on Alcohol, 68*(2), 208–219.

Wagenaar, A. C., Murray, D. M., Gehan, J. P., Wolfson, M., Forster, J. L., Toomey, T. L., et al. (2000a). Communities Mobilizing for Change on Alcohol: Outcomes from a randomized community. *Journal of Studies on Alcohol, 61*(1), 85–94.

Wagenaar, A. C., Murray, D. M., & Toomey, T. L. (2000b). Communities Mobilizing for Change on Alcohol (CMCA): Effects of a randomized trial on arrests and traffic crashes. *Addiction, 95*(2), 209–217.

Weitzman, E. R., & Nelson, T. F. (2004). College student binge drinking and the "prevention paradox": Implications for prevention and harm reduction. *Journal of Drug Education, 34,* 247–266.

Weitzman, E. R., Nelson, T. F., Lee, H., & Wechsler, H. (2004). Reducing drinking and related harms in college: Evaluation of the "A Matter of Degree" program. *American Journal of Preventive Medicine, 27*(3), 187–196.

Wolfson, M., DuRant, R. H., Champion, H., Ip, E., McCoy, T., O'Brien, M. C., et al. (2007). Impact of a group-randomized trial to reduce high risk drinking by college students [Abstract]. *Alcoholism: Clinical and Experimental Research, 31*(6, Suppl. 2), 115A.

CHAPTER 12

The Impact of College Student Substance Use

Working with Students on Campus

Jason R. Kilmer *and* Shannon K. Bailie

College is a time when students are selecting majors, embarking on careers, making friends, starting relationships, and learning about themselves. For some, this is also a time when they are making the choice to drink alcohol or use other drugs. Unfortunately, substance use can be associated with a range of unwanted consequences, and can exacerbate (or even cause) some of the stressors (e.g., anxiety, sleep difficulties, social consequences) students identify as most threatening to their academic success. In this chapter, we review issues related to college student substance use and physical and mental health, the challenges related to connecting students to assistance or services when help seems indicated, and emerging issues related to these domains (particularly for those working directly with students). We also provide an example of a service designed to reach out to students who may be struggling, which emphasizes prevention and early intervention for these overlapping issues.

SUBSTANCE USE AND RELATED CONSEQUENCES

The Monitoring the Future study (Johnston, O'Malley, Bachman, & Schulenberg, 2009) indicates that 82% of college students report that they have consumed alcohol in the past year, and just over two-thirds (67%) report having been drunk in the past year. These rates decrease when the time frame is restricted to the prior month; 69% of students report any alcohol use, and 45% report having been drunk in the past month (Johnston et al., 2009). It is worth noting that approximately one in five college students does not drink alcohol in a given year; these students who choose to abstain can also be considered as targets of prevention programs (with a focus on maintenance of abstinence or delaying the onset of initiation of drinking). Other research has demonstrated that there can be variability in drinking patterns across an academic year (e.g., higher rates during spring break; Del Boca, Darkes, Greenbaum, & Goldman, 2004), and even variability in heavy drinking over one's college career (Schulenberg & Maggs, 2002).

Consequences and risky behaviors certainly can accompany the decision to drink. The American College Health Association's (ACHA) National College Health Assessment includes a range of questions addressing health issues; the sample from the fall of the 2009–2010 academic year involved a referent group of 34,208 students from 57 colleges and universities who provided data on a number of different alcohol-related consequences. Despite efforts to emphasize the dangers of drinking and driving, this risky practice certainly still occurs; within the past 30 days, 15% of college students reported that they drove after drinking any alcohol at all, and 2% drove after having five or more drinks. When the focus shifts to past-year incidence of various consequences or behaviors outside of driving, the impact to students' health and wellness becomes even more evident. As a consequence of drinking within the past 12 months, 22.3% of students responded that they did something they later regretted, 19% forgot where they where or what they did, 10.8% had unprotected sex, and 10.7% physically injured themselves. Additional consequences had lower prevalence rates, but, given the potential impact to the student and his or her community, these rates are troubling when considering the actual number of students affected. For example, in addition to prevention efforts related to substance use, many colleges and universities have identified violence prevention, sexual assault prevention, and suicide prevention as priorities, and it is clear that these issues overlap with alcohol use. As a consequence of drinking, 1.8% of students reported that they physically injured another person in the past year. Further, 1.5% of students reported that they had sex with someone without giving their consent as a consequence of drinking, and 0.3% admitted to having had sex with someone without getting that person's consent as a consequence of drinking. Finally, 1.2% of students reported that they had seriously considered suicide as a consequence of drinking in the past 12 months (American College Health Association [ACHA], 2010). It is evident that these issues do not occur in a vacuum, and efforts to respond to these multiple domains may be necessary.

In considering the context of alcohol use, it is important to recognize that use frequently occurs in conjunction with other substances. Johnston and colleagues (2009) indicated that 35% of college students report past-year use of an illicit substance. When only assessing marijuana use, 32% of students report past-year use; when assessing any illicit drug other than marijuana, 15% report past-year use. Among other substances endorsed by students are Vicodin (6.7% reporting past-year use), narcotics other than heroin (6.5%), amphetamines (5.7%), hallucinogens (5.1%), and tranquilizers (5%). In the United States, more students (32%) report past-year use of marijuana than past-year use of tobacco cigarettes (30%) (Johnston et al., 2009).

MENTAL HEALTH

High-profile incidents such as the horrific shootings at Virginia Tech have brought some extreme examples of mental health struggles in a college setting into the public eye. The reality, of course, is that there is great variability in symptom severity, and some struggles with issues like feeling depressed or feeling anxious may not meet criteria for a diagnosable mood or anxiety disorder (while nevertheless causing challenges for a student). It is clearly the case that with numerous transitions, stressors, and challenges, a range of mental health issues are being experienced by students on our campuses. Blanco and colleagues (2008), using the data set from the National Epidemiological Study on Alcohol and Related Conditions (NESARC), found that almost half of college students (45.8%) met the criteria for past-year prevalence of an Axis I psychiatric disorder, personality disorder, or substance use disorder. Specifically, approximately one in five students (20.4%) met criteria for a substance use disorder, and many students also met criteria for personality disorders (17.7%, although this was assessed on a lifetime basis), anxiety disorders (11.9%), and mood disorders (10.6%). In a separate survey, when students were asked about symptoms related to anxiety, depression, and anger experienced in the past month (independent of any diagnosis), the following symptoms were reported by students: 69.5% were overwhelmed by all that they had to do; 65.8% felt exhausted (unrelated to physical activity); 37.5% felt very sad; 36.1% felt very lonely; 29.9% felt overwhelming anxiety; 25.9% felt things were hopeless; 20.1% felt overwhelming anger; and 15.8% felt so depressed that it was difficult to function (ACHA, 2010).

With the emphasis put on academic success by institutions and students alike, it is not surprising that students identify academics as the top issue from the past year seen as "traumatic or very difficult to handle" (just under half, 44.2%, endorsed this issue) (ACHA, 2010). Of note, then, is that academic struggles and mental health issues often overlap. When asked to select from 31 factors that could impact a student's academic performance, eight categories emerged with prevalence rates greater than 10%. These included: stress (27.8%), sleep difficulties (20%), being sick with a cold, flu, or sore throat (19%), anxiety (18.6%), work (13.6%), Internet use or computer games (12.6%), depression (11.1%), and concern for a troubled friend or family member (10.4%). Heiligenstein, Guenther, Hsu, and Herman (1996) indicated that 92% of depressed students show signs of academic impairment, and Turner and Berry (2000) demonstrated that 70% of students seeking counseling reported that personal problems had affected their academics.

Other issues are also identified as traumatic or very difficult to handle, including challenges with finances, intimate relationships, family, and sleep (ACHA, 2010). Financial concerns are not insignificant, and can be associated with numerous stressors; in fact, one study showed that students who grew up in poor families were significantly more likely to screen positive for depression or anxiety disorders and to report suicidal thoughts (Eisenberg, Gollust, Golberstein, & Hefner, 2007b). Approximately one in six college students reports a lifetime diagnosis of depression (20% of women and 12% of men; ACHA, 2010), and it is possible that students dealing with depression will have other co-occurring issues. Again highlighting the degree to which these domains overlap, it has been demonstrated that co-occurrence of depression with alcohol and other drug use increases the risk of suicide (Ross, 2004).

Unfortunately, not all students struggling with issues like depression are receiving services that could provide assistance or even relief. Eisenberg, Golberstein, and Gollust (2007) screened college students using the nine-item Patient Health Questionnaire (PHQ-9) and identified a subset of students who screened positive for major depression. Almost three-quarters (72%) of the students who screened positive for depression felt that they needed help; however, only 36% of these students actually received medication or therapy of any kind. Analyses of factors related to access indicated less use of services by students who were unaware of or unfamiliar with service options on campus, students who questioned the helpfulness of therapy or medication, and students who were uncertain about their insurance coverage for mental health visits. Further, there was less use by students who reported growing up in a poor family, and less use by those students identifying as Asian or Pacific Islander (Eisenberg, Golberstein, & Gollust, 2007a). Reasons given by students for not obtaining services included the lack of a perceived need at the time, the belief that stress is normal, and the perception that a great deal of time would be needed to get help. Particularly since some of the factors associated with less use of services could be addressed through provision of information (i.e., being unaware of services, questioning helpfulness, and being unaware of what insurance could cover), Eisenberg et al. (2007a) encouraged colleges and universities to consider outreach, education, campaigns, or initiatives to address students' lack of awareness about the availability and potential effectiveness of services and, across various options and services, what is covered by (or not covered by) insurance. They also suggested taking steps to address other issues that may impede students' access to services (e.g., attempting to address attitudes about quality of services, educating students about symptom severity and issuing guidelines suggesting when to ask for help, and providing information about availability of services). They warn, however, that these efforts can only be successful if sufficient resources are available to support the demand for services.

Compared to the disparity between access to services and need for services with depression, the perception of a need for services (and actual access to services) for issues like alcohol use disorders (AUDs) paints a much different picture. Using data from the Substance Abuse and Mental Health Services Administration (SAMHSA), it has been estimated that 12.5% of college students meet past-year criteria for alcohol abuse, and 8.1% meet past-year criteria for alcohol dependence (Wu, Pilowsky, Schlenger, & Hasin, 2007). Yet only 3.9% of full-time college students with an AUD (either abuse or dependence) received any alcohol services in the past year. Unlike the three-quarters of students with depression who felt like they needed help, only 2.4% of those who screened positive for an AUD and did not receive services perceived a need for services. Reasons for not using services included not being ready to stop using substances, having no health care coverage and being unable to afford the cost, being concerned that getting services might give neighbors and others in the community a negative opinion of the individual, and not knowing where to get treatment (Wu et al., 2007). The challenge to prevention and intervention efforts is to find a way to prompt contemplation of change by those who do not perceive a need for counseling or other services—fortunately, such strategies exist, and these brief interventions are discussed elsewhere in this volume (see Cronce & Larimer, Chapter 8, for a review of interventions that include brief motivational enhancement approaches). Although such interventions may be available on many campuses, increasing student access to them by reducing the barriers to seeking help remains an important challenge. In the meantime, however, it is unfortunately the case that although students struggling with the issues described above might be on the radar of professors, student affairs staff, or others within the academic community, over half may not be receiving support services for the issues they are dealing with. Efforts to address this challenge, including screening and outreach; will be discussed later in this chapter.

EMERGING CHALLENGES

Because of the turnover inherent in an academic setting (i.e., population dynamics can shift as students graduate and new students enroll), the campus climate can be ever changing. Increasingly, this climate is being perceived as being more complicated and as presenting more extreme or severe challenges. Two separate surveys of counseling center directors indicate very similar perceptions—94% of directors state that the number of students with severe psychological problems is a growing concern on their campus (Barr, Rando, Krylowicz, & Winfield, 2010), and 93% of directors state that there has been an increase in recent years in the number of students arriving at counseling centers with serious psychological problems (Gallagher, 2009). Furthermore, 71% of directors believe the number of students with severe psychological problems has increased on their campus just in the past year (Barr et al., 2010).

Kettman and colleagues (2007) summarize the research on severity and suggest that there is not much evidence from empirical studies suggesting severity is actually increasing. Instead, they suggest that although there is no general trend, counseling centers on some campuses may be seeing clients with more complex problems or multiple diagnoses. They also suggest that the perception of increases in severity could be impacted by consistent, increased service demand coupled with loss of staff positions, and that this increased demand could also be related to the reduced stigma attached to mental illness (National Center on Addiction and Substance Abuse [CASA], 2003). Although the severity of students' presenting issues seems to have increased, this has not translated into dramatic changes in counseling center staffing. Although the overall number of new positions funded exceeded positions cut across centers (Gallagher, 2009), 67.3% of counseling centers either stayed the same size or lost positions in the year prior to the survey. Gallagher (2009) examined the domains in which increased severity has been observed over the past 5 years. Three-quarters of respondents (75.9%) identified psychiatric medication issues, followed by crisis issues requiring an immediate response (70.6%), learning disabilities (57.7%), self-injury issues (55.7%), illicit drug use (other than alcohol) (46.5%), and alcohol abuse (45%).

Research has emerged on psychiatric medication in college contexts.

Schwartz (2006) indicated that from the 1992–1993 academic year to the 2001–2002 academic year, there had been a five-fold increase in the percentage of students on college campuses who were prescribed medication. It has been suggested that one factor contributing to the perceived increase of severity of psychopathology on college campuses could be the greater availability of medications, as this could allow students to attend college who otherwise might not have done so (CASA, 2003). This idea was recently supported by Hunt and Eisenberg (2010), who suggest that youth access to effective treatments during adolescence may help students function at a level that allows college attendance when enrollment in college would not have previously been as likely. It has also been suggested that students who want to "party" while in college may discontinue their use of medication (hence, impacting symptom severity) or use alcohol and other drugs while still actively taking medications. Either action could compromise effectiveness of the medications (CASA, 2003). Regardless, when students are prescribed medications, conversations about alcohol could address contraindications when necessary (see also McCabe et al., Chapter 2, this volume).

Studies assessing self-harm indicate that students engage in harming behaviors outside of the realm of suicidal gestures or actions. Although 6.1% of students have seriously considered suicide in the past year, and although 1.3% attempted suicide, 5.2% of students report that they intentionally cut, burned, bruised, or otherwise injured themselves (ACHA, 2010). A study by Serras, Saules, Cranford, and Eisenberg (2010) investigated self-harm behavior in a sample of 5,689 students (69.6% of whom were undergraduates). In the past year, 14.3% of the students reported they had hurt themselves without the intent of killing themselves. Among undergraduates only, 15.8% reported past-year self-injury behaviors, with 19.1% of these students identifying cutting as the means of self-injury. Drug use was associated with higher rates of all 12 forms of self-injury assessed in the study. Factors associated with increased odds of self-injury behavior included drug use, cigarette smoking, gambling, depression, sexual orientation (with students identifying as gay, lesbian, queer, or transgender reporting higher rates than students identifying as heterosexual), and undergraduate student status. Although past 2-week "binge drinking" (five drinks in a row for men, four drinks in a row for women) was not a significant predictor of self-injury behavior on its own, frequently engaging in binge drinking (at least three "binge" episodes in the past 2 weeks) was a significant predictor. The authors suggest that prevention efforts targeting those who report frequent binge drinking and drug use could impact those with higher risk of self-injury (Serras et al., 2010).

EARLY IDENTIFICATION THROUGH SCREENING

The sad truth about suicide by college students is that the majority who end their life never utilize services on campus. In fact, of 103 suicides reported by counseling center directors, only 19% were current or former center clients (Gallagher, 2009). How, then, can we attempt to reach the 81% not connected with counseling? When considering college student mental health, Bayram and Bilgel (2008) state that "the solution lies in being aware of it, intervening earlier and providing support with adequate and appropriate services" (p. 671). One opportunity for increasing awareness about those students who are struggling could involve coordinating care between campus health and counseling centers; unfortunately, however, 65% of counseling centers have no relationship with campus health centers (Schuchman, 2007). An additional strategy for intervening earlier involves screening students for mental health or substance use issues when they are already presenting for services in a campus counseling or health center. Particularly in relation to alcohol use, much more can be done in the implementation of such screening efforts. Only 32.5% of health centers routinely screen for alcohol problems; and of these, only 17% use standardized instruments as part of screening (Foote, Wilkens, & Vavagiakis, 2004). Fortunately, efforts to improve screening and referral to services are being made on college campuses.

Martens and colleagues (2007) used the Alcohol Use Disorders Identification Test (AUDIT) to screen students when they presented for appointments in the campus health center or the campus counseling center. They identified 175 students whose AUDIT score suggested risky alcohol use and who agreed to participate in a brief alcohol intervention (the Brief Alcohol Screening and Intervention for College Students, BASICS; Dimeff, Baer, Kivlahan, & Marlatt, 1999). Their study indicated that following the intervention, students reported decreased alcohol use, more accurate perception of drinking norms, and increased use of protective behaviors. (For more information on these types of interventions see Cronce & Larimer, Chapter 8, and Walters et al., Chapter 9, this volume.)

Such efforts have also been used for depression. Chung, Klein, and Greenberg (2010) demonstrated that screening for depression during routine visits in health centers using the PHQ-9 resulted in the identification of over 800 students with depression who were successfully triaged and entered into a database for tracking and follow-up (Kroenke, Spitzer, & Williams, 2001; Spitzer, Kroenke, & Williams, 1999). It is particularly impressive that 35% of the students identified through the screening had self-identified as racial or ethnic minorities, who, as noted by Klein and Chung (2008), typically underutilize mental health services. The authors concluded that they were able to improve clinical outcomes for at-risk, underserved college students through early detection, coordinated proactive follow-up, and better adherence to outcome-based treatment. These promising findings resulted in the launch of the National College Depression Partnership, which involves a diverse group of over 20 colleges and universities applying similar strategies to better identify students who could benefit from counseling services with the assistance and consultation of the original research team. Recent efforts of the partnership have included the implementation of routine screening for alcohol problems (using the three-item AUDIT-C and a single question proposed by the National Institute on Alcohol Abuse and Alcoholism [NIAAA] to assess heavy drinking days) and anxiety (using the Generalized Anxiety Disorder Scale [GAD-7]), in addition to exploring the impact of effective mental health services on learning outcomes.

Larimer, Cronce, Lee, and Kilmer (2004/2005) describe universal screening as one strategy for identifying high-risk drinkers (e.g., screening or surveying all first-year students or all students), though note that a controlled evaluation of the impact of screening and identifying students for referral to brief interventions has not been done outside the context of an intervention efficacy study. They review possible limitations of such an approach, including the impact of distrust from students regarding the intent or purpose of the screening (e.g., fearing a "crackdown"); concern over inaccurate reporting (in cases of underage drinking or if aware that a "high score" results in a referral); institutional liability (if intervention does not occur when information on illegal or risky behavior is in the possession of the institution, and a medical, legal, or judicial situation arises); confidentiality concerns of students (regarding who has access to screening information and for what purposes); and cost of implementation (Larimer et al., 2004/2005). Future research could examine the conditions under which such universal screening strategies can be most successful and for whom they are most beneficial.

EARLY IDENTIFICATION AND INTERVENTION THROUGH OUTREACH: A CASE EXAMPLE

An additional strategy for reaching students who may be showing signs of difficulty with mental health and/or substance use issues is currently in place at the University of Washington in Seattle (with which we are both affiliated) and involves the creation of the Health and Wellness office. The evolution of Health and Wellness at the University of Washington connotes a climate of change not just at the university but within the realm of Student Life (a division closely related to what might be known as Student Affairs at other schools). It became increasingly apparent to Student Life administrators and staff in the 2000s that we were experiencing a major culture shift among college students. The skepticism that greeted administrative involvement in the 1990s made way for a generation that looked to college administrators for collaboration and support. Parents came knocking, demanding more answers and a higher level of involvement than we had previously seen. In response, the University of Washington started to look at what was being offered within Student Life and found that while many top-quality services were provided, departments often conducted their work in virtual isolation. It appeared that across offices (including parallel or related offices), there was confusion regarding the work of the individual components that make up Student Life. Students would often describe the sense that they were being shuttled between services, directed to whichever office they required and given a referral for the next destination, adding to the feeling that the university served the masses and not the individual. In addition, the students who attempted to navigate the channels of the university were in some ways the lucky ones, as the significant barriers to accessing help perceived by students prevented many students from looking for services at all. What emerged from the changing tide of student culture and from a better understanding of what students needed was a more personalized experience for students, including individual assessments and interventions. Below we review the methods of assessment and intervention incorporated in Health and Wellness and the partnerships within the academic community that are crucial to our work with students.

Health and Wellness was founded on a proactive intervention model that seeks out students in need rather than waiting for them to access services. From the beginning, Health and Wellness worked to establish partnerships with entities like our campus health center and the university police, as well as local hospitals and community agencies that may come into contact with students. Health and Wellness provides a central location from which students can explore and access other relevant resources. Most of the outreaches are voluntary and it is explained that working with Health and Wellness, in most cases, is not mandated. Fortunately, once the program is explained, rarely do students decline services. In short, Health and Wellness was born in response to the demand by students and parents seeking more personalized services, but also by the university's understanding that it needed to be more proactive by reaching out to students.

In addition to providing outreach services, Health and Wellness has also become a significant resource for faculty and staff. When students "hit the radar" anywhere on campus, whether they are acting out in the classroom, submitting materials that raise concern, or communicating concerns to their faculty or advisers, faculty and staff are encouraged to contact the office to create an intervention strategy that addresses concerns of both students and the university. Again, connections within Student Life and beyond are a crucial aspect of this service. Intervention strategies are often formed in consultation with mental health experts, attorneys, and any other pertinent resources on or off campus.

The holistic approach to student care requires staff to be versed in a wide range of topics and to look beyond presenting issues to include and incorporate a broader assessment of students in need. Students may first present with alcohol-related consequences but may end up identifying their personal relationships as major stressors contributing to their excessive drinking.

Health and Wellness has established four distinct programs that focus on prevention and intervention, the broadest of which is the Consultation and Assessment Program. In addition, Health and Wellness oversees the Sexual Assault and Relationship Violence Information Service, Alcohol and Other Drug Education, and the Suicide Intervention Program. Students who are connected via one of the Health and Wellness programs receive the support and assessment associated with the broader scope of the consultation program. Often students are struggling with multiple stressors and the team works to defuse the most immediate concern, while paying attention to contributing factors that may continue to pose problems with students if they go unaddressed. The full range of Student Life services is utilized, often drawing on colleagues from other departments for assistance and support of students. The relationships built across campus, within the academic departments, and in the community allow for consultation, collaboration, and the ability to work with students on a truly holistic level.

With alcohol and other drugs, Health and Wellness provides an opportunity to follow up with students when concerns are documented or passed on through a police report, medical transport, professor, family member, or friend, or following an incident on campus in which involvement of judicial/conduct was not indicated. If, for example, it is learned that a student residing off campus was transported to a local hospital for alcohol poisoning, that student will be invited to a check-in with Health and Wellness staff following the incident. This provides the opportunity for staff to discuss substance use with students in a nonjudgmental, nonconfrontational way. During this conversation with the student, who is likely not engaged in counseling, has not formally completed a screening, and has not self-referred for services, concerns can be explored, along with strategies for reducing unwanted consequences. If the student's problem is outside of Health and Wellness's purview, referral and resource information for additional services can be provided.

CASE EXAMPLES: UTILIZING THE HEALTH AND WELLNESS SERVICES

Case Example 1

The following is a case study in which details and names have been changed. The interventions employed are consistent with the approach utilized at the time and in similar cases.

Colin was studying abroad in Croatia on a 2-month program with 12 other students. The faculty member leading the trip was living in an apartment-style housing unit along with the students in the program, and classes were also conducted in this building. Early on, it became clear that Colin, while being a well-liked and successful student on the trip, had an issue with alcohol. When Health and Wellness received a call from the program director, the faculty member was encouraged to have a conversation with Colin using brief intervention strategies. The faculty member was encouraged to discuss Colin's initial experience, character-ized by engaging appropriately with his peers and successfully participat-ing in the academic requirements of the program. Colin acknowledged that he had enjoyed and felt positive about his initial experiences and went on to discuss how his recent episodes were derailing his experience and his relationships. The faculty member worked with Colin to reestab-lish expectations for continued participation in the program, outlined these expectations in writing, and had Colin sign off on them. When the faculty member met with Colin and addressed the concerns, Colin agreed to conduct himself in a manner that did not compromise his safety or the integrity of the program

About a week after this initial meeting, Colin was out with other students in the program; he drank in excess and began to engage in ver-bal confrontations with people on the street. His friends in the program brought him back to their apartments, where Colin's aggressive behav-ior continued to escalate. He began verbally abusing his roommate and other students who had attempted to assist him, and then he physically attacked his roommate. Another student ran down the hall and requested the help of the faculty member, who attempted to intervene and ended up being threatened by Colin. The faculty member called the local police, who came and transported Colin to the local hospital, where he was kept overnight. Health and Wellness was called the next morning by Inter-national Programs and Exchanges to assist in intervention and problem solving. The immediate concern was for the safety of Colin, as well as the program director and other students who were intimidated and fright-ened by him; in fact, many students felt unsafe remaining in the program while he was still in attendance. Colin's brother took charge of getting

Colin back to the United States, and Health and Wellness worked closely with Colin to facilitate a follow-up.

Upon Colin's return to the University of Washington, he met with members of the Community Standards and Student Conduct Office (CCSC), who addressed his Conduct Code violations in consultation with Health and Wellness. Colin was required to participate in an individual assessment with the Alcohol and Drug Education Coordinator.

Through work with Colin, it became clear that he had lost his father 3 months prior to the beginning of the program. He reported that the loss and grief he was experiencing were contributing factors to his alcohol use. Health and Wellness worked to connect Colin to counseling services on campus as well as with his academic adviser. Close contact was maintained with Colin until his graduation. Fortunately, Colin was able to address both his alcohol use and his grief in ways that allowed him to successfully reengage in his academic and social experiences at the University of Washington.

Case Example 2

This next case study involves a student who came to Health and Wellness through the Suicide Intervention Program. Amy was about to enter her sophomore year at the University of Washington. She became intoxicated while attending a party off campus and began to spiral into what she described as an overwhelming sadness. She later reported that she felt she could only stop this sadness by ending her life. Amy attempted to throw herself into oncoming traffic while walking back to her apartment. Her friends intervened and brought her back to her apartment, where they stayed the night with her. Her roommate contacted Student Life the next day requesting help. The roommate was given information on accessing the Counseling Center, as well as Health and Wellness. Health and Wellness chose to reach out to Amy, and Amy scheduled a consultation with a staff member. During that meeting, the Health and Wellness staff member discussed the incident that had occurred and assessed the student's level of suicidal ideation. Amy reported having serious thoughts of suicide while drinking; although she had been drinking socially for several years, these kinds of thoughts had only surfaced recently. She was referred to the assistant director of Health and Wellness, who focuses on alcohol and other types of drug education and prevention, with whom she could meet to address her specific issues with alcohol. In addition, steps were taken to connect her to the Counseling Center.

While this student had acknowledged having suicidal thoughts, she had not put a lot of thought into how her alcohol use was impacting her decisions around self-harm. Once Health and Wellness assessed the level of risk around alcohol and discussed concerns with her, Amy was very willing to engage in a consultation about her alcohol use, in addition to being open to counseling. Amy described a series of barriers that she felt had previously prevented her from accessing counseling services, and stated that the meeting initiated by Health and Wellness alleviated her concerns around finances, confidentiality, and insurance.

CONCLUSION

As colleges and universities consider ways to reach students who may be having difficulty related to health, mental health, or substance use, one possibility could be exploring topics that could serve as a "foot in the door" for discussing health issues with students. Motivational enhancement approaches often identify a "hook" that prompts contemplation of change (i.e., an area of importance to the student for which they recognize potential improvements if changes in a behavior, often substance use, are made). Schools could also consider identifying the areas that students express interest in learning more about and then integrating relevant substance use and mental health information into these educational opportunities. For example, although 61% of students report that they have received information on alcohol or drug use from their institution, only 28% say they are actually interested in receiving such information. However, over half of students express interest in receiving information on stress reduction (63%), nutrition (60%), physical activity (56%), or sleep difficulties (52%) (ACHA, 2010). Perhaps literally giving students what they are asking for could provide an opportunity to highlight ways in which these areas (e.g., stress reduction, nutrition, or sleep difficulties) could be related to, worsen, or be exacerbated by substance use behaviors or mental health issues. It is worth noting that 52% of students also say they would like information on how to help others in distress, so incorporating education or prevention information into this content could be a possible complement to suicide prevention efforts and other strategies for promoting student health.

Additionally, colleges could consider the multiple outlets from which students could receive health information, particularly if there are underutilized resources on campus. For example, over three-quarters (78.2%) of college students report that they get their health information from the Internet, which is the most commonly identified source of health information (ACHA, 2008). However, only 24.9% of college students see the Internet as a believable source of health information. Given these doubts, if schools rely on the Internet for the provision of health information, future studies could evaluate believability of information provided to students through the institutions' websites and from other websites they link to.

One source seen by students as being very believable, though not commonly utilized, is faculty/coursework. In fact, 65.9% of students identify their faculty or coursework as being the third most believable source of health information, behind health center medical staff (89.9%) and health educators (89.8%) (ACHA, 2008). Despite this, only 40.2% of students get their health information from faculty or coursework (ranked 10th behind 9 other resources). Faculty could be the first to identify changes in a student's productivity or the quality of work being turned in, or changes in content (e.g., journal entries becoming "darker" or reflecting distress), or absences from class. Given the credibility of information from faculty, a conversation initiated by the professor could have a real impact, and could result in a student accepting a referral to counseling services, health services, or other campus resources. Finally, parents can and do play an important role. They are seen as a believable source of health information by 65.2% of college students and are the second-most-utilized resource for health information, with 75.5% of students reporting that they get health information from their parents. As prevention and education strategies are implemented, colleges could consider ways to encourage parents to stay connected and engaged with their children, making sure parents are aware of available resources if and when their children discuss difficulties or struggles they are having.

Future research can consider strategies to address the overlap of mental health issues and substance use, in addition to further examining ways to more rapidly identify concerns through screening, outreach, or both. It is clear that these issues are not a challenge for any single college or university; rather, these are important issues faced across institutions. As schools consider solutions or ways to respond to student needs, there are opportunities to build bridges between research and practice. For example, those doing research on prevention efforts, intervention strategies, and the effects of alcohol and other drugs could work with counselors, practitioners, and other "front-line" college staff or faculty to ensure that students are offered empirically supported or evidence-based services. Similarly, counselors, practitioners, and other college staff could highlight dissemination strengths and challenges, in addition to real-world limitations of evidence-based approaches (often tested under more rigorous research conditions), and could identify emerging needs to aid in the formulation of research hypotheses for future study. To bridge the gap between research and practice, students can be offered programs with a strong evidence-base, and research can more rapidly attend to emerging needs identified by practitioners.

ACKNOWLEDGMENTS

The authors thank Amanda Myhre for her editorial suggestions and consultation around the case examples, and Michael Klein for his input on the National College Depression Partnership.

REFERENCES

American College Health Association (ACHA). (2008). *National College HealthAssessment: Retraced Group Data Report*. Baltimore, MD: Author.

American College Health Association (ACHA). (2010). *National College Health Assessment II: Reference Group Data Report*. Baltimore, MD: Author.

Barr, V., Rando, R., Krylowicz, B., & Winfield, E. (2010). *The Association for University and College Counseling Center Directors Annual Survey*. Retrieved from *www.aucccd.org/img/pdfs/aucccd_directors_survey_monograph_2010.pdf*.

Bayram, N., & Bilgel, N. (2008). The prevalence and socio-demographic correlations of depression, anxiety and stress among a group of university students. *Social Psychiatry and Psychiatric Epidemiology, 43*, 667–672.

Blanco, C., Okuda, M., Wright, C., Hasin, D. S., Grant, B. F., Liu, S., et al. (2008). Mental health of college students and their non-college-attending peers: Results from the National Epidemiologic Study on Alcohol and Related Conditions. *Archives of General Psychiatry, 65*, 1429–1437.

Chung, H., Klein, M., & Greenberg, S. (2010). The National College Depression Partnership: Changing how campuses address depression. *NASPA Leadership Exchange, 7*, 16–21.

Del Boca, F. K., Darkes, J., Greenbaum, P. E., & Goldman, M. S. (2004). Up close and personal: Temporal variability in the drinking of individual college students during their first year. *Journal of Consulting and Clinical Psychology, 72*, 155–164.

Dimeff, L. A., Baer, J. S., Kivlahan, D. R., & Marlatt, G. A. (1999). *Brief Alcohol Screening and Intervention for College Students (BASICS): A harm reduction approach*. New York: Guilford Press.

Eisenberg, D., Golberstein, E., & Gollust, S. E. (2007a). Help-seeking and access to mental health care in a university student population. *Medical Care, 45*, 594–601.

Eisenberg, D., Gollust, S. E., Golberstein, E., & Hefner, J. L. (2007b). Prevalence and correlates of depression, anxiety, and suicidality among university students. *American Journal of Orthopsychiatry, 77*, 534–542.

Foote J., Wilkens C., & Vavagiakis, P. (2004). A national survey of alcohol screening and referral in college health centers. *Journal of American College Health, 52*, 149–157.

Gallagher, R. P. (2009). *National Survey of Counseling Center Directors, 2008* (Monograph Series No. 8R). Alexandria, VA: International Association of Counseling Services.

Heiligenstein, E., Guenther, G., Hsu, K., & Herman, K. (1996). Depression and academic impairment in college students. *Journal of American College Health, 45,* 59–64.

Hunt, J., & Eisenberg, D. (2010). Mental health problems and help-seeking behavior among college students. *Journal of Adolescent Health, 46,* 3–10.

Johnston, L. D., O'Malley, P. M., Bachman, J. G., & Schulenberg, J. E. (2009). *Monitoring the Future national survey results on drug use, 1975–2008: Vol. II. College students and adults ages 19–50* (NIH Publication No. 09-7403). Bethesda, MD: National Institute on Drug Abuse.

Kettman, J. D. J., Schoen, E. G., Moel, J. E., Cochran, S. V., Greenberg, S. T., & Corkery, J. M. (2007). Increasing severity of psychopathology at counseling centers: A new look. *Professional Psychology: Research and Practice, 5,* 523–529.

Klein, M. C., & Chung, H. (2008). The College Breakthrough Series—Depression (CBS-D) project: Transforming depression care on college campuses (Part II). College Health in Action, 47(4), 1.

Kroenke, K., Spitzer, R. L., & Williams, J. B. W. (2001). The PHQ-9: Validity of a brief depression severity measure. *Journal of General Internal Medicine, 16,* 600–613.

Larimer, M. E., Cronce, J. M., Lee, C. M., & Kilmer, J. R. (2004/2005). Brief intervention in college settings. *Alcohol, Health, and Research, 28,* 94–104.

Martens, M. P., Cimini, M. D., Barr, A. R., Rivero, E. M., Vellis, P. A., Desemone, G. A., et al. (2007). Implementing a screening and brief intervention for high-risk drinking in university-based health and mental health care settings: Reductions in alcohol use and correlates of success. *Addictive Behaviors, 32,* 2563–2572.

National Center on Addiction and Substance Abuse at Columbia University. (2003). *Depression, substance abuse and college student engagement: A review of the literature.* New York: Author.

Ross, V. (2004). Depression, anxiety, and alcohol or other drug use among college students. Retrieved from the Higher Education Center, U.S. Department of Education, *www.higheredcenter.org.*

Schuchman, M. (2007). Falling through the cracks: Virginia Tech and the restructuring of college mental health services. *New England Journal of Medicine, 357,* 105–110.

Schulenberg, J. E., & Maggs, J. L. (2002). A developmental perspective on alcohol use and heavy drinking during adolescence and the transition to young adulthood. *Journal of Studies on Alcohol* (Suppl. No. 14), 54–70.

Schwartz, A. J. (2006). Are college students more disturbed today? Stability in the acuity and qualitative character of psychopathology of college counseling center clients: 1992–1993 through 2001–2002. *Journal of American College Health, 54,* 327–337.

Serras, A., Saules, K. K., Cranford, J. A., & Eisenberg, D. (2010). Self-injury, substance use, and associated risk factors in a multi-campus probability sample of college students. *Psychology of Addictive Behaviors, 24,* 119–128.

Spitzer, R. L., Kroenke, K., Williams, J. B. W., & the Patient Health Questionnaire Primary Care Study Group. (1991). Validaion and utility of a self-report version of PRIME-MD: The PHQ-9 Primary Care Study. *Journal of the American Medical Association, 282,* 1737–1744.

Turner, A. L., & Berry, T. R. (2000). Counseling center contributions to student retention and graduation: A longitudinal assessment. *Journal of College Student Development, 41,* 627–636.

Wu, L., Pilowsky, D. J., Schlenger, W. E., & Hasin, D. (2007). Alcohol use disorders and the use of treatment services among college-age young adults. *Psychiatric Services, 58,* 192–200.

CHAPTER 13

Campus Recovery Programs

Lisa Laitman *and* Lea P. Stewart

Alcohol and other drug (AOD) use and abuse are serious issues facing college campuses throughout the United States. Many institutions of higher education have developed comprehensive programs to address alcohol use and drive down the rates of high-risk drinking on their campuses. Less attention has been paid to developing programs that assist students facing issues of AOD abuse and dependence. This chapter will briefly highlight the problems of AOD use and abuse on college campuses, describe why providing support to students in recovery from AOD abuse and dependence is important, and summarize the common and unique elements of current recovery support programs. In addition, we will present lessons learned from the recovery program at Rutgers University that others may find helpful in beginning their own campus-based recovery support program.

In the 10 years between 1992 and 2002, the number of adolescent treatment admissions for alcohol-related problems in the U.S. increased by 65%, from 95,000 to 156,000 (Substance Abuse and Mental Health Services Administration [SAMHSA], 2004). This increase, in turn, meant that more young people in recovery wanted to attend college but required support to manage the drinking environment that often exists on a college campus. In addition to adolescents who are in recovery prior to coming to college, 13 to 32% of college students meet DSM-IV criteria for alcohol abuse, and 6 to 8% meet criteria for alcohol dependence (Knight et al., 2002). In 2008–2009, those estimates translated into approximately 1 million college students with alcohol dependence (Misch, 2009). While research on rates of other drug abuse and dependence rates in the college population is rare, Caldeira and colleagues (2008) examined the prevalence of negative consequences of cannabis use in the first-year college student population and concluded that "the prevalence of CUD [cannabis use disorders] and other cannabis-related problems are not trivial" (p. 407).

Clearly, many of these students are in need of treatment and eventually recovery support. Given the estimate of 6 to 8% of the college population meeting diagnostic criteria for alcohol dependence and the addition of students with drug dependence, a college campus with 10,000 students, for example, could expect from 600 to 1,000 students to be in need of treatment and eventual recovery support; yet treatment and other services are rarely available to meet this need and these students remain underserved. For example, Wu, Pilowsky, Schlenger, and Hasin (2007) reported that in 2002 only 4% of full-time college students with an alcohol use disorder had received any alcohol services in the past year. Even today, very few campuses (15 as of 2010) have programs in place to provide comprehensive recovery support for students needing it.

It has often been noted that the college environment is not conducive to recovery nor does it provide the peer support critical to maintaining a sober lifestyle (Botzet, Winters, & Fahnhorst, 2007). This fact is illustrated by reports indicating that high-risk drinking and its consequences are often considered the biggest public health problem on U.S. college campuses today (Boyd, McCabe, & Morales, 2005; Ham & Hope, 2003; Hingson, Zha, & Weitzman, 2009). Since the college environment itself contributes to heavy drinking on campus regardless of the characteristics of the students, college attendance may be a "situational risk" for heavy drinking and its concomitant problems (Jackson, Sher, & Park, 2005; see Vergés & Sher, Chapter 7, this volume). Given the potential toxicity of this environment, it is crucial to provide resources for students who come to college in recovery and to those whose substance dependence develops while they are in college. Recovery support for young people in college not only increases opportunities for a productive adult life but also contributes to recovery success. As Finch (2007a) has noted, "education communities provide a powerful source of influence upon adolescents and young adults, and thus there exists both opportunity and risk" (p. 3).

AN EXPANDED COMPREHENSIVE CAMPUS AOD MODEL

The widely accepted environmental management approach for AOD prevention on college campuses calls for attention to educational programs, changes in the college environment to limit the use of AOD, and programs for early identification, referral, and treatment of problem drinkers (DeJong et al., 1998). This model omits services to students who are in recovery. Given the need for recovery services, and to best meet the needs of students despite staffing limitations and other realities on a college campus (Laitman & Lederman, 2007), an expanded campus AOD model needs to be developed. A truly comprehensive AOD model should include: (1) prevention, (2) policy development, (3) training, (4) screening and brief interventions, (5) short-term counseling, and (6) recovery support. Below we briefly describe the more traditional components of the environmental management model as they relate to the proposed expanded model. This discussion is followed by a description of a campus recovery program that would constitute the recovery support component of the proposed expanded model.

Effective *prevention* efforts follow an environmental management approach that includes strategies such as the enforcement of zero tolerance as well as drinking and driving laws, reducing the availability of alcohol, limiting alcohol advertising and promotions, disseminating social norms campaigns, and developing campus–community coalitions (National Institute on Alcohol Abuse and Alcoholism [NIAAA], 2007). Ideally, *policy development* should begin with an articulation of the expectations and values of a university community in relation to the use and abuse of alcohol and other drugs, which will then serve as the foundation for education and enforcement. Since early intervention can reduce the harm a student (or any individual) may experience (McCrady, 2004), it is important to ensure that professional staff, who are likely to see students on evenings and weekends, when high-risk drinking is more likely to occur, receive adequate *training* to recognize signs of alcohol abuse and acquire information on where to direct at-risk students for appropriate screening, intervention and treatment. *Screening and brief interventions* for AOD programs can be implemented in campus health centers or counseling centers following the SAMHSA Campus SBIRT Initiative recommendations (*sbirt.samhsa. gov/colleges.htm*).

Common screening instruments include: (1) Alcohol Use Disorders Identification Test (AUDIT), a 10-item screening tool developed by the World Health Organization (WHO) to identify persons whose alcohol consumption has become hazardous or harmful to their health; (2) Alcohol, Smoking, and Substance Involvement Screening Test (ASSIST) developed for the WHO by an international group of substance abuse researchers to detect and manage substance use and related problems in primary and general medical care settings; and (3) Drug Abuse Screening Test (DAST), a brief instrument that detects drug abuse or dependence disorders. Additionally, in 2009, the National Institute on Drug Abuse (NIDA) launched an online drug screening instrument for primary care settings, "NIDA MED Assist," which is an adaptation of the ASSIST instrument (*ww1.drugabuse.gov/nmassist*). Referrals for brief motivational interventions with personalized feedback, such as the Brief Alcohol Screening and Intervention for College Students (BASICS; Dimeff, Baer, Kivlahan, & Marlatt, 1999), have been shown to be effective in reducing both the quantity of alcohol use and negative consequences in a number of studies (White, 2006; White, Mun, Pugh, & Morgan, 2007). (For greater detail, see Cronce & Larimer, Chapter 8, and Walters et al., Chapter 9, this volume.) *Short-term counseling* with professionals trained in AOD counseling should be available for students to help them address problems that are not amenable to treatment with brief motivational interviewing. These professionals should also be able to determine, with input from students, if referral for intensive outpatient programs or inpatient treatment is needed. For students who return to campus from treatment for alcohol or drug dependence and/or students who come to campus in recovery, recovery support services are crucial.

WHAT MAKES A COLLEGE CAMPUS ENVIRONMENT DIFFICULT FOR STUDENTS IN RECOVERY?

While many of their peers are engaging in alcohol and other drug experimentation, college students in recovery are learning how to manage abstinence. (See Ham & Hope, 2003, and Jackson et al., 2005, for comprehensive reviews of problematic drinking and its consequences among college students.) Maintaining abstinence is often dependent on restructuring daily life to avoid behaviors and social triggers that may lead to use. While most people in recovery must and do learn how to manage in a culture where many people drink, the college environment presents unique challenges. Although the amount of drinking varies considerably across college campus types, such as residential versus commuter schools or 2-year versus 4-year institutions (Jackson et al., 2005), in general, the college environment has been described as an "abstinence-hostile" one (Cleveland, Harris, Baker, Herbert, & Dean, 2007). As Jackson et al. (2005) note, "because of the nature of the college campus, there is a high concentration of high-risk individuals in a permissive environment, leading to a high concentration of problems not only for the drinker but for others who do not drink and for the larger institution" (p. 108). Most residence halls and off-campus student apartments suffer from a lack of privacy and space, and many roommates do not understand the needs or lifestyle of someone in recovery. In addition to negotiating their way through this environment, young people in recovery must also balance the demands of recovery and academics, a challenge others they live with may not understand (Bell et al., 2009; Misch, 2009).

Though not unique to young adults, the need to fit in, make new friends, and establish a sense of belonging are important components of a successful and satisfying college experience. Developmentally, young adults in early recovery are at a different stage than their peers (Bauer, 1994; Schulenberg et al., 2001). For example, many students in early recovery will comment on the behavior of other students engaged in AOD experimentation as something they did at a younger age (the expression "been there, done that" often is used) (Misch, 2009). Exposure to this culture for someone in early recovery can be overwhelming, and, by trying to avoid it, many students experience a feeling of missing out on a "normal" college experience. By providing access to treatment as well as opportunities for interaction with peers in recovery, campus recovery communities can create social communities that support abstinence, which, in turn, leads to a greater chance of academic success for college students.

ELEMENTS OF CAMPUS RECOVERY PROGRAMS

Currently there are 15 campus recovery programs in the United States. The campuses that have the oldest recovery communities are Brown (1977), Rutgers (1983), and Texas Tech (1986) (Botzet et al., 2007).[1] Subsequent campus recovery programs have adapted elements of existing ones, primarily from the Collegiate Recovery Community developed by the Center for the Study of Addictions and Recovery at Texas Tech University (Cleveland, Harris, & Wiebe, 2010a) and the Rutgers Recovery Housing model, considered the first significant recovery community on a college campus in the United States. Other institutions that have developed recovery communities are Augsburg College, Case Western Reserve University, Washington State University, University of Texas at Austin, University of Virginia, Loyola College (Baltimore, Maryland), Kennesaw State University, University of Pennsylvania, Georgia Southern University, Rutgers-Newark, Grand Valley State University, William Patterson University, Tulsa Community College, Northern State University,

---

[1]In 1989, Wilson Hall was reported to be a structured living environment for students in recovery on the campus of LeMoyne College (Drake & Cosgrove, 1989), but there is no evidence that it currently exists.

and College of St. Scholastica.[2] The following sections focus on common elements of the 15 current campus recovery programs, followed by a discussion of elements that differ among the various programs.

Common Elements of Campus Recovery Programs

Existing campus recovery programs vary in important ways (discussed below), but the common (and essential) characteristics of these programs include: (1) a campus-based professional with responsibility for developing a support network for students in recovery, (2) outreach and publicity about the program, and (3) facilities dedicated to the recovery program.

Campus-Based Professional

A professional with expertise in recovery from addiction can coordinate support services and develop referral and outreach in the campus community, as well as connections with outside resources such as treatment programs, school professionals, and self-help recovery networks. Additionally, this individual should coordinate with staff from health and counseling, academic affairs, campus life, and residence life to ensure the referral of students in need of treatment and recovery support. Students in recovery often face academic challenges that other students do not, and these students may need extra academic support, in part because they may lack foundational knowledge that others received in high school (Harris, Baker, Kimball, & Shumway, 2007). Thus, it is important to provide staff who can advocate for these students by speaking with academic advisers, faculty, and other administrative staff on their behalf. For example, staff may help students who have been placed on academic probation to appeal their suspensions and provide them with support to succeed in their studies (Finch, 2007a).

Program Publicity

Program publicity not only ensures that students and parents are able to locate recovery services, but it also helps others in the community become aware of the institutional value of supporting those in recovery. In addition, publicity can help reduce stigma by making recovery part of the campus vocabulary (e.g., "we have services available to help students ranging from individuals who have made a few poor choices about their

---

[2]In 1992, Central Michigan University had a program called the "Recovering Person's Prevention Project" (R3P) (Rapaport, Minelli, Reyes, & Norton, 1992).

use of alcohol to those who need assistance with alcohol abuse or dependence"). Publicity about campus recovery programs is easily included in a variety of websites and links within other campus websites. Information about campus recovery programs should be included whenever information on alcohol and other drugs is provided. For example, health center websites and counseling center services should clearly state that recovery services are available, not just mention that therapists within counseling address AOD issues. If special campus housing is available for students in recovery, those housing options should be visible on websites that describe general campus housing. Other media that students utilize can also effectively publicize recovery services. For example, campus newspapers and radio stations provide avenues to reach the greater campus community.

Facilities

Facilities dedicated to a campus recovery program serve as a safe haven for students in recovery. They may be buildings, rooms, or offices where students can meet staff or faculty who provide recovery services and/or academic advising, attend support groups, and meet their friends in recovery. There may also be a residential community that provides housing as part of the recovery support process (this option will be discussed in more detail below).

Unique Elements of Campus Recovery Communities

Campus recovery communities are as unique as the campuses in which they reside (White, 2008; White & Finch, 2006). The differences among programs are due in part to the variety of people and administrative units that have developed them, as well as to the culture of a particular campus. Unique aspects of college recovery communities include: (1) the type of housing provided, (2) the role and location of 12-step meetings, (3) the connection between academics and the recovery program, (4) admissions requirements, and (5) development and funding sources.

Type of Housing

As Polcin, Korcha, Bond, and Galloway (2010) note, "many individuals seeking to abstain from alcohol and drugs have difficulty establishing social support systems that reinforce sobriety and finding long-term, stable housing that is free of alcohol and drugs" (p. 357). Thus, one of the important ways to provide support for on-campus students in recovery is through the availability of housing that provides a "safe haven" where students in recovery can live and support each other. One solution to this challenge is to advise students about off-campus housing and to encourage students in recovery to live together (Cleveland et al., 2010a).

Separate on-campus housing for students in recovery may be particularly effective as research indicates that attitudes toward drinking in students' residence halls and floors reliably predict their personal attitudes toward drinking (Bourgeois & Bowen, 2001), with local drinking norms that emerge on residence hall floors often encouraging excessive drinking. In addition, a roommate's alcohol consumption can affect academic performance. Kremer and Levy (2008) conclude that this may be particularly true for male students. Their study revealed that male students who had been randomly assigned to live with roommates who drank alcohol either frequently or occasionally the year before they came to college (self-reported on an entering student survey) had lower GPAs during their first and second years in college than male students assigned to non-drinking roommates. For male students who reported drinking heavily in high school, having a roommate who also reported drinking heavily in high school (and presumably continued this behavior in college) lowered their college GPA by 0.99, a reduction of almost a full point on a 4.0 scale. The researchers posit that roommates who drink excessively may create noise and thus reduce opportunities for study, or perhaps that having alcohol present can induce a desire for alcohol consumption in their roommates. Other researchers have noted the unique challenges faced by female drinkers (McCrady, 2004).

Creating an on-campus recovery housing community requires collaboration and commitment from different departments and resources. The campus AOD professional and others working in conjunction with the students in the recovery community can ensure that values articulated during the policy development process translate into operational terms by giving the community the structure it needs to succeed. Working out these details may be an extensive process and will require the support of administrators who are willing to modify existing housing policies to meet the needs of students in recovery and provide funding to maintain a separate living space. But the benefits of this type of housing can be great. As one student interviewed by Finch (2007a) noted, "the benefits of the recovery house include sober living, sober friends, recovery meetings, and helpful staff.... Being in the presence of students using would be a constant temptation to relapse. Removing me from this dangerous environment has been one of the major benefits of the recovery house" (p. 30).

Although "substance-free" housing has been shown to reduce students' alcohol use (Kremer & Levy, 2008), we believe that its strength is the support provided in this housing rather than the fact that it is substance free. While the term "substance free" refers to an externally enforced system, a recovery community, which is also based on an expectation that the individuals are committed to abstinence, finds its greatest strength in its interpersonal network and the personal commitment to abstinence and recovery that each resident brings to the community. Nevertheless, the term "substance free" can be one that a campus is comfortable using, and this type of special housing can provide the support network that is essential for students in recovery. (For a history of communal living arrangements for individuals in recovery, see Polcin, 2009.)

Role of 12-Step Recovery

Early recovery is a complicated and tenuous period for most people (Woodford, 2010). Transition periods are also difficult times (Ham & Hope, 2003; Schulenberg & Maggs, 2002). Thus, students coming to college in early recovery or coming to college for the first time often need much more support than is available through campus counseling services. Through 12-step meetings they can be provided with a support network that is free and available at times when counseling centers may be closed (e.g., at night or on weekends). Universality, support, and instillation of hope are primary attractions for youth at 12-step meetings. Despite the value of these meetings for individuals living in recovery housing (Polcin & Henderson, 2008), they are often misunderstood by professionals and the community at large. Sometimes seen as cult-like or religious, they may be dismissed before they are completely understood. While no method of treatment is effective for everyone, not recognizing 12-step recovery as a valuable element in a recovery plan is ill advised. Failing to offer 12-step programs deprives young adults of a wonderful peer support network that may enrich their college and recovery experience and can help them to maintain long-term recovery.

Location of 12-Step Meetings

Since students in recovery on a college campus are in many respects no different from other students, having friends their own age to spend time with is vitally important. As noted previously, the college campus poses significant risks to a young person in recovery (Harris et al., 2007) because of the lack of support for abstinence and the fact that so many young people, in their quest to be independent, include drinking and/ or drug use in the expression of that independence. A student who is in recovery and, therefore, not "partying" in this way is often at a loss to negotiate this social environment. Regular participation in 12-step meetings can provide students with emotional and, potentially, social support to overcome these challenges.

Students on campuses that do not have campus recovery programs often attend off-campus 12-step meetings to make sure they have recovery support. However, meeting other college students or people their own age at these meetings is often serendipitous. When off-campus 12-step meetings do not have many college student attendees, students in recovery often finds themselves in a situation where their academic and recovery worlds are separated. This separation is further exacerbated by the fact that the safest course for these students is to avoid the college campus (except to attend classes and access other essential services) or to limit social activities on campus. Creating a campus recovery community and welcoming 12-step meetings to the campus is a deliberate way to ensure that students in recovery meet other students in recovery. Having meetings in which students in recovery meet other students has a synergistic effect that creates other opportunities for on-campus social activities, such as seeing each other in dining halls or attending classes together. These interactions bring recovery and the college experience together in a meaningful way.

Inviting 12-step meetings onto a college campus offers many other benefits (Bell et al., 2009). On-campus 12-step meetings invite a larger recovery community onto campus, providing opportunities to interact with alumni and other mentors who may have longer-term recovery, and thus expanding the possibilities for students to meet others who can be sponsors. These on-campus meetings may also open possibilities to those within the 12-step community to consider attending college. If meetings on campus are known to the university community, faculty and staff may send students who are "newcomers" to these meetings, and these students will be able to avail themselves of the recovery campus community. Since not every student in recovery may live in recovery housing, on-campus meetings provide opportunities for the larger recovery community to meet.

As with the issue of special housing, coordination among different departments and administrative support is necessary to ensure that 12-step groups will be able to host meetings on a campus on a weekly basis year-round. Although the specific traditions of 12-step recovery do not allow for affiliation with an organization or formal program, Alcoholics Anonymous (AA) and Narcotics Anonymous (NA) each have structures to assist institutions in bringing meetings to specific campuses or helping students in recovery to start meetings on campus. Often the most difficult step in negotiating to have a 12-step meeting on campus is obtaining appropriate space that is secure, relatively private, and accessible after normal business hours, since meetings often take place at night or on the weekends. In addition, meetings may involve community mem-

bers, so it is important that administrators be willing to invite nonaffili-
ated individuals onto the campus.

Academic Connection to Recovery Program

As noted previously, established campus recovery communities have
evolved in very unique ways. One of the differences among them is how
each program "creates community" and teaches and reinforces its values to
students in successive generations. Campus life and schedules are often very
complicated, so that finding a time when everyone in an established community can meet together can be difficult. Some campuses (such as Texas
Tech) have found that requiring all students in the community to enroll in a
special course for which students receive academic credit is a way to ensure
that the community has the time necessary to maintain its values (Harris
et al., 2007). Other campus recovery communities have developed a model
that separates academic credit from their recovery programs.

Admissions Requirements

When students in recovery decide to apply to college or return to college,
some will choose campuses that have recovery support communities.
Individuals learn about these communities from sources such as the Association of Recovery Schools (ARS), which has a website (*www.recov-
eryschools.org*) that lists sober high schools and colleges in the United
States that have campus recovery programs. Some treatment programs
have also become familiar with the concept of recovery schools and will
guide young adults looking for colleges in the direction of those schools
that offer recovery support services. Other students may apply and get
accepted at a college and then contact the institution to see if there are
recovery services available at the school. Some students will begin to
take college courses at community colleges near home or near a halfway
house following completion of a treatment program. Taking courses in
this way, usually part-time in the beginning, enables students to make
early recovery their focus and also gives them structure, a sense of direction, and hope for the future.

While different institutions allow for varying recovery time, all
review prospective students on a case-by-case basis and assist families in
making appropriate academic decisions.

Development and Funding Sources

Campus recovery programs have emerged on campuses in a variety of
ways—through academic departments via a faculty member or gradu-

ate student with an interest in addiction and recovery, through health or counseling services, and through existing AOD prevention or counseling programs. More recently, new campus recovery initiatives have received mentoring from existing programs to get their programs started. Contact information about campus recovery programs is available on the ARS website, and many campuses considering developing recovery programs have contacted the established programs listed on the website for technical support. In addition, Texas Tech University's Campus Recovery Community has received funding specifically for replication or for assisting other schools in developing programs (Cleveland et al., 2010a). Treatment programs have offered support as well.

Funding sources for campus recovery programs also vary. Some programs raise much of their own funding from alumni, the recovery community, and other supporters. Other programs are funded by campus resources, whereas others have utilized special grant or state funding sources to enhance their programs.

EVALUATION OF CAMPUS RECOVERY PROGRAMS

Although a growing number of campuses offer recovery communities, research on the effectiveness of the programs at these schools is "thin," primarily including theses and dissertations, single-site evaluations, and unpublished reports (Finch, 2007b; Woodford, 2010). Evaluation of campus recovery programs has focused on identifying key components of successful programs (based on relapse rates and academic performance of students within the campus recovery community), and on designing research to assess those components. Two of the largest campus recovery programs have begun to report some outcome data:

- Texas Tech University's Center for the Study of Addiction and Recovery (CSAR) in Lubbock, Texas, has conducted the most research to date on their campus recovery program (e.g., Bell et al., 2009). For example, researchers at Texas Tech report a relapse rate of 8%, a graduation rate of 70%, and an average GPA of 3.18 for students in their Collegiate Recovery Community (Cleveland, Wiebe, & Wiersma, 2010b; Harris et al., 2007).
- Augsburg College's StepUP Program in Minneapolis, Minnesota, has also been tracking relapse rates of their recovery community. A majority of students and alumni from Augsburg College's StepUP Program who responded to a questionnaire ($N = 83$) reported abstaining from alcohol and drug use, as well as regularly attending self-help groups and having high levels of social support (Botzet et al., 2007).

To date there has not been a full-fledged implementation or outcome evaluation of any campus recovery program. Securing funding for this research has been a major challenge, and many schools have not even put into place procedures for data collection.

RUTGERS RECOVERY HOUSING: A CASE STUDY

The Alcohol and Other Drug Assistance Program (ADAP) at Rutgers was established in 1983 as a result of recommendations by the President's Committee on the Use of Alcohol, which appeared in a report commissioned in 1981 by then president Edward Bloustein. An alcohol/ drug counselor was hired by University Health Services, and ADAP was started to address the needs of high-risk students, including children of alcoholics, and to develop campus recovery support services. A recovery support group for students began in September 1983, and Recovery Housing opened in September 1988, making it one of the earliest campus recovery programs established in the country. Rutgers Recovery Housing was originally developed as a safe haven for students who started recovery through ADAP's on-campus AOD counseling program. Over the years, young adults already in recovery began transferring to Rutgers because of Recovery Housing and its affiliated support services. Many students and families call the ADAP office for information about Recovery Housing months or even a year before they would be coming to college. They may request a tour or an interview, in much the same way that other young people graduating from high school decide which college to apply to and attend. Alternatively, some students apply and are accepted at Rutgers and then contact us regarding the availability of Recovery Housing.

Enrollment in special courses is not required in order to reside in Recovery Housing, but prospective residents must meet certain standards to be accepted and to remain. These arrangements were established through policy discussions with ADAP, Residence Life, and Housing. ADAP staff is responsible for student recruitment and selection, as well as for maintaining the standards of Recovery Housing. This is accomplished through a series of procedures discussed in detail below.

Within the Rutgers program, we have learned that students are most likely to succeed both academically and in recovery if they come to school with at least 3 months of continuous recovery. Being a full-time college student carries significant stress, and balancing the additional pressures of having only a few months of sobriety is often overwhelming. Many students (and people in general) in early recovery are anxious to get on with their lives and are often trying to make up for time lost when they were active in their addictions. We try to evaluate each student applying individually, but in our 22 years of operating Recovery Housing we have learned a few lessons that generalize to many students. When students have less than the time required to enroll in Recovery Housing (3 months is the minimum), we will work with them and their families to find an arrangement that will help them continue looking ahead toward higher education and a college degree, but will also respect the importance of building a solid foundation of recovery. For example, there may be a delay in the admission of a prospective student in this situation; or, alternatively, a student may commute from home, attend Rutgers courses, and participate in campus recovery activities to help prepare him or her for a later admission to Recovery Housing. These students receive counseling from ADAP staff but do not live in Recovery Housing. (As noted previously, not all students in recovery on the campus live in Recovery Housing.)

The structure of the recovery community includes the professional ADAP counselors who are part of counseling services, or CAPS (Counseling, Alcohol and Other Drug Assistance Program and Psychiatry Services). Additionally, a resident assistant (RA) lives in the Recovery House. This individual is a member of the recovery community and has lived in Recovery Housing for at least 1 year as a resident. Students interested in the position apply and are interviewed by ADAP staff. Payment for the position is in the form of a term bill credit and a partial credit toward housing costs. The RA is employed by Residence Life and goes through the same training as other RAs. However, unlike other RAs, the RA in Recovery Housing reports directly to the ADAP staff and can reach the counseling staff at any time, if needed. The primary roles of the RA are to be an in-house resource for the residents, to assist the ADAP staff in organizing activities, and to intervene in emergency or urgent situations. The RA also functions as an initial resource for problem solving.

Recovery Housing does not function as a halfway house, but instead is an on-campus residence hall for students in recovery. The culture is set up to promote independence and the development of responsibility, both for students' recovery as well as for their academic success. The unique guidelines that exist for students who live in Recovery Housing are related to maintaining a community that is AOD-free by choice and defines community behavior to prevent relapse and support recovery and academic success. Emphasis is on self-governance and accountability to the community. For example, all students are required to attend monthly house meetings, to be in counseling with ADAP if they have less than 1 year of recovery or are new to Recovery Housing, to be full-time students, to attend weekly 12-step meetings, and to maintain a relationship with a sponsor. In addition, students are encouraged to reach out to other students if they need help. Although the recovery community is committed to providing an environment that supports recovery from addiction and promotes abstinence from substances, we recognize that relapses do occur. Residents are asked to notify the RA living in the House immediately if they relapse or if they know someone else has relapsed, and ADAP staff is contacted. Staff then work to support the student's effort to return to abstinence and recovery. Students who refuse a new treatment plan must move out of the House immediately.

In 2008, Rutgers and William Patterson University each received a 3-year grant from the New Jersey Department of Human Services Division of Addiction Services (DAS) to develop or enhance campus recovery services. Grant funding for the Rutgers-New Brunswick and Rutgers-Newark campuses supported key improvements, beginning with the hiring of a Recovery Counselor. ADAP clinicians and the newly hired Recovery Counselor, in collaboration with the grant principal investigator (a faculty member and campus dean), were able to improve coordination between student services, counseling services, and academics to the benefit of the students in recovery. The importance of these collaborations was among the "lessons learned" from maintaining on-campus Recovery Housing for over 20 years. Each college campus has a unique organization and values. At Rutgers, we realized that having collaborators from student affairs and academics improved the quality of the experience for our students in recovery.

With the support from this funding, the grant team developed a series of enhancements to reach the larger campus recovery community beyond Recovery Housing. For example, the Recovery Counselor actively engaged alumni of the recovery community. Due to the longevity of the ADAP program, the Rutgers recovery alumni community includes individuals now in the range of 30–50 years of age with up to 27 years of sobriety. ADAP hosted Rutgers Recovery Reunions in 1993 and 2003 to celebrate 10 and 20 years, respectively, of the recovery program. A 25th year reunion was held in November 2008.

Recovery alumni stay in touch with each other all over the country and internationally. Many alumni living in the local area are willing to support the young student community and serve as 12-step program sponsors, mentors, and friends. Alumni support students' recovery and participate in community-building activities including the recently inaugurated annual alumni/student baseball game. While clearly helping students in early recovery, these relationships benefit the alumni since, as Pagano, Friend, Tonigan, and Stout (2004) report, individuals who help others (e.g., by being AA sponsors or carrying the message of AA to others) are better able to maintain their own long-term sobriety.

Additional enhancements have included offering sober social events to the recovery community so that students in recovery can have social interactions that are not organized around alcohol (Bell et al., 2009). Many of these events involve alumni. Planned community events have included Sober Spring Break (for current students), as well as Halloween, New Year's Eve, and Super Bowl parties. These events, as well as participation in intramural sporting events and attending cultural events, emphasize the importance of having fun that fills the time students formerly spent using AOD. Volunteering for speaking opportunities, service work, and internships also serves this function. A new tradition is the Recovery Graduation, which was held for the first time in May 2010. Nine graduates were recognized by over 50 guests including parents, close friends, and sponsors. Graduates were introduced by someone they felt had supported their recovery. All events provide opportunities to bond with others in recovery and to celebrate important milestones. As McCrady (2004) concludes, "having a social network that supports abstinence and that provides other positive functions is associated with better long-term outcomes of treatment" (p. 119).

MANAGING RELAPSE IN A CAMPUS RECOVERY COMMUNITY

Relapse prevention strategies are an integral component of any campus recovery community. How administrators, clinicians, and other personnel associated with the recovery community respond to relapse is vital to the preservation and growth of a healthy community. At Rutgers, procedures for addressing relapse are discussed with all students in Recovery Housing and then are put into writing. Response is not punitive but rather therapeutic and rapid. Clinicians determine responses to individual relapses depending on severity. Following a relapse, those in charge will need to assist in managing the anxiety that relapses create within the recovery community by fostering open and direct communication. Other considerations for campus professionals include balancing confidentiality with transparency. Campus recovery professionals must conduct an administrative review of all relapses. The commitment to having these reviews continually improves the community for all.

CONCLUSION

Addressing alcohol and drug issues within their communities has long been a complex, daunting, and often discouraging process at many college campuses. In the current decade, we have more evidence-based practices, and many campuses have started a dialogue, developed alcohol committees, and allocated resources toward these efforts. However, students with more severe substance abuse and dependence and those students in recovery are often overlooked, and there remain only a very small number of campuses where recovery programs are offered. Providing resources and support services to help those students receive intervention and treatment and then supporting them when they return to campus are critical if a campus plans to reduce the consequences of high-risk AOD use and prevent relapse.

Since a large proportion of college students who meet diagnostic criteria for alcohol abuse or dependence do not seek treatment while they are in college (Knight et al., 2002), providing recovery housing is an excellent way for college campuses to convince these students that recovery and college can be successfully negotiated together. As one alumnus of a recovery community program noted, "living in the recovery house also afforded me the opportunity to live on my own, take care of myself, and have people who supported me in that process. That experience proves more valuable every day as I continue to live a clean and sober life beyond my college experience" (Finch, 2007a).

REFERENCES

Bauer, A. M. (1994, March). *Supportive counseling for students recovering from substance abuse*. Paper presented at the Annual Meeting of the National Association of School Psychologists, Seattle, WA.

Bell, N. J., Kanitkar, K., Kerksiek, K. A., Watson, W., Das, A., Kostina-Ritchey, E., et al. (2009). "It has made college possible for me": Feedback on the impact of a university-based center for students in recovery. *Journal of American College Health, 57*(6), 650–657.

Botzet, A. M., Winters, K., & Fahnhorst, T. (2007). An exploratory assessment of a college substance abuse recovery program: Augsburg College's StepUP Program. *Journal of Groups in Addiction and Recovery, 2*(2–4), 257–270.

Bourgeois, M. J., & Bowen, A. (2001). Self-organization of alcohol-related attitudes and beliefs in a campus housing complex: An initial investigation. *Health Psychology, 20*(6), 434–437.

Boyd, C. J., McCabe, S. E., & Morales, M. (2005). College students' alcohol use: A critical review. *Annual Review of Nursing Research, 23*(1), 179–211.

Caldeira, K. M., Arria, A. M., O'Grady, K. E., Vincent, K. B., & Wish, E. D. (2008). The occurrence of cannabis use disorders and other cannabis-related problems among first-year college students. *Addictive Behaviors, 33*, 397–411.

Cleveland, H. H., Harris, K. S., Baker, A. K., Herbert, R., & Dean, L. R. (2007). Characteristics of a collegiate recovery community: Maintaining recovery in an abstinence-hostile environment. *Journal of Substance Abuse Treatment, 33*, 13–23.

Cleveland, H. H., Harris, K. S., & Wiebe, R. P. (Eds.). (2010a). *Substance abuse recovery in college: Community supported abstinence.* New York: Springer.

Cleveland, H. H., Wiebe, R. P., & Wiersma, J. D. (2010b). How membership in the Collegiate Recovery Community maximizes social support for abstinence and reduces risk of relapse. In H. H. Cleveland, K. S. Harris, & R. P. Wiebe (Eds.), *Substance abuse recovery in college: Community supported abstinence* (pp. 97–111). New York: Springer.

DeJong, W., Vince-Whitman, C., Colthurst, T., Cretella, M., Gilbreath, M., Rosati, M., et al. (1998). *Environmental management: A comprehensive strategy for reducing alcohol and other drug use on college campuses.* Newton, MA: Higher Education Center for Alcohol and Other Drug Prevention. Available at *www.higheredcenter.org/services/publications/environmental-management-comprehensive-strategy-reducing-alcohol-and-other-dru.*

Dimeff, L. A., Baer, J. S., Kivlahan, D. R., & Marlatt, G. A. (1999). *Brief Alcohol Screening and Intervention for College Students(BASICS): A harm reduction approach.* New York: Guilford Press.

Drake, R., & Cosgrove, J. (1989, June/July). Wilson Hall: Structured living on campus in support of recovery. *Adolescent Counselor,* pp. 47–50.

Finch, A. J. (2007a). Authentic voices: Stories from recovery school students. *Journal of Groups in Addiction and Recovery, 2*(2–4), 16–37.

Finch, A. J. (2007b). Rationale for including recovery as part of the educational agenda. *Journal of Groups in Addiction and Recovery, 22*(2–4), 1–15.

Ham, L. S., & Hope, D. A. (2003). College students and problematic drinking: A review of the literature. *Clinical Psychology Review, 23,* 719–759.

Harris, K. S., Baker, A. K., Kimball, T. G., & Shumway, S. T. (2007). Achieving systems-based sustained recovery: A comprehensive model for collegiate recovery communities. *Journal of Groups in Addiction and Recovery, 2*(2–4), 220–237.

Hingson, R. W., Zha, W., & Weitzman, E. R. (2009). Magnitude of and trends in alcohol-related mortality and morbidity among U.S. college students ages 18–24, 1998–2005. *Journal of Studies on Alcohol and Drugs* (Suppl. 16), 12–20.

Jackson, K. M., Sher, K. J., & Park, A. (2005). Drinking among college students. In M. Galanter (Ed.), *Recent developments in alcoholism: Vol. 17. Alcohol problems in adolescent and young adults* (pp. 85–117). New York: Springer.

Knight, J. R., Wechsler, H., Kuo, M., Seibring, M., Weitzman, E. R., & Schuckit, M. A. (2002). Alcohol abuse and dependence among U.S. college students. *Journal of Studies on Alcohol, 63,* 263–270.

Kremer, M., & Levy, D. (2008). Peer effects and alcohol use among college students. *Journal of Economic Perspectives, 22*(3), 189–206.

Laitman, L., & Lederman, L. C. (2007). The need for a continuum of care: The Rutgers comprehensive model. *Journal of Groups in Addiction and Recovery, 2*(2–4), 238–256.

McCrady, B. S. (2004). To have but one true friend: Implications for practice of research on alcohol use disorders and social networks. *Psychology of Addictive Behaviors, 18*(2), 113–121.

Misch, D. A. (2009). On-campus programs to support college students in recovery. *Journal of American College Health, 58*(3), 279–280.

National Institute on Alcohol Abuse and Alcoholism (NIAAA). (2007). *What colleges need to know: An update on college drinking research* (NIH Publication No. 07-5010). Washington, DC: Author.

Pagano, M. E., Friend, K. B., Tonigan, J. S., & Stout, R. L. (2004). Helping other alcoholics in Alcoholics Anonymous and drinking outcomes: Findings from Project MATCH. *Journal of Studies on Alcohol, 65*, 766–773.

Polcin, D. L. (2009). Communal living settings for adults recovering from substance abuse. *Journal of Groups in Addiction and Recovery, 4*(1–2), 7–22.

Polcin, D. L., & Henderson, B. A. (2008). A clean and sober place to live: Philosophy, structure, and purported therapeutic factors in sober living houses. *Journal of Psychoactive Drugs, 40*(2), 153–159.

Polcin, D. L., Korcha, R. A., Bond, J., & Galloway, G. (2010). Sober living houses for alcohol and drug dependence: 18–month outcomes. *Journal of Substance Abuse Treatment, 28*, 356–365.

Rapaport, R. J., Minelli, M. J., Reyes, S., & Norton, P. (1992). *The recovering person's prevention project (R3P): Involving recovering students and community members in alcohol and other drug abuse prevention on the college campus.* Ann Arbor, MI: ERIC Clearinghouse.

Schulenberg, J. E., & Maggs, J. L. (2002). A developmental perspective on alcohol use and heavy drinking during adolescence and the transition to young adulthood. *Journal of Studies on Alcohol* (Suppl. 14), 54–70.

Schulenberg, J., Maggs, J. L., Long, S. W., Sher, K. J., Gotham, H. J., Baer, J. S., et al. (2001). The problem of college drinking: Insights from a developmental perspective. *Alcoholism: Clinical and Experimental Research, 25*(3), 473–477.

Substance Abuse and Mental Health Services Administration (SAMHSA). (2004). *Results from the 2003 National Survey on Drug Use and Health: National findings* (DHHS Publication No. SMA 04-3964). Rockville, MD: Author.

White, H. R. (2006). Reduction of alcohol-related harm on United States college campuses: The use of personal feedback interventions. *International Journal of Drug Policy, 17*(4), 310–319.

White, H. R., Mun, E. Y., Pugh, L., & Morgan, T. J. (2007), Long-term effects of brief substance use interventions for mandated college students: Sleeper effects of an in-person personal feedback intervention. *Alcoholism: Clinical and Experimental Research, 31*(8), 1380–1391.

White, W. L. (2008). The culture of recovery in America: Recent developments and their significance. *Counselor, 9*(4), 44–51.

White, W. L., & Finch, A. J. (2006). The recovery school movement: Its history and future. *Counselor, 7*(2), 54–58.

Woodford, M. S. (2010). Recovering college students: Practical considerations for college counselors. Retrieved from *counselingoutfitters.com/vistas/vistas10/Article_14.pdf.*

Wu, L.T., Pilowsky, D. J., Schlenger, W. E., & Hasin, D. (2007). Alcohol use disorders and the use of treatment services among college-age young adults. *Psychiatric Services, 58*(2), 192–200.

PART V

POLICY ISSUES

CHAPTER 14

The Minimum Legal Drinking Age

21 as an Artifact

Philip J. Cook *and* Maeve E. Gearing

Almost half of all college students are under 21 years old, and are therefore legally prohibited from drinking in every state.[1] Yet most college students drink whether or not they are underage—about 86% of college students who have graduated from high school within the past 4 years report ever having drunk alcohol, 67% drink regularly, and 41% engage in regular binge drinking (Johnston, O'Malley, Bachman, & Schulenberg, 2008). While the underage prohibition evidently has little effect on the prevalence of drinking by college students (given that the overwhelming majority do drink), it nonetheless influences the nature of the alcohol-abuse problem on campuses by pushing it underground (or more precisely, into dorm rooms and other unmonitored places). The administration's response to drinking is limited by the legal fiction of prohibition, so opportunities to promulgate harm-reduction policies are limited. The prohibition has the effect of making scofflaws of millions of college students, which may affect their attitude toward the law in general. It implicitly identifies college-age students as being something less than fully adult, despite the fact that 18-year-olds enjoy the full range of civil rights and responsibilities in all other respects.

In this chapter, we consider the reasoning behind the legal classification and framing of underage drinking, and whether the nationally

---

[1]There are approximately 5 million underage students nationwide, out of 11 million undergraduate and junior college students.

imposed minimum legal drinking age (MLDA) of 21 is justified, by science or by practical considerations. Ultimately, we are led to recommend lowering the drinking age to 18 or 19, based primarily on the social, legal, and cultural standards of adulthood in this country and the realities of young adult drinking. The MLDA does prevent some harms—a fact that we document in what follows—but at an unacceptably high cost.

Reducing the MLDA does not, however, mean endorsing drinking by college students. The consequences of drinking by young people remain severe no matter how the issue is framed. Rather, reducing the legal drinking age means reclassifying college drinking as adult drinking, and thus viewing it not as a distinct problem limited to a youthful population but as part of the much larger problem of alcohol abuse. The repeal of this prohibition would refocus attention on strengthening broad alcohol control measures. It would also allow colleges to pursue forthright strategies to reduce abuse and reduce the resulting harm.

HISTORY OF THE MLDA

The minimum legal drinking age of 21 is an artifact of an earlier age. In this, it is much like other legal anachronisms, such as North Carolina's prohibition on cohabitation (which stood until 2006), or an early-20th-century Texas law requiring married women to be "examined" if they wished to transfer property deeds—it reflects earlier and now-inapplicable mores and social norms ("North Carolina's Anti-cohabitation," 2000; Greer, 1922). Under an MLDA of 21, an 18-year-old soldier cannot toast her own wedding. A 19-year-old juror can sentence someone to death but cannot order a beer at a restaurant. And a 20-year-old student may buy cancer-inducing cigarettes but may not consume a potentially heart-healthy glass of wine with dinner. The story of how the current minimum legal age came about highlights its tenuous philosophical position.

After the repeal of Prohibition in 1933, most states set their minimum legal drinking age at 21 (American Medical Association, 2010). Twenty-one boasted a long history as the age of majority, dating back to English common law of the 13th century (James, 1960). However, even in 1933 many other rights and responsibilities were assigned at earlier ages. Full liability for criminal acts had been mandated for those age 16, 17, or 18 (depending on the state). By 1913, child labor laws in most states had set age 14 as the minimum age of employment; this was raised nationally to 16 for most jobs by the Fair Labor Standards Act of 1938 (Bureau of Labor Statistics, 2000), and set at 18 for certain hazardous occupations. In sum, while 21 held some power as a traditional set point of maturity, it was by no means the agreed-upon age of majority for all rights, as no such age yet existed.

A major shift occurred in the context of the Vietnam War, during which 18-year-olds were being drafted and dying in the service of their country, and the Baby Boom cohorts began asserting themselves politically. In 1968, Congress adopted uniform rules allowing 18-year-olds to serve on juries ("Qualifications for Jury Service," 1968). Most importantly, in 1970, the 26th Amendment was enacted, granting 18-year-olds the right to vote. With this basic marker of citizenship and maturity established, and given the politics of the time, state legislators were inclined to bring other age-based rules into line. A number of states reduced the minimum age for signing binding contracts from 21 to 18.[2] And, between 1970 and 1975, 25 states lowered their MLDA to 18 (Toomey, Nelson, & Lenk, 2009).

One consequence of reducing MLDAs took both public health experts and legislators by surprise. In the late 1970s and early 1980s, evidence began accumulating on the effect of MLDA on traffic fatalities. Research indicated that lowering the drinking age resulted in more drunk driving crashes and more deaths of 18- to 20-year-olds (Cook & Tauchen, 1984). A simple difference-in-difference analysis (Table 14.1), comparing changes in highway fatality rates among 18- to 20-year-olds in states that lowered their MLDA and those which did not, suggests that the reduction in drinking age resulted in an 11-percentage-point increase in young adult traffic deaths—which is in line with estimates based on more sophisticated methods (Cook, 2007).

Lawmakers in a number of states, driven by public concern for safety and by the end of Vietnam-era politics, responded by reversing the downward movement in MLDAs. In 1983, President Reagan formed the Commission on Drunk Driving, which recommended a national minimum legal drinking age of 21 (Exec. Order No. 12,258,1982). While no such law was passed, Congress created a de facto national MLDA of 21 by requiring states to raise their MLDAs as a condition for receiving national highway funds (Pearl, 1985). By 1988, all states had MLDAs of 21 (American Medical Association, 2010).

However, in nearly every other respect 18-year-olds maintained their adult status, including new rights granted following the passage of the 26th Amendment.

---

[2]Every state currently sets 18 as the age of majority and the contract age. The following states, among others, lowered the contract age from 21 to 18 during the early 1970s: California, Delaware, Maryland, Michigan, Minnesota, North Carolina, and West Virginia (*minors.uslegal.com/age-of-majority*, accessed at various times during July 2010).

TABLE 14.1 Effect of MLDA on Traffic Fatalities among 18-to 20-Year-Olds

Change in MLDA	Number of states	Percent change in fatality rate
Reduction from 21 to 18	16	–1%
No change	23	–12%
Difference in difference		11%

Note. Data from Cook (2007).

EFFECTS OF THE MLDA, AND CHANGES TODAY

Thus the newly established status of 18-year-olds as adults was overridden by the concern for highway safety, and that judgment has rarely been questioned in public debate. In recent years, however, a new organization called Choose Responsibility has become a visible advocate for reconsidering the MLDA. John McCardell, former president of Middlebury College, heads this organization, which had some success in 2008 with the so-called Amethyst Initiative, a petition arguing for national debate of the MLDA and use of different policy tools to reduce college drinking.

Pointing to the high prevalence of drinking on college campuses, McCardell argues that the MLDA is ineffective as a deterrent to alcohol consumption. Specifically, McCardell ties the high level of binge drinking to prohibition. Binge drinking (defined as five or more drinks in one session for males, and four or more for females) was found to be extraordinarily prevalent—around 40%—among 4-year college students in all four waves of the College Alcohol Surveys, conducted between 1993 and 2001 (Wechsler & Nelson, 2008). As Wechsler and Nelson (2008) report:

> The drinking style of many college students is one of excess and intoxication. Among drinkers, almost half (48%) report that drinking to get drunk is an important reason for drinking, 1 in 4 (23%) drink alcohol 10 or more times in a month, and 3 in 10 (29%) report being intoxicated three or more times in a month. Binge drinkers consumed 91% of all the alcohol that students reported drinking, and 68% of alcohol was consumed by frequent binge drinkers. (p. 3)

College campuses, with their large populations of underage students, are expected to offer a safe environment to a group who are in most respects deemed adult. Liability is an important factor: in 2000, MIT paid $6 million to settle a lawsuit by the family of a freshman who died of alcohol poisoning during a fraternity pledging event (Levine, 2000). Federal law also governs college alcohol policy. The Drug-Free Schools and Communities Act, passed in 1989, requires all institutions of higher education to create programs to reduce drug and alcohol use and abuse on campus or risk losing federal funding. Such programs must include information on the negative consequences of drug and alcohol use and refer students to available treatment modalities (Faden & Baskin, 2005). The act has been reauthorized every 2 years since 1989 and regularly expanded, most notably in 2002 as part of President Bush's No Child Left Behind Initiative. Now termed the Safe and Drug-Free Schools and Communities Act, the legislation provides funding for anti-alcohol and drug programs but also imposes more regulation on what types of programs universities may promulgate ("Safe and Drug-Free," 2009). More generally, the focus of federal regulations over the past two decades has shifted from urging enforcement of existing drug and alcohol laws to requiring programming to decrease college drinking and adopt a more clearly prohibitionist stance. Modifications in 1998 to the Higher Education Opportunity Act (Amendments, 1965), for example, implicitly encourage universities to notify parents and guardians of student alcohol violations.

A number of college administrators appear to be chafing at the legal restrictions and the difficulties of reducing alcohol-related harms on campus when the legal benchmark is so far removed from reality. By 2010, 135 college presidents had signed Amethyst's call to debate new alcohol policies.

Of course, residential colleges house only a fraction of youth age 18–20, and then only for 8 months per year. A change in the MLDA would affect all youths of this age. Overall trends for this larger group provide additional support for reconsideration of the MLDA. Both population-level drinking patterns and highway safety have changed since the years when states were increasing their MLDAs. Drinking among all age groups, including 18- to 20-year-olds, declined during the 1980s (see Figure 14.1), as did rates of alcohol abuse and addiction. At the same time, the rate of alcohol-related traffic fatalities has decreased dramatically (Figure 14.2). The continued decline in motor vehicle deaths since 1985 cannot be tied to the MLDA, which has not changed during that period. Other changes in law, behavior, and technology get the credit. Thanks in part to the efforts of Mothers Against Drunk Driving and similar groups, penalties for drunk driving have been increased, legal per se limits on blood alcohol content have been established to provide a scientifically verifiable definition of drunk driving, and the use of designated drivers has greatly expanded. Also relevant are general improvements in highway safety, improved safety features on vehicles, better trauma care, and greatly expanded use of seat belts resulting from legal mandates (Zlatoper, 1989; Cook, 2007).

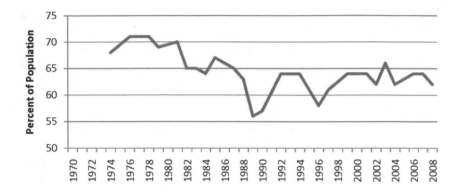

FIGURE 14.1. Self-reported drinking prevalence, all ages. From National Institute on Alcohol Abuse and Alcoholism [NIAAA] (2008).

ARGUMENTS FOR AND AGAINST
LOWERING THE MLDA

Of course, these changes on their own do not justify lowering the MLDA; they only suggest that the cost of doing so has been reduced. In particular, increases in alcohol-related accidents and fatalities, particularly traffic fatalities, would likely be smaller than the increases that were seen when MLDAs were first lowered following the passage of the 26th Amendment.

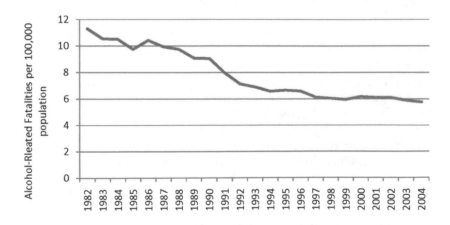

FIGURE 14.2. Alcohol-related traffic fatality rates. From National Institute on Alcohol Abuse and Alcoholism [NIAAA] (2006).

Still, we do not expect that a reduction in MLDAs would be harmless. More 18- to 20-year-olds would drink and they would likely drink more, and alcohol access for high-school-age youth would also increase (Dee, 1999; Cook & Moore, 2001). As a result, it is probable that alcohol-related deaths and accidents would increase among 18- to 20-year-olds.[3]

Finally, there are also potential effects of MLDAs on crime. Alcohol has been found to facilitate aggression and lower inhibitions, resulting in nuisance, property, and violent crime (Leonard, Collins, & Quigley, 2003; Pihl & Peterson, 1993; Martin, 2001; Cook & Moore, 1993; Carpenter, 2005). If a reduction in the MLDA increased alcohol abuse by youth, then increased crime rates might be one result, but there is little direct evidence on this matter.

Thus, available evidence indicates that a reduction in the MLDA would come at the cost of increased alcohol-related harms, although the effects should be less than in the 1970s. In any event, notable benefits must exist to justify lowering the MLDA. Three potential justifications are developed below: that the MLDA is an unacceptable infringement on liberty; that it interferes with a broader, more effective approach to reducing alcohol abuse; and that it interferes with experimentation with potentially effective alternative approaches, especially on college campuses.

Liberty

Perhaps the strongest argument for lowering the MLDA is a philosophical one: at its current level, it is an unacceptable infringement on the liberty of young adults. While 21 may have made some sense earlier in this nation's history as an age of majority, 18-year-olds now have adult status in all other respects. They may vote, serve on juries and in public office, marry without parental consent, serve in the military, work in hazardous jobs, sign contracts, gamble in the lottery (and in casinos in many states), be tried as an adult in criminal court, obtain an unrestricted driving license, and buy tobacco products. Yet they may not drink. In this respect, America is an outlier among developed nations. All European

---

[3]Carpenter and Dobkin (2009), using a regression discontinuity design, find sharp increases in mortality from motor vehicle accidents, suicide, and alcohol poisoning at age 21, suggesting that the current MLDA does offer some protection for those under 21. It is not clear, however, whether this discontinuity is due to a transitory "initiation" effect, which disappears after a few months, or is due to the sustained effect of legal availability. If it is transitory (and the age-trajectory data suggest that it is), then little would be lost from reducing the age—the initiation effect would be moved from the 21st birthday down to the 18th birthday.

nations, Canada, and Mexico have an MLDA under 21, as do most other countries.

By making an exception to majority for alcohol, then, the implicit claim is that 18- to 20- year-olds are somehow different from other adults in this one domain, and that they need to be prevented by law from choosing to drink. What principled arguments could be made in support of depriving this group of the liberty to drink? One type of argument would assert a paternalistic rationale of protecting them against the special hazards associated with alcohol. Another type of argument rests on a claim that drinking is more harmful to 18- to 20-year-olds than to those over 20. Here we assess both arguments.

In his famous harm principle, the 19th-century philosopher John Stuart Mill asserted that government should respect individual choice because liberty is a preeminent concern. Restricting self-regarding behavior (actions that predominantly affect the person making the choice, rather than others) could be justified only in cases where the choice was made without full information or full capabilities. The most important exception to the case for liberty is for children, and more generally for those not capable of making a reasoned decision.

But the justification for paternalism does not apply here. For starters, the law deems 18-year-olds as responsible adults. That age is supported to an extent by developmental science, which increasingly draws sharp distinctions between younger and older adolescents with respect to cognitive and emotional development. Both common sense and law acknowledge the differences between children and adults. Recent court cases have concluded that those under 18 are not fully mature; in *Roper v. Simmons* (2005), *Graham v. Florida* (2010), and *Sullivan v. Florida* (2010), the court relied heavily on scientific evidence to reduce the culpability of young adults. The period between 13 and 18 years of age is one of rapid developmental growth, with measurable increases in the ability to rationally process information, weigh costs and benefits, consider future consequences, and withstand peer influence (Aber et al., 2009). Children should be protected from alcohol; they are biologically prone to risk-taking behavior and are unable to assess the effects rationally (Spear, 2000).

But a line must be drawn between childhood and adulthood, and in many important respects 18 is supported by neuroscience as being an appropriate line. While 18-year-olds are by no means fully mature, research suggests they have close to adult capabilities in perspective, temperance, and responsibility (Steinberg & Cauffman, 1996). According to several studies, preference for risk and immediate rewards (which might drive children toward irresponsible alcohol use) appear to peak between ages 13 and 16, and decrease in the years following (Steinberg, 2008).

Moreover, while 18-year-olds may not be fully developed in some areas, they do not differ significantly in abilities from 21-year-olds in such age-related deficits. Neural connections and cognitive efficiency, for instance, continue to increase through the mid-20s and beyond (Blakemore & Choudhury, 2006).

Similarly, it is difficult to argue that 18- to 20-year-olds are really "different" than their older peers on the basis of their behavior. If frequency of accidents indicates personal irresponsibility (which in turn could justify paternalism), then 21- to 24-year-olds should also be protected. As Table 14.2 shows, 18- to 20-year-olds have rates of both homicide fatalities and motor vehicle fatalities that are comparable to those of 21- to 24-year-olds; rates decrease markedly for those 25 to 29, and even further for those 30 and over. Figure 14.3, meanwhile, shows the lack of obvious changes in fatality rates by multiple causes at age 21; traffic fatalities do not suddenly increase for those now of legal drinking age, and other types of injury death rates do not decrease. At least from evidence of how people act, it is not clear that 21 marks a break with childhood, and it is difficult to argue on this basis that 21 is a better-supported age cutoff for drinking than 18. Either drinking (and other important rights such as marriage, voting, buying tobacco, etc.) should be restricted by age well past where it is now, or alcohol rights should be made consonant with other markers of adulthood. Yet there is no movement to raise the age of adulthood to 21, let alone 25.

So much for paternalism. For adults, the harm principle specifies that actions which place others at risk are candidates for justified regulation. Drinking by 18- to 20-year-olds does have negative externalities (as does drinking by all age groups). For that reason, it is reasonable to ask whether an MLDA would pass a cost–benefit test. For much government regulation, the decision on whether to intervene is based on cost–benefit analysis, where the consequences of a proposed regulation are monetized and summed. Doing a similar analysis for the MLDA is difficult since some of the most important consequences are not valued in the mar-

TABLE 14.2. Death Rates by Age Group, 2007

Age group	Homicide	Motor vehicle accident
18–20	15.7	29.1
21–24	15.8	27.1
25–29	13.0	18.9
30+	5.1	14.7

Note. Rates per 100,000 people. Data from WISQARS (2010).

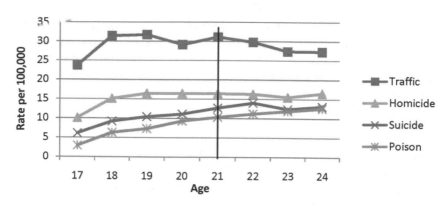

FIGURE 14.3. Fatality rates by age and cause. From WISQARS (2010).

ketplace. Nonetheless it is useful to sketch what a cost–benefit analysis would look like.

Suppose that we were performing this analysis from a regime in which the MLDA were set at 18, and the federal Office of Management and Budget undertook a cost–benefit analysis of a proposal to raise it to 21. If 18- to 20-year-olds are deemed adult, then their interests (as they themselves define those interests) should be counted in this analysis—they have "standing." Presumably most would have to be compensated for the loss of a right to drink legally, and for some the required compensation to make them "whole" would be hundreds of dollars per year. Even if it averaged just $100 per person, the total would be over $1.3 billion per year. That hypothetical compensation is part of the social cost of raising the MLDA. Also included would be the additional costs of enforcing the law, including the costs of arrests and processing of those picked up for underage drinking. Even more important might be the effect of the higher MLDA on public attitudes toward the law—to have a regulation that is destined to be violated by most of the people affected undercuts respect for public authority.

The benefits would include the reduction in injuries, deaths, and property damage to all bystanders, as well as health care costs borne through risk pooling. On the other hand, the direct costs of drinking for 18- to 20-year-olds themselves are internal expenses, assumed to be incorporated in their decision to drink. Most injuries and fatalities from underage drinking are borne by the drinkers themselves, but the external costs may still be significant (Center on Alcohol Marketing and Youth, 2010). The balance between costs and benefits is not clear on the face of it, but quite possibly the increased MLDA would fail the test.

We can estimate one aspect of the benefit from having the MLDA at 21 instead of 18, namely the benefit associated with a lower highway fatality rate. In 2008, there were 34,017 fatal motor vehicle accidents involving 37,261 deaths. Drivers ages 18 to 20 were involved in 4,205 of these accidents. Of those 4,205 drivers, 1,110 (or about 26%) were drinking, as determined either through a blood alcohol concentration greater than zero or through evidence at the scene. Nearly two-thirds (710) of those young adult drunk drivers, meanwhile, died in their accidents. The value of those lives is an internal cost, assumed by the driver when he or she chose to drive drunk. Other people also died in these accidents as well, numbering 460 in 2008. Some of the cost of these lives is internal, and some represents a social cost. Those who were occupants in the vehicle with a drunk driver can be assumed to have accepted the increased risk of such transportation; they are not bystanders, in other words. But those who were in other vehicles, or were pedestrians struck by a drunk driver, are non-consenting victims, and their lost lives are an external cost. The final tally shows that 152 people died as the result of an accident with a drinking young adult driver, but were not themselves in the vehicle with said driver.

To calculate the cost in terms of fatalities from reducing the MLDA, let us assume fatalities increase 20% with the change in law. (That assumption is generally in line with experience from the 1970s.) That would imply an additional 31 deaths. At a cost per life of $5 million, the external traffic fatality cost of a lowered MLDA would be $155 million per year. That and other costs should, in principle, be weighed against the value to youths of being allowed to drink legally. Indeed, the key feature of this analysis is to give standing to the preferences of 18-year-olds, as is logically dictated by the judgment that they are adults. We know for a fact that the overwhelming majority prefer to drink even when prohibited from doing this, and it is a reasonable guess that they would place considerable value on a removal of that prohibition. That value on freedom, whether or not we attempt to monetize it, must be weighed against the costs associated with the presumed increase in drinking and abuse.

Public Health

The philosophical argument is not the only possible justification for lowering the MLDA. Differing interpretations about the nature of college and underage drinking, and its public health causes and consequences more broadly, might also support a reframing of the issue. More specifically, just as we question whether 18- to 20-year-olds are truly different, and somehow less capable, than other adults, so we question whether drinking by this group represents a distinct problem, as opposed to being part of a broader pattern of alcohol consumption and abuse.

Every age group (excepting the very young) has heavy, destructive drinkers and alcoholics (Rehm, Greenfield, & Rogers, 2001). Changes in drinking prevalence by youth, moreover, mirror shifts in adult drinking. Figure 14.4 plots levels of college binge drinking prevalence, defined as having five or more drinks in one drinking episode, along with per capita ethanol sales. Note that *per capita* alcohol sales are dominated by drinking by those over age 20: only one in six drinks is consumed by underage individuals (Bonnie & O'Connell, 2004). As adult drinking declines and rises, so too does college drinking. A number of studies have confirmed the relationship—per capita ethanol consumption (adult drinking) at the state level is significantly related to youth drinking and bingeing, even when alcohol tax rates, minimum purchase age, individual characteristics, and unobserved state characteristics are controlled for (Cook & Moore, 2001). Studies focused solely on colleges have similarly found strong correlations between adult binge drinking rates and college binge drinking rates within states (Nelson, Naimi, Brewer, & Wechsler, 2005; Wechsler & Nelson, 2008).

Thus college drinking, and college problem drinking specifically, is not a phenomenon independent of the broader drinking culture. Treating college-student drinking as distinct from adult drinking ignores the context in which underage drinking occurs and lets adults off the hook, as it were—it releases adults from their responsibility for creating a culture of problematic alcohol consumption. Such responsibility was high-

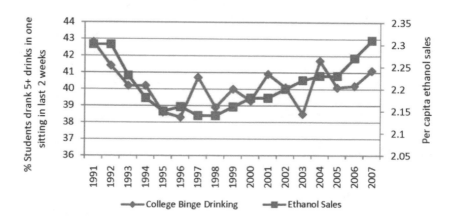

FIGURE 14.4. College binge drinking and adult drinking. From Johnston, O'Malley, Bachman, and Schulenberg (2008).

lighted in the 2004 report *Reducing Underage Drinking*, published by the National Research Council and the Institute of Medicine (Bonnie & O'Connell, 2004). In this report, researchers and public health officials recommended targeting the overall (adult) market to change youth drinking habits through media campaigns and regulation.

A population-level approach toward youthful drinking could be a spur to reduce total consumption and abuse, through which drinking by young people would be reduced as well. Several actions would serve this goal. Raising alcohol taxes is a natural starting point. Excise taxes on beer and liquor have been steadily eroded by inflation since the 1950s; today, the federal beer tax is only $0.33 for a six-pack, whereas restoring the tax to the 1960 level would raise it to $1.20 per six-pack. Even raising the tax to 1991 levels would mean a 62% increase. State excise taxes have followed the same downward path (Cook, 2007).

Given that alcohol consumption and abuse are responsive to price, even a small increase in price could have significant effects on drinking prevalence and consequences. A 2002 review of literature on this topic suggested a 10% increase in the price of alcohol could reduce the number of college students involved in violence each year by 200,000 (Chaloupka, Grossman, & Saffer, 2002). A 2009 study examining changes in beer taxes in Alaska similarly found significant decreases in fatal alcohol-related morbidity from two separate tax increases (Wagenaar, Maldonado-Molina, & Wagenaar, 2009). More generally, raising alcohol excise taxes would reduce the harms attendant on irresponsible alcohol consumption across the board, for adults as well as adolescents.

Policy Design

The Amethyst Initiative argues that the MLDA of 21 is a failure, just like Prohibition in the 1920s, because so many college students, and indeed high school students, drink. While it is true that few teenagers are being "protected" from drinking by the MLDA given that over 80% of high school seniors have drunk, this in itself, does not indicate policy failure. Just as Prohibition reduced drinking, the MLDA does have some effect on drinking among young people (Cook, 2007).

However, the MLDA reduces drinking in a way that is less efficient and less equitable than other policy options. Wide disregard for the law fosters cynicism about alcohol regulation and laws more broadly. The public ambivalence around youth drinking, meanwhile, encourages lax enforcement. Prohibition is a blunt instrument. It reduces public health officials' ability to accurately track consumption and target programs where they are most needed. It forces us to walk on tiptoes around the practical reality of underage drinking. From this perspective, lowering the drinking age would not mean capitulating to high rates of youth alcohol consumption, but rather opening the door to policies that better reflect the reality of drinking.

The repeal of Prohibition resulted in a raft of new alcohol-control policies with more stringent enforcement and less corruption. It also meant a chance for experimentation with alcohol policies in different contexts. Repeal was not an endorsement of alcohol; prominent reformers, many of whom initially campaigned for alcohol bans, instead concluded absolute prohibition was not the best way to reduce drinking. They hoped that repeal would lead to innovation in alcohol policy. In a report issued in 1933, two researchers expressed a common view: that with the change in national policy, "the 48 states will constitute a social science laboratory in which different ideas and methods can be tested, and the exchange of experience will be infinitely valuable for the future" (Fosdick & Scott, 1933). This experimental approach was not implemented, for the most part, but it is not too late, and college campuses are a natural laboratory.

Many policy options are available. At one extreme, the tie between an MLDA of 21 and national highway funds could be severed, and states would be allowed to experiment with different MLDAs and different alcohol policies and programs. A more modest innovation would be to allow states to have more exceptions from an MLDA of 21. Some states do have limited exceptions to the minimum drinking age; in Colorado, for instance, persons under 21 may consume alcohol if their parent or guardian gives consent and supervises such drinking. Military base commanders can declare a holiday from the MLDA for special celebrations (such as the return of a unit from a tour on the front) (Cook, 2007). Such exceptions could be increased to allow residential colleges, military installations, and other institutions to similarly suspend an MLDA of 21 based on the alcohol environment they perceive at their location and their alcohol regulation preferences. Exceptions could be revoked if alcohol-related injuries or fatalities increased beyond a predetermined level.

Other potential innovations include mixed arrangements, where different MLDAs are set for different types of consumption. Prior to the de facto national MLDA of 21, for example, several states set the minimum age for liquor higher than for beer. Such arrangements would decrease incentives to drink high-proof liquor, an incentive created by Prohibition (where the challenge of transporting alcohol undetected encouraged more concentrated forms) (Levine & Reinarman, 1991). A more unusual option might be to create an alcohol licensing system. As researcher Mark Kleiman (1993) details, alcohol could be regulated through consumer licenses, with distribution based on age or completion of alcohol education training. These licenses could then be suspended or revoked if the bearer violated any alcohol regulations, such as providing alcohol to minors, driving while under the influence, or exhibiting public intoxication.

Separate policies could also be targeted specifically at the externalities of alcohol consumption. Current "zero tolerance" drunk driving laws, which make it a violation for those under 21 to drive with any measurable blood alcohol content, could be maintained; allowing 18- to 20-year-olds to drink does not imply allowing them to drink and drive. (These laws could be recast as applying to novice drivers rather than as applying to a particular age group.) Keg registration, dram shop liability,[4] and social host responsibilities could all be mandated or strengthened. All of these options would provide a compromise between liberty and individual and social protection, recognizing the rights of young adults, the responsibilities of society to reduce mortality and injury, and the broad nature of problem drinking.

DRINKING ON COLLEGE CAMPUSES

What would college drinking look like if the MLDA were reduced to 18 or 19? Some, like John McCardell, argue that problem college drinking would be much reduced; he believes binge drinking is driven mainly by the covert alcohol consumption mandated by underage prohibition. Perhaps so, but there is little evidence in support of this view.

Instead, some research suggests there might be some increase in overall drinking, and likely little change in problem drinking. An analysis of changes in drinking on college campuses following the imposition of 21 as the minimum legal drinking age found that underage prohibition decreased alcohol consumption by light and moderate drinkers, but no change was observed in the proportion of heavy drinkers. The proportion of students who experienced most types of negative alcohol consequences (including hangovers and missed classes) also remained constant before and after the MLDA change, although fewer students reported driving while intoxicated (Engs & Hanson, 1988). In reverse, then, we would likely see an increase in the proportion of students who drank, but with little increase in the number of problem drinkers. The current culture on campus that identifies the main use value of alcohol as getting drunk could conceivably be changed for the better, as drinking is incorporated into public social occasions.

---

[4]Dram shop liability is the arcane term used to refer to the liability of commercial servers and sellers of alcoholic beverages for injuries caused by their customers (Cook, 2007).

College administrators, meanwhile, would likely heave a sigh of relief at no longer being required to maintain a prohibition regime. This change would not absolve them of responsibility for working to limit the harms of alcohol abuse on campus. The environmental prevention programs detailed in this volume would be a good start. Stronger regulations by city, state, and federal governments could, in principle, preempt any deleterious consequences of a reduced MLDA.

The biggest gain of changing the MLDA would be greater liberty for young adults, and a new perspective on college drinking, one that embedded it in the broad problem of adult drinking. Reducing the MLDA without strengthening other alcohol control measures would likely increase alcohol-related harms. But even then, the cost of prohibition for 18- to 20-year- olds is arguably greater than its benefits. With legalization would come an opportunity for lawmakers and college administrators to adopt innovative regulations and learn from them.

REFERENCES

Aber, J. L., Atkins, M. S., Benbow, C. P., Brabeck, M. M., Bruner, J., Coleman, H. L. K., et al. (2009). Brief of Amici Curiae in the Supreme Court of the United States in the case of Terrance Jamar Graham v. State of Florida and Joe Harris Sullivan v. State of Florida.

Amendments to the Higher Education Act of 1965. P.L. 105-244 (1998).

American Medical Association. (2010). *Facts about youth and alcohol: Minimum legal drinking age*. Retrieved from *www.ama-assn.org/ama/pub/physician-resources/public-health/promoting-healthy-lifestyles/alcohol-other-drug-abuse/facts-about-youth-alcohol/minimum-legal-drinking-age.shtml*

Blakemore, S., & Choudhury, S. (2006). Development of the adolescent brain: Implications for executive function and social cognition. *Journal of Child Psychology and Psychiatry, 47*(3), 296–312.

Bonnie, R., J., & O'Connell, M. E. (Eds.). (2004). *Reducing underage drinking: A collective responsibility*. Washington, DC: National Academies Press.

Bureau of Labor Statistics. (2000). *Report on the Youth Labor Force*. Washington, DC: U.S. Department of Labor.

Carpenter, C. S. (2005). Heavy alcohol use and the commission of nuisance crime: Evidence from underage drunk driving laws. *American Economic Review, 95*(2), 267–272.

Carpenter, C. S., & Dobkin, C. (2009). The effect of alcohol consumption on mortality: Regression discontinuity evidence from the minimum drinking age. *Journal of Applied Econometrics, 1*(1), 164–182.

Center on Alcohol Marketing and Youth. (2010). *The toll of underage drinking*. Retrieved from *www.camy.org/factsheets/sheets/The_Toll_of_Underage_Drinking.html*.

Chaloupka, F. J., Grossman, M., & Saffer, H. (2002). *The effects of price on alcohol consumption and alcohol-related problems.* Retrieved from NIAAA website, *pubs.niaaa.nih.gov/publications/arh26-1/22-34.htm.*

Cook, P. J. (2007). *Paying the tab.* Princeton, NJ: Princeton University Press.

Cook, P. J., & Moore, M. J. (1993). Economic perspectives on reducing alcohol-related violence. In S. E. Martin (Ed.), *Alcohol and interpersonal violence: Fostering multidisciplinary perspectives* (NIH Publication No. 93-3496, pp. 193–212). Rockville, MD: National Institute on Alcohol Abuse and Alcoholism.

Cook, P. J., & Moore, M. J. (2001). Environment and persistence in youthful drinking patterns. In J. Gruber (Ed.), *Risky behavior among youth* (pp. 375–438). Chicago: Chicago University Press.

Cook, P. J., & Tauchen, G. (1984). The effect of minimum drinking age legislation on youthful auto fatalities, 1970–1977. *Journal of Legal Studies, 13,* 169–190.

Dee, T. S. (1999). State alcohol policies, teen drinking and traffic fatalities. *Journal of Public Economics, 72*(2), 289–315.

Engs, R. C., & Hanson, D. J. (1988). University students' drinking patterns and problems: Examining the effects of raising the purchase age. *Public Health Reports, 103*(6), 667–673.

Exec. Order No. 12,358 (Presidential Commission on Drunk Driving). (1982). Retrieved from *www.presidency.ucsb.edu/ws/index.php?pid=42395.*

Faden, V. B., & Baskin, M. L. (2005). An evaluation of college online alcohol-policy information. Retrieved from *www.collegedrinkingprevention.gov/supportingresearch/onlinealcoinfo.aspx.*

Fosdick, R. B., & Scott, A. L. (1933). *Toward liquor control.* New York: Harper.

Graham v. Florida, 982 So. 2d 43 (2010).

Greer, D. F. (1922). A legal anachronism: The married woman's separate acknowledgment to deeds. *Texas Law Review, 4*(4), 407–423.

James, T. E. (1960). The age of majority. *American Journal of Legal History, 22,* 22–33.

Johnston, L. D., O'Malley, P. M., Bachman, J. G., & Schulenberg, J. E. (2008). *Monitoring the Future national rurvey results on drug use, 1975–2007: Vol. II. College students and adults ages 19–45* (NIH Publication No. 08-6418A). Bethesda, MD: National Institute on Drug Abuse.

Kleiman, M. (1993). *Against excess.* New York: Basic Books.

Leonard, K. E., Collins, R. L., & Quigley, B. M. (2003). Alcohol consumption and the occurrence and severity of aggression: An event-based analysis of male to male barroom violence. *Aggressive Behavior, 29*(4), 346–365.

Levine, D. (2000, September 15). Institute will pay Kruegers $6M for role in death. *The Tech [online addition], tech.mit.edu/V120/N42/42krueger.42n.html.*

Levine, H. G., & Reinarman, C. (1991). From prohibition to regulation: Lessons from alcohol policy for drug policy. *Milbank Quarterly, 69*(3), 461–494.

Martin, S. E. (2001). The links between alcohol, crime and the criminal justice system: Explanations, evidence and interventions. *American Journal on Addictions, 10*(2), 136–158.

National Institute on Alcohol Abuse and Alcoholism (NIAAA). (2006). Total and alcohol-related traffic fatality rates per 100 million VMT, 100,000 population, 100,000 registered vehicles, and 100,000 licensed drivers, United States, 1982–2004. Retrieved from *www.niaaa.nih.gov/Resources/DatabaseResources/QuickFacts/TrafficCrashes/crash02.htm*.

National Institute on Alcohol Abuse and Alcoholism (NIAAA). (2008). Percent who drink beverage alcohol, by gender, 1939–2008. Retrieved from *www.niaaa.nih.gov/Resources/DatabaseResources/QuickFacts/AlcoholConsumption/PercentAlcoholGender.htm*.

National Institute on Alcohol Abuse and Alcoholism (NIAAA). (2009). Apparent per capita ethanol consumption for the United States, 1850–2007. Retrieved from *www.niaaa.nih.gov/Resources/DatabaseResources/QuickFacts/AlcoholSales/consum01.htm*.

Nelson, T. F., Naimi, T. S., Brewer, R. D., & Wechsler, H. (2005). The state sets the rate: The relationship among state-specific college binge drinking, state binge drinking rates, and selected state alcohol control policies. *American Journal of Public Health, 95*(3), 441–446.

North Carolina's anti-cohabitation law under attack. (2000, May 9). Retrieved from *www.usatoday.com/news/nation/2005-05-09-nc-cohab-law_x.htm*.

Pearl, L. D. (1985). The party's over: Controlling drunk drivers. *Urban Lawyer, 17*, 813–827.

Pihl, R.O., & Peterson, J. (1993). Alcohol and aggression: Three potential mechanisms of the drug effect. In S. Martin (Ed.), *Alcohol and interpersonal violence: Fostering interdisciplinary perspectives* (pp. 149–159). Rockville, MD: National Institute on Alcohol Abuse and Alcoholism.

Qualifications for jury service. (1968). 28 U.S.C., Sec. 1865. Retrieved from *www.law.cornell.edu/uscode/uscode28/usc_sup_01_28_10_V_20_121.html*.

Rehm, J., Greenfield, T. K., & Rogers, J. D. (2001). Average volume of alcohol consumption, patterns of drinking, and all-cause mortality: Results from the U.S. National Alcohol Survey. *American Journal of Epidemiology, 153*(1), 64–71.

Roper v. Simmons, 543 U.S. 551 (2005).

Safe and Drug-Free Schools and Communities Act fact sheet. (2009). Retrieved from *www.cde.ca.gov/ls/he/at/safedrugfree.asp*.

Spear, L. P. (2000). The adolescent brain and age-related behavioral manifestations. *Neuroscience and Biobehavioral Reviews, 24*, 417–463.

Steinberg, L. (2008). A social neuroscience perspective on adolescent risk-taking. *Development Review, 28*(1), 78–106.

Steinberg, L., & Cauffman, E. (1996). Maturity of judgment in adolescence: Psychosocial factors in adolescent decision making. *Law and Human Behavior, 20*(3), 249–272.

Sullivan v. Florida, 560 U.S. (2010).

Toomey, T. L., Nelson, T. F., & Lenk, K. M. (2009). The age-21 minimum legal drinking age: A case study linking past and current debates. *Addiction, 104*(12), 1958–1965.

Wagenaar, A. C., Maldonado-Molina, M. M., & Wagenaar, B. H. (2009). Effects of alcohol tax increases on alcohol-related disease mortality in Alaska:

Time-series analyses from 1976 to 2004. *American Journal of Public Health,* 99(8), 1464–1470.

Wechsler, H., & Nelson, T. F. (2008). What we have learned from the Harvard School of Public Health College Alcohol Study: Focusing attention on college student alcohol consumption and the environmental conditions that promote it. *Journal of Studies on Alcohol and Drugs, 69*(4), 481–490.

WISQARS. (2010). Fatal injury data. Retrieved from *www.cdc.gov/injury/wisqars/fatal.html.*

Zlatoper, T. J. (1989). Models explaining motor vehicle death rates in the United States. *Accident Analysis & Prevention, 21*(2), 125–154.

CHAPTER 15

Balancing Cost and Benefits of the Minimum Legal Drinking Age

A Response to Cook and Gearing

Robert F. Saltz *and* James C. Fell

When the voting age in the United States was lowered to 18, several states with higher minimum legal drinking ages decided to match the new voting age. Later, in light of concerns about youthful drinking and especially drinking and driving, federal regulations imposed a de facto national minimum drinking age of 21 (Toomey, Rosenfeld, & Wagenaar, 1996; Williams, 2006). The policy debate over which age is "right" for the minimum legal drinking age (MLDA) did not end there.

In this volume, Cook and Gearing (Chapter 14) take that debate in a slightly different direction by arguing that there is a cost paid for setting the MLDA at an age above the voting age, an age when citizens are granted many other rights and responsibilities. The authors go a bit further and describe how that cost might be estimated (e.g., by imagining the cost of making youth "whole") to place the cost in perspective.

No policy question is ever settled by research alone, as policies represent values as much as empirical support. In that sense, Cook and Gearing are right to address the value we may place on "liberty" and draw attention to the cost we may be paying to maintain an MLDA of 21. In this brief response to their chapter, however, we seek first to quickly summarize the wealth of evidence that supports the main argument that a higher MLDA saves many lives in the United States each year so that readers will appreciate the reasons why many support the age 21 MLDA.

We conclude with only a short discussion aimed more directly at Cook and Gearing's argument.

States were given the responsibility for setting controls for alcohol sales and consumption along with the repeal of Prohibition (the 21st Amendment to the U.S. Constitution) in 1933. Most states at that time set the MLDA at 21 years of age. Later, when the national voting age was lowered to 18 by the 26th Amendment in 1971, many states lowered their drinking age to 18 or 19; this change occurred in the early 1970s (Toomey et al., 1996). The early 1980s saw the founding of Mothers Against Drunk Driving (MADD) and the Presidential Commission on Drunk Driving (see Volpe, 1983). MADD, the Commission, and several political leaders and agencies argued for establishing a national MLDA of 21 in order to reduce the prevalence of drunk driving among the younger population and to avoid differences in state MLDAs that could encourage older teens to drive distances in order to legally drink. As a result, a de facto federal MLDA of 21 was established by tying the requirement to set 21 as the minimum age to states receiving federal highway construction funds (Fell & Voas, 2006; Williams, 2006).

Since the passage of that law, the number of drinking drivers in fatal crashes among 16- to 20-year-olds has declined by 62% (National Highway Traffic Safety Administration [NHTSA], 2008) whereas the number of nondrinking drivers in fatal crashes among the same age group rose by 9%. The fact that many states had lowered and then raised their MLDA allowed researchers the opportunity to study the effects of moving the age in each direction, while having good statistical controls for other events and influences that might have had an effect on youth at the same time. Dozens of studies have been published on the effects of these changes, and reviews of that literature are nicely summarized by Wagenaar and Toomey (2002) and by Shults and colleagues (2001). The latter article concludes that according to the best estimate of the law's effects, alcohol-related crashes among youth increased by 10% when the MLDA was lowered, and then decreased by 16% when the MLDA was raised to 21. A recent comprehensive analysis of the MLDA's effect on traffic crashes, alongside other control measures meant to lower traffic deaths (e.g., zero tolerance laws, administrative license revocation, seat-belt laws), found that raising the MLDA was independently responsible for a 16% decline in the ratio of drinking to nondrinking driver fatalities among those under 21, while other measures, (e.g., zero tolerance laws, administrative license revocation, seat-belt laws) independently added to those effects (Fell, Fisher, Voas, Blackman, & Tippetts, 2009).

The NHTSA has estimated that 800 or more lives have been saved each year since the minimum drinking age was raised to 21 (NHTSA, 1998, 2010). In his history of public health successes, Hemenway (2009)

discusses raising the MLDA and states that "this natural experiment is
the most well-studied alcohol control policy in U.S. history.... [The benefit of higher MLDA] holds even when there has not been strong enforcement of the law."

The effects of the age 21 MLDA on driving fatalities are more
impressive given that enforcement of MLDA has been, at best, uneven.
Wagenaar and Wolfson (1994) estimate that only two of every 1,000
occasions of underage drinking result in an arrest, and that only five of
every 100,000 occasions of underage drinking result in action against
a commercial outlet. The effects of raising the MLDA, in other words,
could be even greater if it were uniformly enforced. Direct community
intervention studies such as the Communities Mobilizing for Change on
Alcohol (CMCA) project (Wagenaar et al., 2000) and the Sacramento
Neighborhood Alcohol Prevention Project (SNAPP) study (Treno, Gruenewald, Lee, & Remer, 2007) have demonstrated that enhanced enforcement can reduce underage drinking and associated problems beyond the
effect of "business as usual." As summarized by Saltz in Chapter 11 of
this volume, the enforcement of laws related to MLDA (e.g., prohibiting
sales to minors) was a component in more than one efficacious college
drinking prevention intervention.

In almost all the cited research, the focus has been on traffic deaths,
not only because they represent the greatest threat to life among this age
group, but also because alcohol-related traffic deaths are better measured
(e.g., via NHTSA's Fatality Analysis Reporting System [FARS]) than other
harms. As estimated by Hingson, Zha, and Weitzman (2009), beyond the
estimated 1,800 annual alcohol-related deaths among college students,
other major consequences include 590,000 unintentional injuries, more
than 690,000 assaults by another student, and more than 97,000 vic-
timizations through sexual assault or date rape. Twenty-five percent of
college students reported that drinking had in some way impaired their
academic performance.

Despite this overwhelming evidence in support of keeping the
MLDA at 21, some wonder whether lowering the age would achieve
some kind of cultural shift in the way young people and their parents
view alcohol and incorporate it into their everyday lives. The argument is made that a "prohibitionist" stance with regard to drinking
among 18- to 20-year-olds actually increases the risk of so-called binge
drinking, an argument cited by Cook and Gearing in this volume. This
perspective often looks to the European countries as models of how
alcohol might be better integrated into the culture of drinking. Unfortunately for this view, the evidence here does not support the hypothetical
benefits of a younger drinking age. Cross-national surveys of 15- and
16-year-olds show that youth in nearly every European country drink

at higher levels than their U.S. counterparts (Hibell, Andersson, & Bjarnasson, 2004).

Finally, we have the benefit of another country's experience in lowering their drinking age. In 1999, New Zealand lowered its drinking age from 20 to 18, partially as a result of similar claims that doing so would enable youth to drink in "safer" environments. The result, according to a recent study, was a dramatic increase in automobile crashes (Kypri et al., 2006). The rate of traffic crashes and injuries increased 12% for 18- and 19-year-old males and 14% for males ages 15 to 17. For females, the effect was even greater: rates increased 51% for 18- to 19-year-olds and 24% for 15- to 17-year-olds. Note here a very important consequence of this policy change: not only were newly legal drinkers suffering greater harms, but so were those younger than the new MLDA, who arguably had greater access to alcohol via their slightly older peers.

We wish to conclude this brief piece with a response to a few of the most general points raised by Cook and Gearing in Chapter 14, not only because space restricts how much we can include, but also because it would be unfair to go into details without the opportunity of a longer dialogue. First, Cook and Gearing seem to argue that a reduction in alcohol-related harm (especially traffic crashes) implies that we can relax the MLDA, as though the two phenomena were unrelated. The empirical evidence, only some of which we highlighted above, strongly supports the fact that these reductions derive, in large part but not exclusively, from having raised the MLDA to 21.

A second, related argument is made that because we have seen a reduction in alcohol-related crashes across the age span, raising the MLDA cannot be given credit. This argument supposes that the United States has not been engaged in a multipronged attack on alcohol-impaired driving across the entire age span. Our success with those over 21 is real (a 33% reduction in drinking drivers involved in fatal crashes), but we have had even greater progress with those under 21 (a 62% reduction in drinking drivers in fatal crashes per the National Highway Traffic Safety Administration data cited above).

Third, Cook and Gearing argue that the continued declines in crashes among those under 21 since the raising of the MLDA means that these declines have nothing to do with raising the MLDA. Again, raising the drinking age is but one measure this country has taken to lower crashes, so other measures would still be operative since the MLDA was raised to 21. More important, we have seen that enforcement of the MLDA has been inconsistent and sometimes nonexistent. Thus, we would expect the raising of the MLDA to have a greater impact over time as the higher drinking age becomes perceived as more legitimate and is more fully supported by enforcement.

The arguments by Cook and Gearing described above seem to take the position that many things could have accounted for the downward trends that we have observed in traffic fatalities and that we cannot know the relative contribution of the age 21 MLDA among the other prevention measures. The value of the article by Fell and colleagues (2009) is that it capitalizes on variation in the use of various alcohol control measures to not only establish the independent effect of raising the MLDA (as cited above), but also to show the relative magnitude of other control measures. Lowering the blood alcohol concentration for intoxication, for instance, was itself associated with an additional 8% reduction in fatal crashes. Zero tolerance laws for minors reduced crashes an additional 5%, as did administrative license revocation (Fell et al., 2009).

Cook and Gearing also argue that if the age 21 MLDA were effective, we would see a large jump in the crash rates for those who just turned 21. The fact that no such jump has been observed may be due to many different things. Lower enforcement of the MLDA would reduce the effect of turning 21, for instance, but a more intriguing possibility is suggested by research findings published by O'Malley and Wagenaar (1991). They found that a higher MLDA in a given state was associated with lower risk of alcohol-related harm even after drinkers there turned 21, suggesting that delaying the onset of legal alcohol consumption may have benefits beyond the teenage years. Those turning 21 are likely to be more mature and drink with lower risk than those turning 18.

While these points are based on how one interprets the results of empirical research, Cook and Gearing make several additional conceptual comments that are important to address. First, they say that we should not focus exclusively on underage drinkers but should be working to reduce alcohol-related harm across all ages. This is certainly a point on which we all agree, and studies such as Nelson, Naimi, Brewer, and Wechsler (2005) show that college student drinking does seem to reflect drinking norms of the adult population. Fortunately, we do not have to choose between focusing on underage drinkers versus the adult population. Some prevention and policy measures can be effective across the board (e.g., DUI enforcement), while simultaneously also enforcing the age 21 MLDA.

We also have some disagreement on another general point made by Cook and Gearing. They argue that setting the MLDA at 21 means that college prevention specialists are somehow handicapped in their efforts. This argument would seem to fly in the face of all the successful strategies identified in this volume. From programs similar to the Brief Alcohol Screening and Intervention for College Students (BASICS; see Cronce & Larimer, Chapter 8, this volume) to parental interventions, to community-level interventions, college administrators have access to a growing number of prevention strategies available that seem perfectly functional whatever the minimum drinking age might be. We would argue that the higher legal drinking age serves as just one more lever that college communities can put to use in their efforts to protect the health and safety of college students and every other member of their communities.

Taking the broadest view, we agree with Cook and Geary when they recognize that policy represents "a compromise between liberty and individual and social protection." We just disagree with their view that the cost of an MLDA of 21 is unacceptably high, and about where the best point of compromise lies.

REFERENCES

Fell, J. C., Fisher, D. A., Voas, R. B., Blackman, K., & Tippetts, A. S. (2009). The impact of underage drinking laws on alcohol-related fatal crashes of young drivers. *Alcoholism: Clinical and Experimental Research, 33*, 1208–1219.

Fell, J. C., & Voas, R. B. (2006). Mothers Against Drunk Driving (MADD): The first 25 years. *Traffic Injury Prevention, 7*, 195–212.

Hemenway, D. (2009). *While we were sleeping: Success stories in injury and violence prevention.* Berkeley: University of California Press.

Hibell, B., Andersson, B., & Bjarnasson, T. (2004). *The 2003 ESPAD Report: Alcohol and other drug use among students in 35 European countries.* Stockholm: Swedish Council for Information on Alcohol and Other Drugs.

Hingson, R. W., Zha, W., & Weitzman, E. R. (2009). Magnitude of and trends in alcohol-related mortality and morbidity among U.S. college students ages 18–24, 1998–2005. *Journal of Studies on Alcohol and Drugs* (Suppl. 16), 12–20.

Kypri, K., Voas, R. B., Langley, J. D., Stephenson, S. C., Begg, D. J., Tippetts, A. S., et al. (2006). Minimum purchasing age for alcohol and traffic crash injuries among 15- to 19-year-olds in New Zealand. *American Journal of Public Health, 96*(1), 126–131.

Nelson, T. F., Naimi, T. S., Brewer, R. D., & Wechsler, H. (2005). The state sets the rate: The relationship among state-specific college binge drinking, state binge drinking rates, and selected state alcohol control policies. *American Journal of Public Health, 95*(3), 441–446.

National Highway Traffic Safety Administration (NHTSA). (2008). *Fatality Analysis Reporting System (FARS) 1982–2005.* (Last accessed: April 2011). Available from *www-nrd.nhtsa.dot.gov/Pubs/810942.pdf*.

National Highway Traffic Safety Administration (NHTSA). (1998). *Traffic safety facts 1998* (DOT HS 808 953). Washington, DC: U.S. Department of Transportation.

National Highway Traffic Safety Administration (NHTSA). (2010). Traffic safety facts September. (DOT HS 811 383). Washington, DC: US Department of Transportation.

O'Malley, P. M., & Wagenaar, A. C. (1991). Effects of minimum drinking age laws on alcohol use, related behaviors and traffic crash involvement among American youth: 1976–1987. *Journal of Studies on Alcohol, 52,* 478–491.

Shults, R. A., Elder, R. W., Sleet, D. A, Nichols, J. L., Alao, M. O., Carande-Kulis, V. G., et al. (2001). Task Force on Community Preventive Services: Reviews of evidence regarding interventions to reduce alcohol-impaired driving. *American Journal of Preventive Medicine, 21,* 66-88.

Toomey, T. L., Rosenfeld, C., & Wagenaar, A. C. (1996). The minimum legal drinking age: History, effectiveness and ongoing debate. *Alcohol Health and Research World, 20,* 213-218.

Treno, A. J., Gruenewald, P. J., Lee, J. P., & Remer, L. G. (2007). The Sacramento Neighborhood Alcohol Prevention Project: Outcomes from a community prevention trial. *Journal of Studies on Alcohol and Drugs, 68*(2), 197–207.

Volpe, J. A. (1983). *Presidential Commission on Drunk Driving, final report.* Washington, DC: U.S. Government Printing Office.

Wagenaar, A. C., Murray, D. M., Gehan, J. P., Wolfson, M., Forster, J. L., Toomey, T. L., et al. (2000). Communities Mobilizing for Change on Alcohol: Outcomes from a randomized community trial. *Journal of Studies on Alcohol, 61*(1), 85–94.

Wagenaar A. C., & Toomey, T. L. (2002). Effects of minimum drinking age laws: Review and analyses of the literature from 1960 to 2000. *Journal of Studies on Alcohol* (Suppl. 14), 206–225.

Wagenaar, A. C., & Wolfson, M. (1994). Enforcement of the legal minimum drinking age in the United States. *Journal of Public Health Policy, 15*(1), 37–53.

Williams, A. F. (2006). Alcohol-impaired driving and its consequences in the United States: The past 25 years. *Journal of Safety Research, 37*(2), 123–138.

Index